Treating Survivors of Childhood Abuse

Treating Survivors of Childhood Abuse

~

Psychotherapy for
the Interrupted Life

MARYLENE CLOITRE
LISA R. COHEN
KARESTAN C. KOENEN

THE GUILFORD PRESS
New York   London

©2006 The Guilford Press
A Division of Guilford Publications, Inc.
72 Spring Street, New York, NY 10012
www.guilford.com

Printed in the United States of America

This book is printed on acid-free paper.

Last digit is print number: 9   8   7   6   5

Library of Congress Cataloging-in-Publication Data
Cloitre, Marylene.
    Treating survivors of childhood abuse : psychotherapy for the interrupted life / Marylene Cloitre, Lisa R. Cohen, Karestan C. Koenen.
        p. cm.
    Includes bibliographical references and index.
    ISBN-10: 1-59385-312-2   ISBN-13: 978-1-59385-312-9 (pbk.)
    1. Adult child sexual abuse victims—Treatment. 2. Psychotherapy. I. Cohen, Lisa R.
II. Koenen, Karestan C. III. Title.
    [DNLM: 1. Stress Disorders, Post-Traumatic—therapy. 2. Child Abuse—
therapy. 3. Survivors—psychology. 4. Adult—psychology. 5. Psychotherapy—
methods.   WM 170 C643t 2006]
    RC569.5.A28C48 2006
    616.85′83690651—dc22
                                                                        2006007900

This book is dedicated to

Caleb

for his inspiring optimism and capacity for love

and to all other children for whom we hold
the enduring wish that they grow up to be
their best possible selves

A survivor ultimately has two psychological possibilities: to shut down or to open up. Usually the survivor does both. . . . The protean self opts for opening out. . . . This includes the basic satisfaction, even joy, in being alive, in not having died, along with the sense of having undergone an experience that is illuminating in its pain. Survival also implies persevering, holding on, maintaining one's existence . . . a physical and mental strength. That sense of victory over destruction is evident in gatherings of survivors . . . where one hears clearly the words, even if actually unspoken: "We are here! We're alive! We have won!"

—ROBERT JAY LIFTON (1993, pp. 81, 82)

About the Authors

Marylene Cloitre, PhD, is the founding director of the Institute for Trauma and Stress at the New York University Child Study Center and is also NYU's first Cathy and Stephen Graham Professor of Child and Adolescent Psychiatry. Dr. Cloitre's primary clinical and research interests focus on the developmental consequences and treatment of childhood abuse in adults and adolescents. She has published widely on this topic and has received several grants from the National Institutes of Health and other agencies for evidence-based intervention and prevention programs addressing the psychological and social effects of trauma in adults and children. Dr. Cloitre is currently a member of the Board of Directors for the International Society for Traumatic Stress Studies and was a member of the American National Committee to Develop Treatment Guidelines for PTSD. She received her BA in philosophy from McGill University and her PhD from Columbia University.

Lisa R. Cohen, PhD, is a Research Scientist with the Social Intervention Group at the Columbia University School of Social Work, where her work focuses on developing and testing treatments for women with PTSD and substance use disorders through grants funded by the National Institute on Drug Abuse. She also conducts research on the impact of trauma on parenting and its intergenerational implications. Dr. Cohen maintains a private psychotherapy practice in New York City specializing in the treatment of complex trauma disorders. She received her BA from the University of Pennsylvania and her PhD in clinical psychology from Yale University. She was a postdoctoral fellow at the Anxiety and Traumatic Stress Program at the Payne Whitney Clinic of New York Hospital–Cornell Medical Center.

Karestan C. Koenen, PhD, is an Assistant Professor of Society, Human Development, and Health and Epidemiology at the Harvard School of Public Health. She uses a developmental approach to understanding the epidemiology of trauma exposure and stress-related mental disorders such as PTSD and depression. Her research is funded by the National Institutes of Health, and she has received the Chaim Danieli Young Professional Award from the International Society for Traumatic Stress Studies and the Robins–Guze Young Investigator Award from the American Psychopathological Association. Dr. Koenen is also an experienced clinician, specializing in empirically validated treatments for PTSD. She received her BA from Wellesley College, her MA from Columbia University, and her PhD from Boston University.

Acknowledgments

First, we wish to acknowledge our clients, who have inspired us with their courage in coming to treatment, confronting their traumas, and daring to hope for the possibility of a life different from the one they have known. We wish to thank Stephanie Cherry, Sharon Feeney, Tamar Gordon, Dawn Hughes, Karen Heffernan, Jill Levitt, and Chase Stovall-McClough, who as students, postdoctoral fellows, and colleagues contributed to the development of this treatment as long-term members of the research team.

We also thank Elissa Brown, Paul Frewen, Ruth Lanius, and Elizabeth Power, who read parts of the manuscript and gave feedback with humor, energy, and appreciation of the task at hand. We wish to acknowledge innovators in psychotherapy intervention research, from whom we have learned much. We thank Marsha Linehan, who developed intervention strategies that have profoundly influenced our work and our effectiveness as trauma therapists. We give special thanks to Edna Foa, who gave generously and always of her knowledge and insights and who has served as a role model in the scientific inquiry of posttraumatic stress disorder intervention. With pleasure and deepest gratitude, we thank the pioneers in the field of complex trauma, who by their example and encouragement have guided and inspired our efforts: John Briere, Christine Courtois, Judy Herman, and Bessel van der Kolk.

Lastly, we would like to thank those individuals who have been especially important in our professional development and personal growth: Susan and George Cohen, Diana Fosha, Fran Grossman, Denise Hien, Nick Jollymore, Harold Koplewicz, Kathleen and Austin Koenen, Alba Ludmer, Shaun Purcell, and Ron Taffel.

Preface

WHAT IS THE INTERRUPTED LIFE?

There is an avalanche of data that tell us something survivors of abuse already know themselves: Functioning in day-to-day life is much harder for them than for those who have experienced a safe and secure childhood. Perhaps less well known to them are the reasons why. Throughout this book we highlight and specify ways in which childhood abuse can derail the normal course of development and deprive the individual of important learning experiences that foster healthy and effective life skills. These include basic and complex skills such as the capacity for sustained attention, the capacity to express feelings effectively and appropriately, the capacity to use emotions as a guide for action, and the capacity to relate well to others and to enjoy relationships. Interventions for children and youth who have experienced abuse are sensitive to these consequences and include strategies that repair and enrich emotional and social competencies, with the goal of realigning the young client back on the normative trajectory of development.

But what of the adults who lived through an abusive childhood without help? Those who come to treatment often express concern about long-standing emotion management and relationship problems. And yet, there is no program or intervention that addresses their concerns. Instead, the suffering of the adult survivor is typically organized by diagnostic status and symptom categories. The interpersonal and other difficulties are viewed as secondary to evident symptomatology: If the depression or anxiety is resolved, these other difficulties are expected to dissipate. The scientific community's careful tracking of the compromised social and emotional competencies caused by maltreatment ends with studies of teens and young adults. There is a remarkable disconnect between the observations made by child mental health professionals and the clinical world that treats the adults who were once abused children.

This book provides a treatment program that takes into account the long trajectory of disadvantages experienced by many abuse survivors that precedes their arrival into the therapist's office. The concept of the "interrupted life," which guides this treatment, refers to the disruption caused by abuse to self-regulation and interpersonal capacities that otherwise would have been expected to develop. The treatment is intended to provide the survivors with emotional and social skills they did not have the opportunity to obtain due to the diminished presence of a competent, caring, nurturing parent and the burden of managing the abuse, often alone or in secrect. The first module of this treatment, Skills Training for Affective and Interpersonal Regulation (STAIR), has been explicitly developed to generate and strengthen social and emotional resources for effective living.

A treatment for trauma would be incomplete if it did not address the equally profound although more recognized problem of posttraumatic stress disorder (PTSD). PTSD symptoms and associated disturbances such as depression, dissociation, anger, and feelings of shame and loss are indicators that there is "unfinished business" in the processing of traumatic experiences. Traumatic events, by their very nature, overwhelm the individual's capacity for understanding and analysis. The challenge to understanding is made even greater because the emotions associated with the abuse—terror, humiliation, and betrayal—are extremely painful and thus often avoided. Traumatic memories, when they remain unprocessed, are expressed through intrusive memories and reexperiencing, which interfere with the capacity to live meaningfully and fully in the present. Moreover, this processing work is a prerequisite to the integration of such memories into one's autobiographical narrative, the existence of which provides a coherent sense of self and one that is continuous across time. The inability to experience oneself as coherent and existing through time is another way in which life is "interrupted" for the trauma survivor.

Narrative Story Telling (NST) provides a structure and strategy for approaching, managing, and organizing traumatic experiences that have been unaddressed but are still quite alive with emotional power. NST begins with the emotional processing of fear memories using traditional imaginal exposure techniques (Chapter 6). However, this work is extended in two ways. First, we have developed and systematically employed "contextualization" strategies, grounded in recent models of autobiographical memory, to organize and construct a "narrative of self" (Chapter 7). Second, through these strategies, the client and therapist are able safely and effectively to explore and organize a sense of self around two critical affective themes that often burden the abuse survivor: shame and betrayal (Chapter 22) and loss and grief (Chapter 23).

Finally, the phrase "psychotherapy for the interrupted life" has a third meaning, one that alludes to a particular hope for the client. It recognizes that the management and consequences of abuse create circumstances in which the gifts and talents an individual may have had were irrelevant, unrecognized, or underdeveloped. In regenerating important life skills and a coherent and revitalized sense of self, we hope that the clients can, in essence, resume the realization of their hidden potential.

WHO CAN BENEFIT FROM THIS BOOK?

This book provides an evidence-based treatment for mental health providers who work with survivors of childhood abuse. These survivors include women and men who have experienced sexual abuse, physical abuse, and neglect. The treatment was originally developed for women, but it also has been successfully used with men and with clients of varied ages (including children and adolescents) who have experienced maltreatment in early life and multiple forms of interpersonal violence (see Chapter 8).

This book is also for survivors themselves. We hope that each survivor may "see" something of themselves in the descriptions and stories told in the book and, more important, find the interventions and ways of approaching problems relevant to them. Ideally, survivors perusing the book can come to know what they need or want and be better prepared to search for an effective therapy that is appropriate for them.

THE TREATMENT PHILOSOPHY

The "orientation" of the treatment is a blend of principles from the cognitive-behavioral and the attachment–interpersonal–object relational traditions evolving from the work of Bowlby (1988), Sullivan (1970), Mitchell and Greenberg (1983), and Safran and Segal (1990).

The intervention techniques rely heavily on those from the cognitive-behavioral therapy (CBT) tradition. These include, for example, strategies for evaluating beliefs about oneself and the world, and use of role playing to facilitate new learning and behavioral changes. They also adhere to a philosophy implicit in CBT: that with practice, new ways of behaving, feeling, and thinking are possible. In this way, CBT is a remarkably practical and optimistic psychotherapeutic tradition.

The theoretical framework of the treatment falls squarely within the interpersonal tradition, particularly as it has evolved from the work of Bowlby. The use of this framework emphasizes the importance of early life attachments and the long-term consequences that disturbances in caretaking relationships have in adult functioning. The cognitive-behavioral strategies are the means by which the client identifies these problems and works toward change. For example, problems in relationships related to early abuse are described through the attachment concept of "internal working models of relating." This concept is operationalized in the practical form of "interpersonal schemas," a familiar tool used in many cognitive therapies, used here to assess and change ideas about self and other.

HOW TO USE THIS BOOK

This book is intended to provide therapists with the skills, competence, and confidence to effectively treat survivors of childhood abuse. We have provided a session-by-session guide to a treatment that is grounded in theory, tested in its benefits, and repeatedly refined over 15 years with feedback from our clients. The book provides practical "nuts-and-bolts" guidance for all the technical aspects of the treatment. Equally important, the book is organized and written to highlight the rationale for the treatment and the primary goals behind each intervention so that the clinician can use STAIR/NST guided by the principles of the treatment as they fit the particular client rather than feel compelled to follow the phase, session, and interventions in a lockstep fashion.

The book is divided into three parts. Part I characterizes the effects of abuse in the context of an attachment–developmental framework; Part II describes the theoretical and empirical bases for the treatment rationale and outcome data reporting the benefits of the therapy; and Part III provides session-by-session descriptions of the treatment preceded by assessment and treatment guidelines. The book as a whole is intended to convey *a way of thinking* about abuse survivors that can facilitate effective therapy. Theory, research, and clinical service are unified under the theme that recovery from childhood abuse requires recognition and redress of a life history in which terrible things have happened, and, equally important, recognition and redress of a life history in which in which many important normative events and experiences have been absent or diminished.

In Part III, the Phase 1 STAIR targets the generation of social and emotional resources, while Phase 2 NST aims to resolve PTSD and other symptoms. Many survivors have both types of problems and so will benefit from the use of both treatment components, but therapists can consider using only one or the other as suits the needs of the particular client at a particular time. Such judgments are aided by a review of treatment guidelines (Chapter 8), strategies for evaluating when to transition from skills training to narrative work (Chapter 18), and a review of the summaries provided in each session chapter. These "at-a-glance" summaries identify what matters most in the session (e.g., the development of emotional awareness) and why it matters. This is intended to liberate the therapist from the assumption that, in order to be successful, the session must be completed as described. Rather, the theme should prompt the therapist to ask: How significant is this problem for my client? How skilled is my client in each of these activities? Which of these strategies address my client's current problems? Ideally, the therapist and client will work together to answer these questions. The selection of the interventions and the specific goals that are targeted are the result of a collaborative effort.

It is well known that the therapeutic alliance influences and enhances the benefits of any treatment, and this is particularly true for abuse survivors (see Cloitre et al., 2004). For this reason, the nature and role of the therapeutic alliance is integrated into several chapters of the book. Chapter 8 provides an overview of the value of the therapeutic relationship and strategies for building a good working relationship, particularly in the context of potential ruptures common in work with abuse survivors. Several sessions identify specific therapist attitudes and behaviors that support and facilitate effective implementation of the session interventions, for example, those related to emotional awareness (Chapter 11) and narratives of shame and loss (Chapters 22 and 23).

Finally, we hope the book is written with awareness of the need for the therapist to manage his or her own mental and physical health. We have highlighted the importance of therapist self-care and provided several references on the topic (see Chapter 8 and Appendix A). We hope that the philosophy and guidelines for treatment that are set out provide compassion and understanding for their clients' condition and in doing so protect and empower therapists in their work.

Contents

PHASE I. Skills Training in Affective and Interpersonal Regulation (STAIR): Building Resources

CHAPTER 1

∽

The Trauma of Childhood Abuse
A Resource Loss Model

Childhood abuse is not a diagnosis but a life experience.
—Frank W. Putnam (2004)

WHY A TREATMENT FOR CHILDHOOD ABUSE TRAUMA?

The treatment described in this book is the result of more than a decade of listening and responding to the needs and concerns expressed by treatment-seeking women with histories of childhood abuse. It has undergone rigorous empirical evaluation, and it is the first treatment specifically designed for childhood abuse survivors that has been demonstrated as efficacious, feasible, and, most important, acceptable to such survivors. Community studies indicate that one in five women has experienced either sexual or physical abuse, with many experiencing both (e.g., Edwards, Holden, Felitti, & Anda, 2003; Schoen, Davis, & Collins, 1997). In clinical settings, 40% or more of women in treatment report an abuse history (e.g., Briere & Runtz, 1987; Cloitre, Tardiff, Marzuk, Leon, & Portera, 1996). It is rather astonishing that until this time, no demonstrably effective treatments have been developed specifically for this population. The motivation for this book was derived from the observation that the substantial presence of abuse survivors in mental health settings was completely at odds with the absence of programs that effectively addressed their needs.

What constitutes "childhood abuse"? According to federal law, such abuse is broadly defined as an "act or failure to act on the part of a parent or caretaker which results in death, serious physical or emotional harm, sexual abuse or exploitation; or an act or failure to act which presents an imminent risk or serious harm" (http://nccanch.acf.hhs.gov/pubs/factsheets/Whatiscan.cfm). Over the past several decades, there has been significant debate about the potential mental health consequences of childhood abuse. We have heard by turns that it is a critical life experience or, alternatively, that it is irrelevant; that it brings on irreparable character problems or can build personal strength; that it is associated with multiple psychiatric disorders or is really just an excuse for poor behavior. Who would not be confused? Although understanding has been slow in coming, childhood abuse is now known to be at least one thing: a traumatic experience. Like other identified traumas, such as combat and rape, it is most frequently associated with posttraumatic stress disorder (PTSD) and, to a lesser extent, major depression.

The reliable association of PTSD and major depression with childhood abuse has served to legitimize such abuse as a trauma and provides an accurate characterization of some of its psychological consequences. However, the impairment and psychic suffering caused by this phenomenon are enormous and go beyond that implied by a psychiatric diagnosis. Moreover, traumatized clients coming to treatment will almost inevitably ask for and need help with resolving impairments in life functioning, in addition to the diagnosis-specific difficulties that may be present. One of the goals of this book is to provide a framework for thinking about the effects of trauma in a coherent way—one that includes, but goes beyond, diagnostic categorization—and, in doing so, to help the therapist and client develop an effective treatment plan.

Below, we provide a "resource loss model" as the framework for understanding trauma in general and childhood abuse in particular. Resource loss is a critical and universal feature of all traumas: Life after a trauma is diminished. Depending on the trauma, the lost resources may be both psychological (such as sense of security, optimism, and social support) and material (such as a home, family, schooling or employment, and a community within which to prosper). In addition, certain types of traumatic events and their harshest consequences befall those who are already in circumstances with limited resources. Trauma often comes to people with fewer financial resources. For instance, hurricanes and floods are experienced by individuals who cannot afford to live in areas outside of hurricane paths and floodplains. Similarly, interpersonal violence is experienced more often by those who have fewer physical and psychological resources to protect themselves, such as children, elderly individuals, and injured persons. Forcible rape among females, for example, is not randomly distributed across the lifespan, but occurs predominantly in the vulnerable years: in childhood and youth. Over two-thirds of all such rapes are experienced by those under the age of 18 (Kilpatrick, Edmunds, & Seymour, 1992).

In addition, those who are most vulnerable to trauma due to limited resources will, for the same reasons, have more difficulty recovering. The irony of trauma is that recovery requires the presence of resources greater than those the victim often had in the first place. Rebuilding a house destroyed by a hurricane requires more than bricks, mortar, and the owner's own toil; it also requires a team of roofers, bricklayers, plumbers, and painters. Just as the homeowner's own resources are not enough, the resources of a trauma survivor are often insufficient without an additional investment from the outside. This is particularly true of child victims: Childhood is a time when the individual is vulnerable to victimization, and once victimization occurs, he/she has even fewer psychological and social resources than before with which to negotiate a recovery process.

Lastly, the traumatized state is not static. If resource regeneration does not occur, the result is not stasis, but rather continued resource loss and degeneration (see Monnier &

Hobfall, 2000). The unrepaired or partially repaired house will be buffeted by wind, risk further decay or be entirely destroyed in the onslaught of another hurricane. Similarly, without resource recovery, the trauma survivor's psychological and social trajectory will be vulnerable to the vicissitudes of ordinary life stressors and additional traumas. The risk of downward trajectory is particularly relevant and evident among those abused in childhood. The mandate of childhood is growth: physical, psychological, and social. Trauma reduces the resources necessary not only for trauma recovery but for the developmental tasks intrinsic to childhood. As a result, the achievement of such tasks is often compromised, with impairments—evident in poor life functioning—accumulating into adulthood.

The resource loss model thus informs our understanding of trauma recovery. Trauma recovery requires resource recovery. Accordingly, the principle of intervention to which this program adheres is one of recovery of resource losses—in particular, the rehabilitation of the psychological, emotional, and social capacities whose development have been interrupted by abuse.

We now describe our resource loss model framework for defining trauma, vulnerability to trauma, its psychosocial consequences, and the characteristics of effective intervention. We catalogue the losses associated with childhood abuse, some of which are common to all traumas and others of which are specific to the abuse experience. In addition, we describe PTSD and risk for PTSD within the context of this model. We conclude with implications for intervention, which leads to the central concern of the remainder of this book: the successful treatment of the adult survivor of childhood abuse.

A RESOURCE LOSS MODEL OF CHILDHOOD ABUSE TRAUMA

Definition of Trauma

"Trauma" has been defined in medicine as a circumstance in which some part of the body has been suddenly damaged by a force so powerful that the body's natural protections are unable to prevent injury and the body's natural healing abilities are inadequate to resolve the injury without medical assistance (*Stedman's Medical Dictionary*, 2000). The word "trauma" is, in fact, derived from the Greek for "wound." As noted by Chris Brewin (2003), Freud (1920/1955) was the first to define the term "psychic injury" by analogy to physical injury. Psychic trauma was described by Freud as an event that "penetrates a kind of mental skin designed to protect a person from excessive external forces; trauma was essentially a 'breach in an otherwise efficacious barrier' " (Brewin, 2003, p. 4). The breach is the result not only of the strength and impact of the external force, but of the inability of the organism or affected area to deflect, absorb, neutralize, or compensate for the injury.

Following this analogy, we describe psychological trauma as a circumstance in which an event overwhelms or exceeds a person's capacity to protect his or her psychic wellbeing and integrity. It is a collision between an event and a person's resources, where the power of the event is greater than the resources available for effective response and recovery. Deterioration in functioning occurs, and intervention or resources beyond those the individual has available are required for recovery. Psychological trauma, like physical trauma, represents a complex relationship between an event and a response. The objective characteristics of a potentially traumatic event—its force, strength, or "dose"—can be quantified, but the impact of the event cannot be determined without taking into account the vulnerabilities of the particular individual who sustains the injury.

Childhood Abuse as the Prototypical Trauma: An Event That Overwhelms Resources

This analysis has significant implications for our understanding of childhood abuse as a major trauma. To continue the medical analogy, it is well known that certain toxic chemicals and environmental pollutants have a significantly greater impact on children than on adults, even when the amount of exposure or "dose" is the same. Children's immature development makes them vulnerable to the effects of such toxins. The impact on their bodily systems is more potent than that experienced by adults, and the effect of a toxin on one system has negative effects on other related and vulnerable developing systems.

Now let us consider, for example, a child who is subjected to sexual abuse. Within the *Diagnostic and Statistical Manual of Mental Disorders*, fourth edition, text revision (DSM-IV-TR), sexual abuse is categorized as a trauma because it is "an event [involving] . . . serious injury, or a threat to the physical integrity of self" (American Psychiatric Association, 2000, p. 467). The experience of "threat to physical integrity" in sexual abuse is in the transgression against the child's entire body. Physical contact with a child for sexual purposes uses the body of the child without his or her meaningful consent. This act is one in which the perpetrator takes ownership of another's body, which, by definition, is the essential and basic territory of the self. Furthermore, sexual abuse often, if not typically, co-occurs with physical abuse (e.g., Briere, 1992; Diaz, Simatov, & Rickert, 2000). Thus a typical picture of childhood abuse is one in which there are repeated exposures to multiple forms of bodily violence. An effective response to this circumstance requires internal and external resources of a kind and quantity not typically within children's grasp.

The internal or personal resources with which children can protect themselves are limited by the simple fact of their life stage. Their levels of cognitive-affective and physical development place significant limits on their capacity to recognize, avoid, or escape perpetrators of abuse. Explicit or implied suggestions that sexual activity with a caretaker or other adult is good or that physical abuse is deserved are difficult for children to oppose or resist. They tend to be naive or confused by the threat hiding behind the blandishments and compliments of perpetrators of sexual abuse. Their small size also makes them easy targets for physically abusive adults.

In addition, children's external resources are far more limited than those of adults. When adults experience a trauma such as a rape or motor vehicle accident, or when they witness violence, they are more likely to have a place of safety to recover and or a social support network on which to rely on for care as needed. In contrast, children have little choice about where they live or on whom they depend. Their home, the traditional source of safety, is also very often the source of their injury. In such cases, the individuals on which the children depend are those who are committing the transgressions against them. The necessary alternative in this situation, of telling someone about a caretaker's abuse, can be frightening in its implication of loss of home and caretaker, or attendant sense of betrayal, regardless of the danger posed by the abuse. Even getting access to agencies and institutions that aim to protect children is difficult or impossible for a child to do alone, as it legally requires the accompaniment or aid of other adults.

The resource limitations of children confronted with sexual and physical abuse lead us to define childhood abuse as a trauma in all of its essential characteristics. Children who are abused are individuals who are helpless in the face of repeated, unavoidable, and inescapable transgressions against their bodies. A child's resources are no match for the immediate and consistent threat of physical or sexual assaults by an adult, particularly when that adult is a parent or other caretaker.

From Resource Limitations to Resource Loss

The resource limitations the child experiences in confronting the trauma are defined by his or her life stage and yield a circumstance in which the child rarely succeeds in warding off or neutralizing sexual or physical threats. In addition, once the trauma occurs, its presence creates a cascade of resource losses that continue during its typically chronic course and have significant consequences long after the abuse ends.

The most immediate consequences of abuse are the losses of physical safety and physical integrity. Less evident, but equally profound and perhaps fairly unique to childhood abuse, are the losses of many psychological and social-developmental opportunities and advances, which are diminished or negated as either direct or indirect results of the abuse. Childhood abuse is a trauma perpetrated by an adult, usually an important caretaker upon whom a child depends significantly for psychological and material resources. It occurs during a time of life when many developmental tasks, involving the growth of emotional and social competencies, are being completed; these tasks require sustained contributions by the caretaker, family, and community. Under conditions of abuse, these very necessary resources are often deficient or disturbed, compromising the child's ability to complete these tasks successfully. Lastly, it is critical to note that recovery from the effects of abuse, like recovery from all traumas, requires the investment of additional "repairing" resources. But for children and adolescents, this investment often requires the initiative of the caretaker—and if the caretaker is the perpetrator of the trauma, he or she is motivated to ignore, hide, or deny the abuse. This aspect of abuse, the silence and stigma associated with it, adds to further resource loss (i.e., the support and intervention of the community). All of these losses and the absence of intervention in a time of development conspire to create substantial functional impairment among adult survivors.

Acknowledging all these circumstances, we have catalogued the potential resource losses that childhood abuse engenders in both the short and long term. They include (1) loss of healthy attachment, (2) loss of effective guidance in the development of emotional and social competencies, and (3) loss of support and connection to the larger social community.

Loss of Healthy Attachment

One of the most devastating aspects of childhood abuse is that the perpetrator of the trauma is almost always a parent or other important caretaker. The implications of this circumstance as a resource loss are staggering. The attachment of a child to a parent or other primary caregiver creates the base for learning about the essentials of living. This attachment is a resource from which springs the evolution of effective agency, self-definition, and autonomy. This attachment is intended to provide sufficient safety and security for the child to explore and learn about the world, and to grow in confidence and autonomy. Ideally, a caretaker provides a secure base or home for "refueling" of resources to explore the world. This secure base involves the caretaker's availability to act as a facilitator to the child's growing capacities in self-management and effective interaction with the social and physical environment.

Abuse undermines the development of all these powerful psychological and social assets. Sexual and physical abuse are essentially a betrayal of the assumption of care by the parent for the child (see Freyd, 1996), and in every aspect of the betrayal of parenting responsibilities, there is a defined loss.

There is a profound loss of a sense of security and personal safety; associated with this is a restricted capacity for curiosity and exploration about the world. There is also the loss of a healthy trajectory of affective organization. The developing capacity for self-soothing is challenged by physical and sexual violations, and guidance from the abusing caretaker is often absent, irregular, or deviant. Moreover, there is significant disturbance in the development of a sense of autonomy and agency. Rather than recognize and protect the necessary but vulnerable authority of the child as an agent of his or her own experience, the abusive caretaker acts in such a way that the child becomes an extension of the caretaker's own sexual and aggressive impulses. The betrayal of the attachment bond often leads to loss of trust in intimate relationships, with long-term consequences in the management of future interpersonal relationships. Lastly, to the extent that such violations elicit feelings of shame and guilt, they create a loss of the capacity for self-love and positive self-regard.

Loss of Opportunities for Social and Emotional Development

Childhood abuse derails the development of important life skills, particularly emotional and social competencies that lead to effective self-management and interpersonal relationships. Children who are abused often come from families in which parents or caretakers are often themselves limited in emotional expression and interpersonal functioning (Chattin, Kelleher, & Hollenberg, 1996; Hein & Honeyman, 2000; Nash, Hulsey, Sexton, Harralason, & Lambert, 1993; Ray, Jackson, & Townley, 1991), and so are less than ideal role models for learning such skills. In addition, abuse within the home setting creates paradoxical and conflicting information about acceptable and effective rules for living. For example, standard rules of sexual and physical behavior are applicable in general but not in the home. These inconsistencies, often unexplained, can create inappropriate social behaviors that lead to peer rejection and loss of confidence in the survivor's own perceptions and judgments about social realities.

The diminished emotional and social competencies associated with abuse are further exacerbated or result in continued social/emotional injury and loss in the larger social environment during both childhood and adolescence. For example, compared to their peers, abused children have difficulty with social engagement and especially with conflict negotiation, are more uncomfortable with high levels of emotion, expect little social support from adults in resolving social difficulties (e.g., Cummings, Hennessy, Rabideau, & Cicchetti, 1994; Schwartz & Proctor, 2000; Shields & Cicchetti, 1998; Shipman, Zeman, Penza, & Champion, 2000), and are less confident and report lower self-esteem (e.g., Feiring, Taska, & Lewis, 1998; Spaccarelli, 1994). In adolescent years, those with abuse histories, are more likely than their peers to drop out of school, engage in substance abuse and delinquent behaviors, and experience interpersonal violence both as victims and as perpetrators (e.g., Giaconia et al., 1995; Kilpatrick et al., 2003; Lipschitz, Rasmusson, Anyan, Comwell, & Southwick, 2000). Perhaps, as the ultimate behavioral expression of all that ails them, compared to their peers, adolescents with abuse histories are 2 to 5 times more likely to attempt suicide (Garnestski & Dieksha, 1997; Gianconia et al., 1995).

In adulthood, individuals with a history of childhood abuse often report a profound sense of lost opportunities in realizing desired goals in both their work and personal lives. Kessler (2000) reported that in the general population, individuals with PTSD related to chronic interpersonal violence at an early age are more likely than those with other types of PTSD to fall short in achieving expectable life milestones in employment, marriage, childbearing, and earnings. Indeed, there is often an accumulation of repeated relationship failures, domestic violence and other forms of revictimization (e.g., Polusny & Follette, 1995), chronic substance abuse (Najavits, Weiss, & Shaw, 1997), and impaired parenting (e.g., Hien & Honeyman, 2000).

Loss of Perceived Support of the Community

It has become clear that welcoming children into the larger community enhances their development, including self-esteem, social skills, and physical well-being (www. searchinstitute.com). The support of the community is expressed in the explicit valuing of children as community members; this valuing is demonstrated by acknowledgment of their presence in the community, concern about their experiences, expression of positive regard, and active efforts to provide them with appropriate roles. Abused children often do not experience full and positive engagement in the community. This can occur in many ways and for many reasons. The abused children may be hampered in integrating themselves if their emotional resources are primarily absorbed by the demands of the home environment (managing abusive parents and experiences). Their lesser social and emotional regulation skills, as described above, may make them less attractive to peers, teachers, coaches, religious leaders, or other important figures of influence. Furthermore, silence about the abuse may create a feeling of alienation and a loss of any authentic sense of relating to peers, teachers, or other members of the community.

Lastly, the stigma of abuse and general discomfort about recognizing its presence may keep community members at a distance from an abused child or youth. The tendency to "blame the victim" (see Matsakis, 1998) emerges from the distress that is elicited by recognizing and responding to victimization. It forces recognition of malfeasance toward a vulnerable person, and in the case of childhood abuse, adult malfeasance toward an innocent person. Abused children make the rest of us uncomfortable, because they challenge our belief system that the world is benevolent and that we are all competent to take care of ourselves. The desire to maintain this illusion leads us to expect an unrealistic level of competence in children to defend themselves.

The alternative to "blaming the victim," which is to recognize the existence of abuse, leads to other kinds of difficulties. There may well be confusion and uncertainty about how to intervene and reluctance to do so. Indeed, recent data indicate that, while 9 in 10 Americans regard childhood abuse as a serious problem, only 1 in 3 reported abuse when confronted with an actual situation (www.childrensinstitute.org/publications.html). The impulse to intervene in the activities of a family where a child is being victimized by a parent or other caretaker conflicts with traditional beliefs about the integrity and autonomy of the family unit. Strategies for intervention have been developed through family courts and the development of agencies that monitor the safety of children, but there is a sustained tension between these interventions and beliefs about the privacy and authority of the family unit and its potential superiority as a context for caring for children.

Finally, as exemplified by the development of safety-monitoring agencies, abused children, like all traumatized individuals, require the extension of social and community resources. Such resources include money, time, and effort. If such resources become scarce, sympathy for these children may yield to feelings of resentment or indifference. Those with more resources may lose patience with those who have fewer of them. Thus the consequences of childhood abuse as a resource loss ripple out to the community in which an abused child lives and needs to be supported. Reactions to the diminution of resources often lead to conflict and reduced integrity of the community and its members. The integration of the abused child into the community is strained. Stigma remains, and the child still feels alienated and out of the mainstream. The alienation generated by the silence is transformed into alienation generated by resentment.

PTSD as a Consequence of Inadequate Resources

Resource limitations may also play a key role in the development of PTSD. Recent longitudinal studies (e.g., Shalev, 1997; Shalev, Tuval-Mashiach, & Hadar, 2004) have suggested that the first or immediate reactions to a trauma are those described in the PTSD diagnosis. Individuals exposed to trauma feel hypervigilant, have poor concentration, feel irritable, and can't sleep. They do not seem to be fully present in place and time. Images and thoughts about the event are constantly replayed in their minds. Remarkably, for most people, the course of recovery progresses substantially within a few days to a few weeks. The reality of the unexpected event begins to be assimilated: The specifics of the incident are organized into a sequence of events, and some kind of evaluation of the meaning of the event and its impact on the person's view of the world and of the self begins. But for a subset of individuals, the reactions persist, and PTSD emerges from the sustained and unremitting presence of normal posttraumatic reactions.

We propose that the development of PTSD, and perhaps other long-term psychiatric symptoms such as depression, can be explained within the context of the resource loss model: In those who develop enduring symptoms, the resources required to recover from the trauma are insufficient relative to their need. The analogy to the process of recovery from physical trauma can describe this idea. Once an injury has been sustained, the recovery from an injury varies from person to person. The recovery depends in part on the status of individuals, such as the health and maturity of their immune systems. It also depends on the nature and quality of the health services they receive, and on other environmental resources, including a support network that can relieve the individuals of responsibilities they cannot manage themselves (food, clothing, and shelter). In brief, natural recovery from trauma calls on and is facilitated by a variety of internal and external resources.

Brewin, Andrews, and Valentine (2000) have provided the most comprehensive assessment yet conducted of risk factors contributing to PTSD among adults. The majority and certainly the most influential of these factors can be understood as "low-resource" phenomena. These include past adversity, previously diminished mental health, lack of social support, and low education. Other risk factors that have been identified as contributing to negative impact following trauma include maladaptive coping strategies such as denial, giving up, or substance abuse, and environmental factors such as an unstable family and environment (Norris, Perilla, & Murphy, 2001; Shalev, 2002). These risks can be viewed as the absence or limited availability of personal and environmental resources to cope with adversity.

It may come as little surprise that children who are abused suffer many of these resource limitations and resource losses. Indeed, as might be expected, rates of abuse-related PTSD are higher than those of PTSD related to traumas that have a more circumscribed influence on a child's extant and developing resources. In addition, adults who have experienced childhood abuse are more vulnerable to developing PTSD when they experience traumas in adulthood, even when they have never had PTSD before. The strength of childhood trauma as a risk factor for adult PTSD is consistent with the suggestion that childhood abuse represents the risk deriving not only from the abuse, but also from the short- and long-term resource losses that occur in its wake.

PTSD among Children

The most pertinent question concerning resources and the risk for PTSD among traumatized children is to what extent the children's caretakers are resources for them. It was first noted during World War II that children exposed to bombings did rather well if their parents did well by them and were psychologically healthy themselves (Carey-Trefzer, 1949). Children look within their immediate environment, and particularly to their caretakers, to gauge safety and interpret the level of threat in a particular situation. That is, children use their parents as anchors or reference points to understand the meaning of traumatic events, understand cause and effect, experience safety and support, obtain comfort, and receive guidance in effective coping. A consistent finding in the trauma literature is that rates of PTSD in children exposed to the same stressor, such as violence in war-torn countries, vary with the warmth, psychological stability, and coping capacities of the parents (e.g., Laor et al., 1997; Scheeringa & Zeanah, 2001).

This observation leads to alarming implications for children whose trauma is generated by their parents or other caregivers. The sense of safety that is obtained from calm and concerned caretakers following a traumatic incident is not available to such children. Let's take the example of a child who has been injured in a traffic accident. A parent's explanations about what happened and why create an understanding of cause and effect. The concerned parent's sense of confidence and realistic appraisal of the low probability of recurrence of that event assures the child about his or her relative safety. The traumatic event is shared by the family and perhaps also by the larger community, creating a network of social support. People visit the child, bring gifts, write cards, and generally wish the child well in his or her recovery.

This situation contrasts rather starkly with that in intrafamilial sexual or physical abuse, where a child's source of safety is his or her source of danger. Moreover, the event is chronic and unending. The caretaker also rarely makes explanations about the events that are accurate or realistic (e.g., he or she may say that it happens "because you deserve it" or "because you want this"). Few people know about the trauma, and no one comes to visit or brings cards wishing a speedy recovery. The trauma is secret, hidden, and confusing. There is also chronic uncertainty about the next sexual or physical assault event, which can lead to a continued sense of alarm and sustained symptoms of hyperarousal. The alternating experiences of intrusive reexperiencing and avoidance/numbing, which under different circumstances might be resolved through repeated efforts at mental organization and appraisal of the meaning of the event, are repeatedly disturbed by similar additional events and misinformation by adults, and by the continuing toll these traumas take on the child's diminishing personal emotional and cognitive resources.

Rates of PTSD associated with traffic accidents and burns among children seen in outpatient and inpatient services range from 14% to 27% (DeVries et al., 1999; Keppel-Benson, Ollendick, & Benson, 2002; Stoddard, Norman, Murphy, & Beardslee, 1989). In contrast, PTSD rates for children with sexual and physical abuse seen in outpatient and related services range from 34% to 58% (Adam et al., 1992; Ackerman et al., 1998; McLeer, Callaghan, Henry, & Wallen, 1994; McLeer, Deblinger, Henry, & Orvaschel, 1992; McLeer et al., 1998; Wolfe, Sas, & Wekerle, 1994). Apart from war violence, situations of chronic violence, loss of multiple resources (including the death or disappearance of parents), sexual abuse, and physical abuse are associated with the highest rates of PTSD in children across all traumas. The use of different measures and different environments across these studies calls for caution in drawing this conclusion incontrovertibly. However, at least one investigator, Philip Saigh, has used the same clinical method and measure to identify rates of PTSD across different traumas. Saigh and Bremner (1999) report the rates of PTSD for specific types of trauma as follows: accidents, 11%; war, 29%–33%; and physical and sexual abuse, 65%. In addition, studies of adolescents, for whom there are more well-controlled and more numerous investigations, report results consistent with the conclusions about children.

PTSD among Adolescents

Studies of traumatized adolescents that have explicitly queried for the presence of abuse have indicated that childhood sexual abuse is more likely to produce PTSD than other traumatic stressors. In four methodologically rigorous studies, PTSD related to specific traumatic events was identified, and sexual abuse was consistently the top-ranking PTSD-producing traumatic event (Dubner & Motta, 1999; Giaconia et al., 1995; Horowitz, Weine, & Jekel, 1995; Lipschitz, Winegar, Hartnick, Foote, & Southwick, 1999a). For example, Lipshitz et al. (1999a) reported that 60.5% of inpatient adolescents with sexual abuse had PTSD, compared to those with the two other most frequently occurring stressors—namely, exposure to family violence (50% PTSD rate) and physical abuse (28% PTSD rate). When study participants were compared by PTSD status (those with vs. without PTSD), a history of childhood sexual abuse was almost always present in the PTSD-positive group, independent of whether it had been identified as the most stressful event: 91% of the PTSD-positive patients had a history of childhood sexual abuse, compared to 32% of those without PTSD. In summary, a conservative estimate would suggest that 50% or more of adolescents who have experienced childhood sexual trauma have full-blown PTSD.

Adults with PTSD Related to Childhood Abuse

As might be expected, by adulthood the lifetime prevalence of PTSD is higher than that reported among children and adolescents. The DSM-IV field trials for PTSD identified the prevalence of PTSD in a combined community and clinical sample as 77% for those who had experienced childhood sexual abuse, 45% for those with physical abuse, and 85% for those with physical and sexual abuse (Roth, Newman, Pelcovitz, van der Kolk, & Mandel, 1997). Other studies report similar rates of DSM-III-R-diagnosed PTSD among adults with histories of childhood abuse, ranging from 69% to 73% depending on the sample (community or clinical) (Cloitre, Scarvalone, & Difede, 1997; O'Neill & Gupta, 1991; Rodriguez, Ryan, Rowan, & Foy, 1996; Rowan & Foy, 1993). As might be expected from this summary, comparisons with the rates of other disorders have identified PTSD as the most frequently occurring Axis I disorder associated with a history of childhood abuse among adults (Cloitre et al., 1997).

Implications for Treatment

PTSD symptoms are the direct and evident results of a trauma. But along with the *presence* or positive signs of psychiatric symptoms, childhood abuse trauma often produces a form of negative symptoms—that is, the *absence* of substantive emotional and social competencies.

The treatment philosophy described in this book affirms that recovery from childhood trauma requires the rehabilitation of resources and life skills that were derailed or denied in the skirmish of survival in a chronically abusive environment. The treatment is at heart a resource recovery program, with an emphasis on reclaiming and building emotional and social competencies. We adhere to the notion that resources above and beyond those necessary for basic survival must be recruited and accumulated in order to recover from the damages inflicted by a trauma. In addition, like many other researchers, clinicians, and survivors, we have found that emotional processing of the trauma is a powerful if not a critical component in trauma recovery.

Accordingly, we have developed a two-phase treatment program in which the development of resources and emotional processing of the trauma are equal and balanced partners. The first phase of the treatment, Skills Training in Affective and Interpersonal Regulation (STAIR), is dedicated to building emotional and social competencies as resources. The second phase of the treatment, Narrative Story Telling (NST), involves the emotional processing of the traumatic events in the context of a safe and supportive environment. The ordering of the phases is purposeful: Resource development precedes the trauma-processing work, because the intention is that the former prepares and strengthens the client to succeed in the latter.

We have proposed that in the course of a life that includes chronic exposure to traumatic events, the development of PTSD is the result of insufficient resources with which to heal from the trauma. In the same way, we propose that in the course of therapy, confronting the pain of multiple traumatic memories requires the presence of emotional and interpersonal resources to be successful and healing. The treatment is in essence a recapitulation of the appropriate order of development in the ideal case: The fortunate person is provided with the advantage of the accrual of multiple and diverse resources as he or she faces their life challenges.

~

CHAPTER 2

Attachment

When Protector and Perpetrator Are One

Attachment theory starts from the power of adults to protect and provide security for their children. In abuse, this fundamental biosocial contract between adults and children is ruptured: adults use their power for their own ends rather than those of the child.

—JEREMY HOLMES (2001, p. 95)

THE POWER OF THE ATTACHMENT BOND

By far, a child's parents or other caretakers are his or her most important resources. Parents provide safety. They provide instruction on how the world works and how to function in it. They stand between the child and the vicissitudes of life until the child is ready to face these independently. Parents extend the child's awareness of external resources to those in the larger world, and oversee the child's ability to use these resources on his or her own behalf: in maintaining safety, in solving problems, in finding friends and a supportive environment, and in experiencing pleasure and joy. Parents also build the child's internal resources. A parent helps a child develop a sense of competence through regular instruction and feedback. More importantly, the parent mirrors back not only success in a learned skill, but something more ineffable and more valuable: pride in the child's accomplishment. The infrastructure of the child's self is built on the parent's internalized view of him or her: that of being well regarded and valued. These perceptions are the foundations of self-esteem, confidence, and self-love, which allow the developing child to do well. This positive view of self provides the child with the capacity to confront new situations with the expectation of doing well, and to meet new people with the expectation of being well regarded. It also allows the child to approach difficulties with the belief that solutions can be found and that personal limitations can be managed.

Perhaps it is inevitable that the proximity of a child to a caretaker, intended to secure the child's continued growth, is also his or her Achilles heel: The primary sources of injury and harm to children are their caretakers. For example, recent reviews of nearly 3 million cases of documented child abuse in a single year in the United States indicated that 80% of the sexual abuse perpetrators were parents (Golden, 2000). Such circumstances pervert the resource relationship between parent and child. The child's need for physical proximity to the caretaker, and dependence on the caretaker for safety, result in experiences of physical transgressions. The bond with the caretaker becomes an affective and cognitive contradiction: The source of safety is also a source of danger. The explanations for effective functioning in the world at large are suspended, irrelevant, or contradicted at home. The person responsible for building the child's self-regard also breaks it down with physical intrusions or assaults. The parent who creates bridges between the child and his or her social world also severs those connections with secret sexual transgressions. As a result, the child's feelings of safety and control, positive regard, competence, and connection to the larger world are compromised.

The attachment literature has demonstrated that the connection between caretaker and offspring is a critical dynamic that supports the survival and growth of the child. In this design of care, it is expected that threats to safety are generated beyond the shadow of the caretaker, and that when threatened, the child returns to the safety of home base. Evolution of the fight-or-flight reaction is viewed as consistent with a system of safety in which protection is anchored to a home base. The fight-or-flight response is effective for refueling in the short term and for longer-term resource building in the affiliative/protective network of home base. But this arrangement is not a "fail-safe" system, as demonstrated by circumstances in which parents/caretakers themselves become the threat via physical and sexual abuse of their offspring. The consequence of such circumstances is that for at least some period of time, a child inevitably experiences a relationship in which perpetrator and care provider are one.

The power of the attachment bond remains apparent, even in the context of abuse. This has been demonstrated in several research literatures. For example, among nonhuman species, offspring will remain in physical proximity to their parents or designated caretakers, even when contact with the caretakers is associated with significant physical pain and aversive experiences (see Hofer, 2003). The evolution of this circumstance is presumably related to the biosocial net cost of such relationships: Any caretaker is better than none, particularly when the offspring have little capacity to function independently. Among humans, the rate of maturation is relatively slow and the dependence of children on adult caretakers is sustained, with several years of guardianship required to monitor and support the children's constant cognitive, social, and emotional growth.

One of the more perplexing consequences of early life abuse is that attachment to an abusive caretaker can be more powerful than that which occurs within nonabusive bonds. Although this is a devastating consequence of abuse, it is not difficult to understand once the dynamics of childhood abuse are understood. As Freyd (1996, p. 71) notes, "The child is charged by life" to sustain the attachment to parents, and so to sustain him- or herself. A vicious cycle that begins with the child's inherent dependence on the parent is established. In healthy circumstances, development progresses with increasing autonomy and the prerequisite resources to succeed in this independence, all of which are supported by the caretakers. However, autonomy is stymied in circumstances of abuse, because injury and diminished capacity actually increase rather than decrease dependence. Research with nonhuman species has shown that maltreatment actually *increases* attachment, because the more an individual is injured or terrorized, the stronger his or her need for protection and comforting. Allen (1995, p. 157) describes the bond in terms of a three-part cycle: The worse the injury, the greater need for care and security, and so the tighter the bond.

This dynamic operates with children under circumstances of intrafamilial abuse. The children grow more helpless and less competent. Typically living in relative social isolation and naïve to alternatives, the children continue to turn to their parents for help. In addition, children assume that their parents have their best interests in mind, despite the abuse. Frightened and confused, they are seeking safety and security; the provision of any shred of care, affection, or attention will draw them closer to their parents.

ABUSE-GENERATED INTERPERSONAL SCHEMAS: "TO BE ATTACHED MEANS TO BE ABUSED" AND "ABUSE IS ONE WAY OF ATTACHING"

One of the most alarming legacies of childhood abuse is repeated victimization (see Cloitre, 1998). This includes relatively high rates of bullying and scapegoating experiences in childhood (e.g., Shipman et al., 2000), of sexual assaults and date rape among adolescent girls and young women (e.g., Gidycz, Hanson, & Layman, 1995; Krahe, Sheinberger-Olwig, Waizenhofer, & Koplin, 1999), of domestic violence among women (Messman & Long, 1996; Polusny & Follette, 1995), and of particularly high rates of repeated sexual assaults among women with significant psychiatric illness (Cloitre, Tardiff, Marzuk, Leon, & Portera, 1996). These observations have led some to hypothesize the presence of masochistic tendencies or "self-defeating personality syndromes" among abuse survivors. The philosophy on which the treatment described in this book is based assumes an entirely different set of principles. In our view, the aspects of revictimization that come from habitual modes of interpersonal relating are actually based on a healthy impulse to engage. This impulse, however, has been wildly misdirected by the disturbing influence of abuse. Engaging with other people and staying in relationships are learned behaviors. When significant learning experiences come from an abusive context or abusive people, the interpersonal expectations and social behaviors that result are likely to be negative. One goal of the present treatment is to help survivors maintain the desire for connection, but to change their behavioral patterns of relating and the people with whom they relate.

The treatment uses the notion of an "interpersonal schema," derived from the work of John Bowlby and other attachment theorists, as an explanatory construct for understanding how healthy impulses go wrong. The identification of schema theory within an attachment model is theoretically very important, because it provides a value-neutral explanation of revictimization within the context of general principles of interpersonal behavior.

Some Aspects of Attachment Theory

Bowlby (1969) and others have suggested that several biologically based mechanisms support the propensity to maintain closeness to the available caretaker and function to maximize survival. Their nature and complexity are in accord with the point at which they emerge during the course of behavioral, cognitive, and affective development. One mechanism is the development of "interpersonal schemas" or "working models of relating." These schemas have been described as cognitive–affective structures that organize information which, based on experience, specify and anticipate the contingencies for maintaining relatedness to the caretakers (Safran, 1990a, 1990b; Safran & Segal, 1990). Multiple schemas develop through time, based on differing interpersonal events of consequence with different important people. Schemas are also amenable to revision as a result of changing circumstances. There is some evidence, however, that the first and oldest of interpersonal schemas, formed within the context of attachment relationships, play a central role in shaping future thoughts, feelings, and behaviors in the interpersonal domain (Main, Kaplan, & Cassidy, 1985).

Among the earliest and prototypical schemas are those pertaining to specific behaviors that will elicit the approach or proximity of the caretaker. Under advantageous circumstances, this proximity yields a response of care and concern. In turn, the expression of care elicited by the child is experienced by the caretaker as intrinsically satisfying. However, the interpersonal schema for attachment that emerges in an abusive caretaking setting will deviate from this proposed dynamic of mutual satisfaction. For example, in a physically assaultive home, proximity—a condition for care—may also elicit physical assault. Thus care and physical assault become paired. In sexually abusive homes, proximity can elicit sexual activity. Such contingency experiences, whatever their particulars, may lead to the following schemas of interpersonal relatedness: "To be interpersonally engaged means to be abused" and "Abuse is a way to be connected."

The Self-Fulfilling Nature of Schemas

Because schemas are assumed to be the templates that guide future expectations and behaviors, it is easy to see how negative patterns set down in childhood can guide an adult toward repeating activities that are maladaptive in adulthood. The schema model suggests that reliance on past experiences to anticipate the future is a typically adaptive strategy for living, and that the resultant tendency to repeat one's history is normative. Indeed, for those who have had positive attachment experiences, the self-fulfilling aspect of schemas works to their advantage: Expectations of positive regard tend to elicit positive responses. For abuse survivors, however, reliance on past experiences means reliance on deviant patterns of relating. This tends to lead the survivors to function in social environments in ways that elicit similar deviant patterns, or to find that patterns for relating that were adaptive in an abusive environment are no longer effective in healthier social contexts.

The first time we observed this principle in action with disastrous results concerned a case of a female soldier in the Army who had been sexually assaulted by a fellow soldier.

The two had been romantically involved. When the woman decided to break off the relationship, her boyfriend responded with rage and physically assaulted her. He also threatened to make her life miserable for the duration of their time on the base. Fearful of continued physical reprisal from him, she bought groceries and sundries from the post exchange and brought them to him at his barracks. His response was one of outrage: He sexually assaulted her and enlisted the help of a bunkmate in this act, which was repeated several times. During this woman's first visit at our clinic, the interviewer asked, in a gentle, supportive, but curious way, why she had gone to the boyfriend's barracks. She answered with surprise, "Why, this is what I knew to do when I got beat." It had always worked to save her from trouble before. The child of severely abusive parents, this woman had learned that the most effective way to appease her brawling parents was to take over the tasks of the household—to go for groceries, do the cooking, and clean the house.

The woman was acting in a way that was intended to help herself. However, the actions that had previously worked well now, in a changed environment, failed her; in fact, they contributed to the repetition of an old scenario she was trying to escape. The rules guiding effective living in an abusive environment needed to be changed now that she had left it.

Dimensions of Abuse-Related Interpersonal Schemas: Repeated Experiences of Others as Cold and Controlling

Our empirical inquiry (see Cloitre, Cohen, & Scarvalone, 2002a) into the general characteristics of the interpersonal schemas of abuse survivors has been derived from a well-established system of categorizing types of self–other interactions (Kiesler, 1983; Leary, 1957). It is a model intend to capture the full range of potential interpersonal interactions as based on two independent dimensions that are assumed to be present in all human interactions: an affective/affiliative dimension (warm to cold) and a control dimension (high to low). We compared the interpersonal expectations of women with histories of childhood abuse, women with childhood abuse and adult revictimization experiences, and women who had never experienced abuse or other forms of interpersonal victimization. When asked to recall the responses of their caretakers to them in a variety of emotional and social circumstances, the survivors described their caretakers as predominantly cold—and, among those survivors with repeated victimizations in adult life, cold and highly controlling. In contrast, the never-abused group reported their caretakers' reactions to them as warm and responsive to their situation and with respect for their autonomy.

When asked to think about an important person in their lives now (e.g., their current best friend), the most common type of interpersonal attitude and behavior expected was, for each of the study groups, a match to the type described for the caretaker. The group who had never experienced trauma had the largest number (60%) of women who expected those in their current lives to behave in ways similar to their caretakers—that is, as warm, responsive, and open to them, and as willing to follow their lead. In contrast, the majority of those with abuse histories described their current relationships as cold and their significant others as emotionally unresponsive, controlling and domineering. The self-fulfilling

AFFILIATION

	High	Low
High	*Warm and controlling*	*Cold and controlling* Revictimized: 35%
Control	*Warm and not controlling* Never traumatized: 60%	*Cold and not controlling* Childhood abuse only: 50%
Low		

FIGURE 2.1. Most frequently repeated schemas for each type of childhood history, as measured by percentage of matches in "expected responses from others" between parent/caretaker and current best friend. Data from Cloitre, Cohen, and Scarvalone (2002a).

prophecy thus appeared to operate among both the traumatized and the nontraumatized respondents, with the only difference between the groups being the particulars of their life experiences and expectations.

These results are consistent with interpersonal schema models of behavior, which describe generalization from predominant schemas as a basic human cognitive–affective tendency. It also supports our analysis of revictimization as a consequence of a general principle of functioning, rather than as a pathological behavior associated with abuse survivors. Still, the implications for the two groups differ. Among those who are not traumatized, routine schema-guided actions may be an effective strategy for living, as the expectation for positive interactions creates a bias toward positive outcome. In contrast, trauma survivors are burdened with the necessity of recognizing and changing their patterns of relating if they are to improve their functioning and escape their traumatic past.

WHEN THE PROTECTOR FAILS TO PROTECT

Our research (Cloitre et al., 2002a), consistent with the bulk of epidemiological studies of childhood abuse (see Finkelhor, 1994; Russell, 1983; Wyatt, Loeb, Solis, & Carmona, 1999), indicates that sexual abuse is most often perpetrated by males in caretaking roles or positions of authority. Still, we know from the theory and research of Bowlby and other attachment specialists that the capacity for relatedness is modifiable, and that the presence of "even just one" positive care figure can produce a "protective shield" around a child and mediate negative outcomes (Lieberman & Amaya-Jackson, 2005). This leads to the question of the role of the mother or other critical caretakers in an abused child's system of care as a factor mediating or contributing to the child's immediate or long-term outcome. The topic is remarkably understudied. The complexity and sensitive nature of the situation may contribute to the dearth of investigation. For example, research on disclosure of abuse suggests that telling a mother or someone else with power to intervene about the abuse is not related to symptom status in the short or long term (e.g., Blieberg, 2000; Wyatt, Guthrie, & Notgrass, 1992). Disclosure may be positive only when the telling leads to a protective and supportive response. Responses of agitation, denial, and even upheaval in the family system may negate any benefit that might accrue (see Alaggia, 2002; Heriot, 1996).

Among abuse survivors who seek treatment, we have found either that they have typically experienced abuse from multiple caretakers, or that nonabusing caretakers are neglectful, are absent, or simply deny or avoid recognition of the abuse. In our schema study (Cloitre et al., 2002a), sexual abuse was perpetrated most often by a male family member (88%), and abuse of some kind (physical, verbal, or sexual) by the mother was reported in half of the sample. The characterizations of the paternal and maternal caretakers did not differ: Both father and mother figures were reported as either cold and distant or cold and controlling, and there were no significant discrepancies between the abuse characteristics and schemas for the two types of figures.

The limited writing and research on the topic of the parent who is a witness to abuse rather than an active agent of it suggests that passivity in the face of abuse is itself harmful (e.g., Herman, 1992). Indeed, our own clinical experience suggests that the failure of a parent to care for and safeguard a child appears to have its own specific impact on the interpersonal beliefs and attitudes of survivors (e.g., "When I am in trouble, I know I need to take care of things myself"). This is most salient in clients' narratives about the passive or neglectful parent who turns a blind eye to the presence of physical or sexual abuse in the home. Anger and a sense of betrayal are directed toward the parent who did not intervene: the father who silently watched the mother batter their children, or the mother who denied the sexual intrusions of the father, stepfather, or boyfriend.

Steven Gold (2000) makes the important point that the significant impact of the passive bystander parent is often overlooked:

> It is not unusual to hear therapists voice the conviction that resentment directed toward non-offending parents of others who did not prevent or stop the abuse is undeserved, or represents displaced hostility that, in actuality, is related to the perpetrator. This follows logically from a trauma model framework which assumes that the abuse itself is cardinal in its impact. However, this viewpoint negates a child's fundamental need to be valued and cherished enough to be protected, supported, and affirmed, particularly by parental figures and other caretakers . . . the anger toward non-offending parties may also reflect the fact that failing to stop the abuse was just one of the myriad of ways in which parents and other caretakers abrogated their responsibilities to nurture validate, and safeguard the client in childhood. (p. 31)

Consistent with this perspective, we view the neglectful parent as representing a variation of a disturbed attachment relationship. The primary function of the attachment relationship is to ensure the safety of the child. The absence of this most simple but essential dimension from the child's relationship with the parent/caretaker is an instance of a separate and independent psychological trauma. An attachment compromised by neglect, inconsistency, or hostility/distance also has a significant impact on a child's capacity to manage abuse, even when the abuse is not perpetrated by the primary caretaker; indeed, it may create vulnerability to sexual abuse by other adults in the child's larger system of care (see Chapter 3).

SUMMARY AND IMPLICATIONS FOR TREATMENT

The overriding theme of this chapter has been the impact of abuse on the capacity for interpersonal relatedness when abuse is perpetrated by a primary caretaker. We have articulated the outcome of this experience through the shorthand of the schema "To be connected means to be abused." This shorthand refers to the tendency of survivor relationships to consist of victim–perpetrator bonds and dynamics. These dynamics are expressed directly in repeated abusive relationships (e.g., date rape, domestic violence) and high rates of revictimization. They are also reflected in chronic and pervasive problems with intimacy: Suspicion, anger, and mistrust erode relationships, leading to patterns of relationships that are short-lived or end badly.

We have also suggested that a sense of self develops in the context of relationships to others. When abuse occurs, both the sense of self and the capacity for relating are disturbed. So feelings of self-love and compassion are in part the results of having been loved and protected, and the capacity to love someone is related to one's own capacity to feel lovable and loving. Feelings of security are instilled by trust-inspiring caretakers, and these in turn allow risk taking in relationships.

All these ideas are realized in the treatment in a practical way through the notion of the "interpersonal schema." The schema is a conceptual tool with a specific structure and is included in many of the interventions in our treatment program. During Phase I, therapists and clients work to identify problematic interpersonal schemas. These are often variations of "To be attached means to be abused" and, once organized, reveal and clarify deep-seated beliefs involving feelings and themes of fear, despair, shame, and grief. The schemas articulate negative beliefs about self and expectations of others, which limit the range of perceptions the clients can have of themselves and of experiences with others. Alternative schemas and associated experiential exercises are proposed. These alternative schemas become the basis for exploring, testing, and practicing alternative ways of relating to others and experiencing new personal possibilities.

Interpersonal schema analysis is part of both phases of treatment and creates a conceptual bridge between the two phases. During the narrative work of Phase II, therapists and clients identify the core interpersonal schemas embedded in the narratives. The abuse-related schemas embedded in the narrative are contrasted with the newly emerging schemas that have been proposed in Phase I. This contrast reminds the clients that the narrative represents contingencies for living that belong to the past and need not be continued in the present. The new schemas represent the opportunity for living in the present and ideas for shaping a possible future. This contrast helps move clients from a view of themselves as victims with limited options, to a sense of themselves as adults with new resources, new choices, and new ways to think through and plan for the future.

CHAPTER 3

~

Development in the Context of Deprivation

Growing up in an abusive household is like learning to run under water.
—AUGUSTEN BURROUGHS (2003)

T he context in which a chronically abused child lives is directly contrary to the kind of environment required for healthy development. The child strives to move forward in a setting that, like water rather than air, lacks the essential resources needed to support growth. The treatment presented in this book is based on the understanding that the reduction, loss, or absence of normative social experiences is a critical feature of chronic childhood abuse, equivalent to and potentially more powerful than the traumatic events themselves. The first component of our treatment program is dedicated to providing the opportunity for survivors to explore and systematically address specific social and emotional skills difficulties that have a negative impact on their functioning, future opportunities, and quality of life. The goal of this treatment component is to help survivors develop emotional and social competencies whose progress was interrupted when resources for appropriate learning were deficient or unavailable as a result of the abuse.

Most people who have experienced trauma, or known someone who has experienced trauma, understand the potent psychological effects such events can have. The successful management of both daily tasks and major life challenges results from having specific emotional and social skills. These include the abilities to know what one feels, to communicate those feelings effectively to others, to solve problems effectively, to recognize the value of practical and emotional social support, and to know how to recruit such support when it is needed. These are all skills that grow, are elaborated, and are reinforced during the childhood years of physical, cognitive, emotional, and behavioral development. The development of these skills is compromised by the intrusion of trauma and the context of an abusive home. We describe below the specific developmental disturbances that have been documented among those who have experienced childhood abuse. Tracking these problems has helped us understand the particular competencies that have been compromised by abuse, and has allowed us to develop a program with interventions and activities formulated to address them.

The compromised competencies also have pernicious effects on abused persons' confidence, particularly their confidence in their perceptions and judgments about themselves and about others. They second-guess their own emotional reactions, fearing (sometimes accurately) that their "emotion sensors" have been damaged or disturbed. Abuse survivors also often second-guess their appraisals of situations and the motives of others, because their learning experiences have deviated from the norm. They do not trust either themselves or others.

One overarching theme in the treatment we have developed for adult survivors is facilitating the rebirth and growth of their confidence in themselves. This confidence generates the freedom to engage effectively and fluidly in day-to-day life and the belief that they can respond effectively to future hardships.

CHILDHOOD ABUSE INTERRUPTS DEVELOPMENT

Intrafamilial trauma during childhood creates a burden that both distracts from and distorts the achievement of typical developmental goals of the childhood and adolescent years. A highly traumatized childhood often involves putting energies into strategies for maximizing physical and psychological survival. In the case of childhood sexual and physical abuse, such strategies are often physical activities that reduce the risk of exposure to the assaults, or psychological strategies such as numbing, denial, dissociation, or distorting the meaning of the event when physical escape is not possible. There is a significant literature on the psychological mechanisms used for coping with chronic intrafamilial abuse. In contrast, there has been relatively little discussion of the deprivation of normative developmental experiences and the consequences of this deprivation for adult functioning.

Emotional and Sensory Development

Sexual or physical abuse disturbs the development of a coherent and integrated experience of the body. This is so in part because the immature body of the child is overwhelmed by the unmodulated, uncontrolled, and undifferentiated sensations of arousal that occur during sexual and/or physical abuse. Perhaps more important is that children are almost always abused by parents or caretakers, and abusive caretakers fail in the fundamental tasks involving the guidance of children in the modulation of arousal. An effective caretaker modulates a child's emotional arousal by providing appropriate doses of soothing and stimulating activities (Stern, 1985). Doing this not only maximizes comfort and security; it facilitates the child's learning how to self-soothe and to selectively orient him- or herself to both the external and internal environment. This learning in turn contributes to the accumulation of additional experiences of discrimination and categorization—between self and other, as well as across different kinds of emotions and emotional exchanges (see Gergely & Watson, 1996; Nichols, Gergely, & Fonagy, 2001).

Through a caretaker's tone of voice and later through language, the learning of self-soothing and affective discrimination continues. For example, parents ideally contribute to healthy emotional development in their children by accurately labeling feelings the children express. A mother might say to a distressed child, "You're upset because you missed seeing your friend today." This statement gives a label to a feeling, describes the experience, and ideally explains the source of the feeling. A typical report from an adult survivor of childhood abuse describes a scene in which a parent slaps him or her and follows the slapping with the statement "That did not hurt." The child experiences a discrepancy between the internal experience and the label. As a result of such events, abused children often experience confusion, distrust of their sensory perceptions, and a limited capacity to describe and accurately differentiate their feeling states.

Furthermore, abusive caretakers are poor guides to emotional modulation because they have limited emotion regulation skills themselves. Compared to the parents of never-abused children, the parents of abused children are significantly more likely to have drug and alcohol problems, to experience substantial mood disturbance, to have been in trouble with the law, and to experience jail time and mental health hospitalizations (Hien & Honeyman, 2000; Shearer, Peters, Quaytman, & Ogden, 1990; Sheridan, 1999; Widom, 1999). Such parents are poor role models for "learning by observation" the behaviors and attitudes that lead to effective emotion modulation. What abused children observe are the relative absence of emotion modulation, and the negative consequences of this absence—such as a deteriorating family environment, acrimony in the family, legal difficulties, hospitalizations, and substance-related problems.

The presence of poor affect regulation development in abused children is behaviorally evident as early as the toddler and preschool years (e.g., Cicchetti & White, 1990; Shields & Cicchetti, 1998). For instance, early maltreatment, including both sexual and physical abuse, is associated with high levels of negativity and anger in toddlers and lack of self-control in preschoolers (Erickson, Egeland, & Pianta, 1989). In the preteen and adolescent years, those with abuse histories are much more likely to engage in impulsive behaviors, including sexual and drug-related activities and reactive aggression (Lipschitz et al., 1999b, 2002; Kilpatrick et al., 2003).

In adulthood, difficulty with emotion regulation is one of the primary reasons for seeking mental health treatment (Levitt & Cloitre, 2005). Problems with modulating feeling states have been identified by several other researchers. Some describe this population as "emotion-phobic" (van der Kolk, 1996); others note significantly higher levels of hostility and anxiety compared to other clinical samples (Zlotnick et al., 1996), and chronic problems with depression and with anger management (Briere, 1988; Browne & Finkelhor, 1986).

In sum, childhood abuse survivors learn the negative consequences of unregulated feelings. What they do not learn is that emotional states can be controlled and well regulated, can support relationships, and can even be a source of pleasure. One goal of our treatment is to address this deficit and introduce the experience and management of feelings as positive and life-affirming.

Cognitive Development: Experience of Agency

Understanding of cause and effect is demonstrated in infants as early as 12 months, and integral to this development is the experience of the self as an agent or cause of events (see Gergely, 2004; Gergely & Watson, 1996). Caretakers play a critical role in this process. They draw out connections of cause and effect through movement and tone of voice, as well as by directing children's attention to changes in the environment that are causally related. In particular, a caretaker draws attention to a child's actions as having consequences in the environment, including effects on that most important and powerful figure of the social world—the caretaker. The child's sense of agency develops and is reinforced by the caretaker's directed responses to his or her expressed needs. The child experiences the self as an initiator of action or the cause of an effect (i.e., "If I do something, I get a response").

Conversely, caretakers diminish children's sense of agency by remaining unaware of, neglecting, or ignoring the children's signals. In fact, caretakers who sexually or physically abuse children nullify their experience of agency, since these events occur without regard to their needs or despite their protest. An abused child is given the message "You don't exist" or "You don't count."

A sense of agency is experienced in part through expressions of feelings. A child cries, and the caretaker responds; the child stops crying, and the caretaker changes behavior once again. This type of experience contributes to the child's sense of ownership of and authority over his or her feelings. It also encourages feelings to become valid reference points from which action is initiated and is expected to be successful. Abuse by caretakers includes the experience of having feelings ignored, dismissed, or distorted. Survivors who have experienced chronic abuse often not only do not know their own feelings, but also do not expect their feelings to matter or to be respected. They do not use their feelings as points of initiative or justification for action (e.g., "I feel this way, so I better do something about it").

A sense of agency is also created through interpersonal experiences—particularly recognition by a caretaker who follows and supports the child's actions, responds to these in a complementary fashion. This happens in play or in "mirroring-back" behaviors, where the caregiver reflects back, amplifies, or elaborates the actions of the child. For example, a child may slap her hand down on a table, creating a smacking sound and look to the caretaker, who responds by clapping with delight, simultaneously reinforcing and praising this instances of cause ("your hand") and effect ("makes noise"). The self-enhancing power of experiences in which the child takes the initiative and is followed by the caretaker is undercut by experiences of abuse. Abuse expresses the perpetrator's power to initiate and sustain action, regardless of the will or intention of the child. This kind of experience denies the child's recognition of the self as an autonomous being, and may convey to the child that he or she is merely an extension of the abuser's will. In adulthood, survivors often report feelings of incipient "annihilation" during experiences of conflict. This experience may be the result of lapses in recognition of the survivors' agency, and transgression of their autonomy during their abusive childhood. It is thus not surprising that survivors often struggle with power dynamics in interpersonal relationships—sometimes feeling overly dependent and passive, and other times exerting great effort to be "in control" of a relationship.

Our program's interventions help clients become better at identifying feeling states and more effective in interpersonal relationships. In many of the session chapters describing Phase I of the treatment (Chapters 10–17), the instructions to the therapist include not only how to teach clients a particular skill, but also what attitude to bring to the task and how to give feedback, so that the therapist acknowledges clients' experiences in a supportive, affirming, and accepting manner. We hope that in the process, clients will not only learn the names of their feelings, but also experience themselves as the authors of their own feelings and agents of their meaning and use; and that in the task of adopting new interpersonal positions and responses with the therapist, they will experience "being seen" by the therapist as persons in their own right and so will experience themselves as persons in their own right.

Interpersonal Development

As implied above, interpersonal development incorporates the management of feelings in relation to others. Interpersonal development across childhood and adolescence involves at least three key tasks: learning and implementing interpersonal models for establishing relationships, learning how to resolve conflicts, and developing flexibility in interpersonal expectations and behaviors.

Relationships with parents, other caretakers, and siblings create the first models for relating to others and are used as templates to guide expectations and prime behaviors in the development of relationships that follow. These first relationships are essentially characterized by the reliance of the young on elders, particularly primary caretakers, as sources of safety and nurturance. Over many years of clinical practice and research, we have found that the interpersonal models adapted by those abused in childhood assume that relationships are essentially adversarial, that vulnerability leads to exploitation, and that intimacy leads to pain and betrayal. These assumptions become most evident at times of conflict, when differences between individuals can threaten an abuse survivor's sense of control, autonomy, and recognition of needs.

Social-observational studies of maltreated preschool and school-age children have found an association between abuse and maladaptive internal models of attachment (Carlson, Cicchetti, Barnett, & Braunwald, 1989; Main, Kaplan, & Cassidy, 1985; Solomon, George, & DeJong, 1995). In addition, such internal models of attachment have been found to be associated with aggressive and fearful peer relationships and externalizing symptoms in school-age children (e.g., Lyons-Ruth, Alpern, & Repacholi, 1993). Although empirical investigation of the role of specific internal working models and behavioral problems among abused children is just emerging, the presence of interpersonal and social impairment among children and youth with a history of abuse is well established. Childhood victimization is associated with social behaviors such as peer rejection and bullying in the school years (Shields & Cicchetti, 1998; Schwartz & Proctor, 2000). Among adolescents, it is associated with increases in both aggression and social avoidance, as well as significant increases in criminal and delinquent behaviors and early sexual activity (Giaconia et al., 1995; Horowitz et al., 1995; Malmquist, 1986; Pynoos et al., 1987).

Consistent with these observations, adult abuse survivors report significant interpersonal problems. In a large study on the effects of childhood physical and sexual abuse in adult women, 91% of the respondents described significant problems in relationships (van der Kolk, Roth, Pelcovitz, & Mandel, 1993). The most frequent difficulties were sensitivity to criticism, inability to hear other viewpoints, difficulty in standing up for themselves, and a tendency to quit jobs and relationships without negotiation. Our own research is consistent with these findings: Among treatment-seeking women, the majority reported significant problems with intimacy, being too controlling, acting too submissive, being inappropriately assertive, and being insufficiently sociable (Cloitre, Scarvalone, & Difede, 1997; see also Chapter 4).

Taken together, these studies suggest that central difficulties arise in emotion-laden situations that involve the management of conflict or balance in power in the relationship. These behaviors are quite understandable when viewed from the perspective of the lessons learned about relationships in abusive homes. The hypersensitivities to conflict reported by adult survivors are a legacy of these experiences. The interpersonal schemas that abuse survivors most frequently rely on reflect expectations that others will respond to them in a cold, controlling, or distant manner (Cloitre et al., 2002a). Their current behaviors may in part be premptive maneuvers to avoid the negative outcomes that they expect, or reenactments of familiar interpersonal roles.

The interpersonal schema study discussed in Chapter 2 (Cloitre et al., 2002a) also reported that the schemas of abuse survivors tended to be limited in number and fairly rigidly applied across different people and different situations. For example, when abuse survivors were confronted with hypothetical situations in which the behavior of another person was most likely to be warm and inviting, the survivors still responded with expectations of the other to be cold, hostile, and controlling. In addition, the particular relationship with the significant other did not seem to make a difference to the expectations of the survivors: Mother, father, significant other, and best friend were responded to in the same way, regardless of the appropriateness of that expectation for each person in that situation.

Part of the normative trajectory of social development involves refining and adding interpersonal rules for relating, depending on the contexts and the individuals involved. For example, children learn when aggressive behaviors are appropriate (e.g., on the basketball court) and when they are not (e.g., with a toddler sibling); when obedience to an adult is appropriate (e.g., with a teacher in the classroom) and when it is not (e.g., with a stranger in an elevator); and so on. Parents help guide this knowledge with specific teaching about diversity in interpersonal expectations within and beyond the family, and provide children with opportunities to explore their emotional reactions as they experience these different interpersonal scenarios. Our data suggest that this sensitivity is not well developed among treatment-seeking abuse survivors.

The treatment program we have devised includes a strong emphasis on expanding the number and kind of interpersonal schemas a client has available for consideration. Models of interaction (schemas) are proposed in which the client's overtures of warmth will be met with warmth, and overtures of appropriate assertiveness will be met with recognition and respect. Furthermore, development of these models is grounded in an understanding of their context-sensitive nature—that is, the concept that different types of relationships (work vs. romantic vs. parenting relationships) require different expectations or different actions and reactions. Key goals of the treatment involve helping the abuse survivor develop alternative ways of relating to people from those that emerge from abuse, and develop sensitivity to the diversity in the nature, character, and context of relationships.

WHEN ABUSE HAPPENS OUTSIDE THE HOME: THE INFLUENCE OF IMPOVERISHED CARETAKING AND LEARNING EXPERIENCES

Individuals who experience sexual and physical abuse as children often have primary caretakers who do not or cannot effectively respond to their attachment mandates as caretakers and have impaired parenting skills. This is directly the case when the abuse is perpetrated by the caretakers. However, clinical experience and substantial research suggest that individuals who come to treatment with a history of abuse outside the home often report parenting or environmental difficulties that predate or are separate from the abuse experiences. Many (e.g., Conte, Wolfe, & Smith, 1989; Gold, 2000; Finkelhor, 1980) have suggested that beyond the fact of the abuse itself, the presence of problematic attachment, disturbed parenting behaviors, and certain types of living environments create vulnerability to abuse and other interpersonal traumas outside the home, and in general make recovery more difficult.

A substantial literature indicates that problematic attachment can occur with a nonabusing parent because the parent is too preoccupied, distant, or distressed to be reliably responsive and nurturing. Other factors might include the presence of psychiatric problems, including those that are consequences of the caretaker's own trauma history, such as PTSD or depression. Environmental pressures such as limited income and poor health or injury among family members may also contribute to the caretaker's difficulties. In such circumstances, the caretaker may not have the ability to provide a sufficient "secure base" for the child, guidance in developing competencies, protection from significant threats, or the nurturing capacity to help the child recover from traumas.

In addition, studies of the families of abuse survivors have certain similar characteristics, regardless of whether the abuse occurred inside or outside the home. These include being high in rigid behavioral control, and low in adaptive emotional expressiveness (Nash et al., 1993; Ray et al., 1991). Translated into terms of daily living, relationships among family members tend to be circumscribed within specific roles (often of an authoritarian nature), and there is little flexibility or range in expression of emotions. In addition, the experience of limited and rigid role relationships tends to limit the ability of survivors to learn the subtle but critical life lesson that different people and different contexts require diverse ways of relating and different sets of interpersonal expectations.

Gold (2000) has suggested that the typical characteristics of these families are likely to produce or mold expectations and behaviors in children that leave them vulnerable to exploitation and abuse by predatory adults. For example, a caretaking environment that is cold, unaffectionate, and unresponsive to a child's emotional needs may result in a child who hungers for warmth, recognition, support, and validation. Such a child may be particularly vulnerable to the attentions, blandishments, and flattery of a child molester. Family systems that are high in authoritarian and controlling behaviors toward children may elicit and shape interpersonal styles marked by unassertiveness, deference, and appeasement. This creates an interpersonal dynamic that allows a child to be easily intimated and coerced by demanding adults. A family that is low in organization, cohesion, and expressiveness can reduce clarity about appropriate adult behaviors and reduced confidence in perceptions of threatening adult behavior, further reducing the likelihood of a child's avoiding or escaping from adult intrusions (see Gold, 2000, pp. 24–25).

In our own clinic population, parents are the primary perpetrators of abuse in 80% of cases (e.g., Cloitre, Stovall, McClough, & Zorbas, 2005). The remainder of clients (those whose abuse has been perpetrated by a nonfamily member) report some form of maltreatment in the home—typically verbal abuse and neglect, or some combination. These statistics and our own clinical experiences have led us to surmise that negative family contexts, and cold and distant relationships with caretakers in particular, are associated with victimization outside the home. Children seek out or are comforted by the presence of alternative caregivers—in the form of babysitters, coaches, teachers, religious or community leaders, or more generally individuals who make themselves available to give attention to neglected children.

In short, a survivor of childhood abuse has almost always grown up in a family that provides little in the way of skills necessary for adaptive or adequate functioning. The difficulties in emotion management and interpersonal relating described above are known to emanate from intrafamilial abuse, but also can be risk factors creating vulnerability to abuse and additional types of trauma outside the home.

SUMMARY

In this chapter, we have noted that difficulties in emotion regulation and interpersonal relationships are present at each developmental stage among those abused in childhood, including toddlerhood, the middle years, and adolescence. These data suggest that the similar problems seen in adults who come to treatment may have their origins in the developmental years. They also suggest the entrenched and enduring nature of such difficulties.

One critical goal of the STAIR component of our treatment program is to provide clients with a clear analysis of their problems in these areas, and to respond to gaps in their social and emotional competence by building and reinforcing emotion management and social skills. In this way, the treatment is conceptualized as the provision or rehabilitation of basic and life-enhancing social and emotional competencies with which survivors of abuse often have not had sufficient experience.

The role of poor emotion management in interpersonal difficulties cannot be overstated. The reasons for interpersonal conflict are often readily identified as emerging from distressing and unmanageable feelings. Anger leads to words that are later regretted, to strained or ruptured friendships, and sometimes to physical violence. Feelings of anger, hurt, sadness, and humiliation are often out of proportion to the events that elicited them. Even when justified, such feelings may be expressed in ways that do not lead to a satisfactory conclusion or a sustained human connection. Alternatively, emerging positive feelings such as happiness, pride, or pleasure can overwhelm an abuse survivor's ability to function in a situation; the consequence may be that emotionally intense feelings and situations are avoided, leading to social withdrawal and isolation.

STAIR was developed with the view that individuals communicate powerfully if not primarily through the expression of feelings—verbal or nonverbal, intended or not. As a result, the interpersonal interventions exercise clients' awareness of and behaviors related to the expression and modulation of emotion. Simply put, feelings are often about others or about the self in relation to others. One goal of STAIR is to help clients develop an expanded repertoire of emotional expressiveness that effectively and adaptively communicates to others.

CHAPTER 4

∽

Treatment Rationale

Psychotherapy is not really about symptom relief; its essential purpose is to help a person function in the world, and ideally, to function well.

—ANONYMOUS

Treatments for PTSD have been available since childhood abuse was formally recognized as a traumatic event in 1980 (American Psychiatric Association, 1980). Why not simply adapt available PTSD treatments for childhood abuse survivors? Our experience as clinicians informed us that such an approach would be insufficient. The women who came to our clinic sought help for self-identified and long-standing emotion management and relationship problems, and with work and career goals. Often clients would acknowledge the presence of PTSD symptoms when asked, but would dismiss them as the reason for entering therapy. Some reported that they had hit "rock bottom" and could no longer deny the level of functional impairment in their lives. These clients were often unemployed or working at jobs far lower than their education or abilities warranted, had lost one or more jobs per year for several years, and/or had intimate partners who were threatening to leave or who had already left.

We found that these problems were not random assortments of life difficulties. Rather, they reflected specific and enduring disturbances in emotion regulation and interpersonal capacities. The common sources of these problems in day-to-day life functioning appeared to be severely limited emotional and social competencies. Such clients did not know how to manage emotional distress effectively or deal with fluctuations in negative emotional states. Similarly, the many failed relationships they reported were the results of limited expectations that relationships could involve mutual trust, respect, and support, and limited skills in creating such relationships (including the selection of appropriate partners and friends) and the skills to maintain healthy relationships and end bad ones. All these limited competencies conceptually represented a good fit with characteristics of "derailed development" as predicted by attachment theory. Still, it was clear that the journey from theory to intervention was not very well mapped.

Our goal in developing Skills Training in Affective and Interpersonal Regulation (STAIR) and Narrative Story Telling (NST) has been to create a treatment program that supports recovery from the difficulties caused by caregiver-related trauma in the developmental years. The formulation and testing of STAIR/NST have been based on evidence emerging from the clinical, trauma, memory, and developmental literatures. This chapter describes the systematic empirical investigation that yielded the rationale for this treatment, as well as the empirical outcomes of the treatment. Our goal in providing this historical review is to allow readers to evaluate critically what makes sense to them, and to adapt effectively the strategies described in the second half of the book in a principle governed as to the particular needs of individual survivors.

LISTENING TO CLIENTS: WHAT DO THEY REALLY WANT?

The very first empirical effort in our initiative was to determine what survivors were most concerned about and wanted treatment for. A phone survey of 98 childhood abuse survivors inquiring about treatment was conducted by members of our clinic staff. They found that the most common reasons for seeking services were interpersonal problems (67%), emotion management problems (31%), and symptoms of PTSD (59%).

It clearly did not seem sufficient to provide treatment for the one set of problems for which we had effective therapy—the PTSD symptoms. It was only one of three problem sets cited as a treatment need. Nor did we wish to assume that targeting this one problem set would automatically resolve the other two. Indeed, this seemed unlikely. Certainly, PTSD symptoms do disrupt functioning; for example, sexual intimacy can be quickly disturbed when certain touches or sensations are traumatic reminders of sexual abuse and trigger flashbacks, acute physical discomfort, and fear. But many of the observed emotion management and relationship problems seemed to derive from other aspects of the experience of childhood trauma—particularly disturbances in emotional and social learning experiences. We wished to provide treatment that directly responded to the most evident needs expressed by childhood abuse survivors beyond those of PTSD.

WHAT MAKES CLIENTS' FUNCTIONING IN DAY-TO-DAY LIFE SO DIFFICULT?

We were committed to the ideal that good treatment required us to attend to our clients' complaints and that to take seriously the factors having the greatest apparent impact on their day-to-day functioning. Indeed, one traditional way to identify the presence of significant mental health problems is to assess the impact of the problem on a client's functional status. The diagnostic statistical manual (DSM), for example, the compendium of formally accepted psychiatric disorders in the United States, stipulates that functional impairment must be associated with symptoms as a requirement for a psychiatric diagnosis (American Psychiatric Association, 2000).

In an effort to organize a trauma treatment around functional capacity, our team analyzed the data from the face-to-face assessment interviews of the first consecutive 167 treatment-seeking women with childhood abuse. We conducted a series of statistical analyses to determine to what extent each of the three symptom sets—PTSD symptoms, emotion management problems, and interpersonal problems—made a significant contribution to functional impairment. The importance of this task was reinforced by the treatment literature on the mood and anxiety disorders indicating that while various treatments were successful in resolving disorder-specific symptoms, significant functional impairment persisted (e.g., Agosti & Stewart, 1998; Coryell et al., 1993; Rapaport, Endicott, & Clary, 2002; Serretti et al., 1999). These data were taken to suggest that functional impairment not only is a direct result of diagnostically defined symptoms, but has other sources.

The results of our own investigation indicated that functional impairment was related not only to PTSD symptoms, but also to emotion regulation difficulties and interpersonal problems (see Cloitre, Miranda, Stovall-McClough, & Han, 2005). Analyses were conducted conservatively, maximizing the opportunity for PTSD symptoms to be associated with functional status. To the extent that PTSD and the other symptom sets shared the predictive weighting of functional status, the predictive weighting was credited only to PTSD only and not the other two factors. After age and other sociodemographic factors were accounted for, PTSD symptoms accounted for 20% of functional impairment. Emotion regulation difficulties in and of themselves accounted for an additional 4%, and interpersonal problems for yet another 18% of functional impairment (see Figure 4.1). In sum, emotion regulation and interpersonal difficulties combined accounted for essentially the same proportion of functional impairment as PTSD symptoms. This indicated an important organizing framework for developing the treatment. In order to reduce functional impairment among trauma survivors, we needed a treatment that focused on ameliorating emotion regulation and interpersonal difficulties as well as PTSD symptoms.

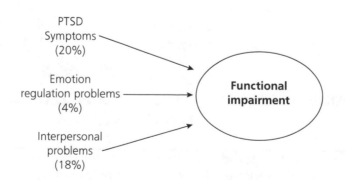

FIGURE 4.1. Contributions of PTSD symptoms, emotion regulation difficulties, and interpersonal problems to functional impairment. Data from Cloitre, Miranda, Stovall-McClough, and Han (2005).

The extent to which these three factors together accounted for functional impairment—a total of 42% of impairment—gave us confidence in advocating for resources of time, money, and effort to be spent on developing an intervention that took these problems seriously. To put the relative explanatory power of this model into perspective, we considered the translation of statistical results into funding resources for physical health problems salient to women. For example, researchers' investigations into the causes of breast cancer have found that family history accounts for 10% of breast cancer cases (e.g., Yang et al., 1998) and is a significant predictor of the disease. Several million dollars have been spent disseminating this information and providing prevention and early detection interventions. By comparison, the research described above has captured a much greater proportion of the sources of the problem of interest. In this context, the results of the study become more compelling.

DO THE PROBLEMS OF CHILDHOOD ABUSE SURVIVORS DIFFER FROM THOSE OF ADULT-ONSET TRAUMA SURVIVORS?

In the previous chapters, we have described scenarios suggesting that problems in emotion management and interpersonal functioning may have their source in disturbed attachment and social learning. The salience of these early life experiences, their influence on adolescent and later-life emotional and social development, and their cumulative impact over decades suggest that such problems may be more severe among childhood abuse survivors than among those who have had experienced their firsst significant trauma in adulthood. The most compelling support for this view are studies that have directly compared individuals with childhood-onset trauma to those with adult-onset trauma (e.g., survivors of rape or natural disasters) and found that childhood abuse survivors are consistently more troubled, particularly in the domains of affect modulation, anger management, and interpersonal relationships (Cloitre et al., 1997; van der Kolk et al., 1993; Zlotnick et al., 1996).

Results from a study by Cloitre et al. (1997) found that while rates of PTSD were similar among women who sought treatment for rape in adulthood versus childhood sexual abuse (70% vs. 75%, respectively), those with childhood sexual abuse as their primary concern reported significantly more affect regulation difficulties and had more significant interpersonal problem profiles. Both groups were compared on these measures to a comparison group of women of similar age and background who had never been traumatized and had no psychiatric diagnosis (see Figures 4.2 and 4.3). Women who had experienced childhood abuse showed much more pronounced problems in affect regulation than either of the other groups, while the rape survivors looked rather similar to the trauma-free comparison group. Affect regulation was measured by alexithymia (difficulty identifying and labeling feelings) and dissociation. We also included lifetime suicide attempts, following Marsha Linehan's (1993a) notion that suicide attempts often represent a way of controlling and ending chronic and acute states of extreme distress—a commonly endorsed reason for suicide attempts among childhood abuse survivors (see Brodsky, Cloitre, & Dulit, 1995).

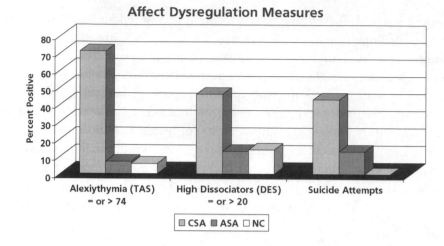

FIGURE 4.2. Differential impact of trauma, depending on life stage: Emotion regulation. TAS, Toronto Alexithymia Scale; DES, Dissociative Experience Scale; CSA, group with childhood sexual abuse; ASA, group with adulthood sexual abuse (rape); NC, never-abused comparison group. Data from Cloitre, Scarvalone, and Difede (1997).

A similar pattern was obtained in the assessment of reports of interpersonal problems: Childhood abuse survivors consistently reported more problems than either the rape survivors or the nontraumatized comparison group. Of particular interest was that the childhood abuse survivors reported significant problems in all aspects of interpersonal problems queried, including problems with being assertive and with being submissive, as well as problems with being *too* controlling. Although these may look like contradictory endorsements, our work with this population suggests that the reporting is accurate and reflects these survivors' overall problems in managing power dynamics in relationships:

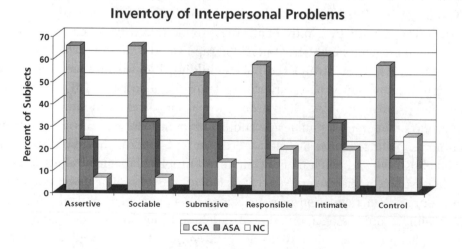

FIGURE 4.3. Differential impact of trauma, depending on life stage: Interpersonal functioning. CSA, ASA, NC as in Figure 4.2. Data from Cloitre et al. (1997).

being insufficiently assertive in situations in which they should have a strong voice, but being too controlling in situations that do not warrant such. Sustained problems in managing power and control in relationships are also consistent with our research on interpersonal schemas among childhood abuse survivors, which indicated a rigidity in perceptions of power and control, reflected in a predominant schema of human relationships as based on dynamics of control (Cloitre et al., 2002a; see also Chapter 2).

Some studies have reported that there are no or few differences between clients with adult onset traumas (e.g., rape survivors) and those with chronic childhood traumas (e.g., Resick et al., 2005), suggesting the adequacy of a "one-size-fits-all" treatment approach. However, these types of studies have focused on symptoms that are shared among trauma survivors such as anxiety, depression, and low self-esteem. The problematic aspects salient to the childhood abuse survivor, such as alexithymia, emotion regulation disturbance, chronic suicidality, and problems maintaining enduring relationships are often not assessed. Indeed, childhood abuse survivors who have such problems particularly as manifest in substance abuse, disordered eating, and self-harming behavior are frequently excluded from the studies in which these comparisons are made. Spinazolla, Blaustein, and van der Kolk (2005), for example, reported that over 50% of trauma survivors seeking treatment in research studies are excluded, many of these for the difficulties associated with the childhood abuse. As a consequence, the conclusion that childhood and adult trauma survivors are similar is based on selectively screened and substantially biased samples.

DEVELOPMENT OF STAIR/NST: MATCHING INTERVENTIONS TO TARGETED PROBLEMS

The research described above produced a symptom profile of childhood abuse survivors. Their difficulties have been organized into three core sets of disturbances associated with childhood abuse that contribute to functional impairment. A characterization of these symptom sets in terms of typical behaviors and client complaints is provided in Box 4.1. We wished to develop a treatment program that could target this range of symptoms. We felt strongly that a maximally effective treatment for childhood abuse survivors would include skills training with the goal of ameliorating emotional and social skills deficits. What, then, were we to do with the PTSD symptoms? There was evidence that skills training could lead to some reduction in PTSD symptoms, but that such an approach had limited effectiveness (Foa, Dancu, Hembree, Jaycox, & Meadows, 1999a; Resick, Jordon, Girelli, Hutter, & Marhoefer-Dvorak, 1988). Indeed, overall, exposure interventions had been shown to be superior to other forms of forms of cognitive and behavioral therapies for resolving PTSD symptoms (Foa, Keane, & Friedman, 2000; Foa & Meadows, 1997). There was also consistent evidence that when a client successfully engaged in exposure therapy, the long-term benefits after treatment ended were superior to those found for other treatments (Foa et al., 1999a).

Given that each type of intervention was intended to address different sets of problems, that childhood abuse survivors had both PTSD symptoms and the other two sets of

---

BOX 4.1
General Symptom Profile of Childhood Abuse Survivors

SYMPTOMS OF PTSD

- *Reexperiencing symptoms*: Nightmares, flashbacks, intrusive thoughts/images related to the trauma
- *Avoidance and emotional numbing*: Avoidance of thoughts, people, places, or activities that produce reminders of the trauma; loss of interest in things that used to give pleasure; feeling numb
- *Hyperarousal*: Difficulties with sleeping and concentration; exaggerated startle response; irritability

EMOTION REGULATION PROBLEMS

- Emotional reactivity (fear, rage, avoidance) to minor stimuli
- Difficulty in "getting back down to baseline" or restoring sense of equilibrium
- Tendency to dissociate under stressful circumstances
- Engaging in self-injurious behaviors (self-cutting, burning)
- Coping through excessive use of alcohol or drugs

INTERPERSONAL PROBLEMS

- Difficulty with intimacy and trust
- Sensitivity to criticism
- Inability to hear other viewpoints
- Difficulty in standing up for oneself
- Tendency to quit jobs and relationships without negotiation
- History of repeated victimization (e.g., domestic violence, date rape)

---

problems, and that there was no evidence that one type of intervention could achieve the goals of the other, we determined to develop two distinct modules of treatment. The first module of treatment would focus on the development of modulated emotional expression and an enhanced repertoire of interpersonal behaviors. The immediate goals of this module, STAIR, were to vigorously and directly address problems in affect and interpersonal problems and to help clients improve their functioning in daily life. The second module would focus on the emotional processing of the trauma, and was intended to resolve the PTSD symptoms. The therapy with the most evidence and with the best outcomes in PTSD reduction was prolonged exposure (Foa et al., 1999a; Resick, Nishith, Weaver, Astin, & Feuer, 2002). We modified prolonged exposure and adapted it to the needs of abuse survivors (Cloitre, Koenen, Cohen, & Han, 2002b), and we developed a series of interventions wrapped around it, called NST.

The sequencing of STAIR before NST was intended to enhance the effective use of exposure treatment through the development of affect management skills. We also reasoned that the STAIR phase would allow a period of symptom stabilization and the development of a therapeutic alliance, which might facilitate success in the trauma-processing module.

A summary of the interventions for STAIR/NST is provided in Box 4.2. Detailed descriptions of the reasoning behind the selection and development of the specific interventions for STAIR and for NST are provided in the next two chapters (Chapters 5 and 6, respectively).

BOX 4.2
Overview of STAIR/NST with Symptom Targets

PHASE I: SKILLS TRAINING
FOR AFFECTIVE AND INTERPERSONAL REGULATION (STAIR)

Symptom Targets: Emotion Regulation Difficulties, Interpersonal Problems

- *Emotional awareness*: Identification and labeling of feelings, self-monitoring of emotions; focused breathing
- *Emotion regulation*: Psychoeducation on emotional responding in physiological, cognitive, and behavioral channels; strategies of focused breathing, attention shifting, positive imagery, positive self-statements; working with fear and anger, pleasurable activities, and positive emotions
- *Emotionally engaged living*: Goal identification; distress tolerance; pros and cons; using positive feelings as guide to decision making and action; acceptance of negative emotions

Changing Relationship Patterns

- Understanding the self-fulfilling nature of trauma-based schemas
- Taking an opportunity to change; revising interpersonal expectations
- Agency in relationships; focus on appropriate assertiveness, changing schemas, practice in role play
- Felxibility in relationships; focus on different actions and reactions for different situations; generating mutiple schemas, role play different actions in similar situations but with relationships of differing intimacy and power differentials
- For different situation; generate multiple schemas, role play different actions in similar situations but with relationships of differing intimacy and power differentials

PHASE II: NARRATIVE STORY TELLING (NST)

Symptom Targets: PTSD Symptoms, Emotion Regulation Difficulties, Interpersonal Problems

- Narratives of traumatic memories with focus on fear, shame, loss
- Using postnarrative grounding strategies to orient client to present
- Identifying interpersonal schemas in narratives; contrasting narratives from these schemas with alternative interpersonal schemas based on current situation and goals
- Practice new behaviors, exercise emotional awareness, contrast the present with the past, redirect attention and energy to the present

WHY A PHASE-BASED TREATMENT?

One might consider that skills training could be provided simultaneously with more traditional trauma-focused work. But we decided against this for several reasons.

Giving Clients Time to Learn

First, the empirical literature indicated that when coping interventions and trauma processing of trauma were conducted simultaneously within a session, the benefits of the treatment were no greater than the benefits of treatments that just provided one or the other component of treatment. Some treatment researchers (e.g., Foa et al., 1999a) have suggested that the limits on effectiveness may be the result of "information overload," in which clients cannot absorb the substantial amount of information provided in the limited time typically available for treatment.

Preparing Clients for Narrative Work

Second, we wished our clients to have a maximal skill set with which to engage in the narrative work. While many trauma survivors are able to accomplish exposure to their traumatic events, there is a substantial clinical literature reporting concern that abuse survivors may come to the work with fewer resources than are optimal for the emotional effort involved. For example, Steven Gold (2000) comments:

> Adults with adequate adaptive skills that have been disrupted by the impact of a single traumatic event enter treatment with an array of personal capacities (e.g., coping skills, judgment, a sense of efficacy) and environmental resources (e.g., social support, financial reserves) that are nowhere near as likely to be accessible to survivors of extended child abuse. The former group, therefore, even if they are highly symptomatic individually, has firmly rooted strength to draw upon that greatly bolster their capacity to face and productively process trauma. The latter group, however, lacks these advantages. Consequently, even the routine stressors of daily adult living tax their capacities and can be destabilizing. It is unreasonable to expect that they are in a substantially better position to productively assimilate traumatic experiences than when those events originally occurred. (p. 58)

Indeed, several clinical reports indicate that clients who have compromised capacities in tolerating distress and difficulty securing good relationships with their therapists may experience symptom exacerbation during exposure or drop out of the therapy (McDonagh et al., 2005; Pitman, Altman, Greenwald, Longpre, & Macklin, 1991; Scott & Stradling, 1997; Tarrier et al., 1999) or not obtain as good an outcome as clients without such problems (Foa, Riggs, Massie, & Yarczower, 1995d; Ford, Fisher, & Larson, 1997; Ford & Kidd, 1998; Funari, Piekarski, & Sherwood, 1991). The implementation of STAIR prior to trauma processing was intended to address this concern. STAIR, which develops and strengthens emotional and relational capacities, will ideally serve to stabilize and prepare clients for the trauma-processing treatment component.

Respecting the Power of the Therapeutic Alliance

Lastly, we were sensitive to the importance of the therapeutic relationship. The working relationship between the therapist and client is the single most important factor predicting good treatment outcome (Horvath & Symonds, 1991; Martin, Garske, & Davis, 2000). This is a remarkably durable phenomenon. It has been observed in interpersonal (e.g., Kruptnick et al., 1996), cognitive (e.g., Muran, Segal, Samstag, & Crawford, 1994), and dynamic (e.g., Stiles, Agnew-Davis, Hardy, Barkman, & Shapiro, 1998; Yeomans et al., 1994) therapies, as well as in a range of therapy problems or goals (e.g., alleviating depression or anxiety, treating alcohol or substance use).

It is clearly important for the therapist and client to develop a rapport and good understanding of each other before engaging in the emotional processing of the trauma. Many trauma therapists have alluded to the difficulties any trauma survivor has in tolerating the interpersonal nature of therapy—that is, "the [need] to . . . trust another person with his or her pain" (Turner, McFarlane, & van der Kolk, 1996, p. 538; see also Pearlman & Saakvitne, 1995; Lindy, 1996). This difficulty would seem further exacerbated in exposure-based treatments, which require a significant and sustained amount of emotional disclosure. We wished to maximize the client's sense of being understood and supported by the therapist, and, just as important, the therapist's and client's mutual recognition that the therapist is familiar with the client's strengths and vulnerabilities and will attend to them accordingly during the narrative work.

BENEFITS OF THE PHASE-BASED APPROACH

Our research with STAIR/NST has supported the notion that a preparatory phase of treatment contributes to good outcome in trauma-processing work. Specifically, we found that two characteristics of STAIR significantly influenced the success of the narrative work: a strong and positive therapeutic alliance, and the development of good emotion regulation skills (Cloitre et al., 2002b). While STAIR produced many positive and important improvements for the clients, such as decreases in anxiety and depression, only improvement in negative mood regulation and the strength of the therapeutic relationship were significantly related to PTSD reduction in the narrative phase (see Table 4.1). These results suggested the relative specificity of the resources that support good processing work, as well as the value of organizing the treatment components in a chronological fashion.

TABLE 4.1. Phase I (STAIR) Predictors of Success in Phase II (NST) as Measured by PTSD Symptom Reduction

Phase I variables	R	p	Effect size[a]
Therapeutic alliance (WAI)	−.64	.03	Large
Improved negative mood regulation (NMR)	−.47	.03	Medium–large

Note. WAI, Working Alliance Inventory; NMR, Generalized Expectancy for Negative Mood Regulation Scale. Data from Cloitre, Koenen, Cohen, and Han (2002b).
[a]An effect size of 0.10 is small; one of 0.30 is medium; one of 0.50 is large.

TREATMENT OUTCOME

A randomized controlled trial of STAIR/NST found that, compared to a Minimal Attention Wait List, the treatment program was successful in producing very substantial reductions in PTSD symptoms (Cloitre et al., 2002b). In addition, there was significant improvement in experiencing and modulating emotions (as measured by increased ability to identify and name feelings, improved mood regulation, and decreased dissociation). Moreover, there was significant and sustained reduction in three central mood disturbances: anxiety, anger, and depression. Lastly, interpersonal problems were significantly reduced, and role functioning in home, work, and social domains was improved. All of these gains were maintained at 3- and 9-month follow-ups. In addition, the follow-up data indicated continued improvement at the 3-month mark in PTSD symptom resolution, and continued significant improvement in interpersonal functioning at the 9-month mark (see Figures 4.4 through 4.7).

EXPERIENTIAL ASPECTS OF STAIR/NST

As we spent time working with our clients, we came to appreciate an experiential aspect of sequencing skills training before the narrative work for which we have no data but our own clinical observations. We noted that the skills work, in combination with a positive relationship with the therapist, provided the clients with increased confidence and perceptions of themselves as persons who were competent, well regarded, and esteemed. These new self-perceptions seemed to provide the clients with a way of thinking about themselves that made the confrontation of the past less difficult and overwhelming. The confidence in engaging in the narrative work seemed to come not only from the clients' awareness of their own capacity to manage the feelings the trauma memories engendered, but also from their knowledge that they were no longer exactly the persons they described in their narratives.

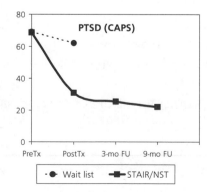

FIGURE 4.4. Reduction in PTSD symptoms. CAPS, Clinician-Administered PTSD Scale. Data from Cloitre, Koenen, Cohen, and Han (2002b).

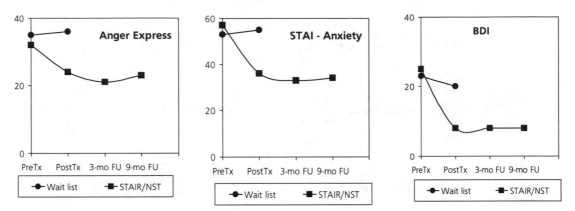

FIGURE 4.5. Reduction in negative emotions: Anger, anxiety, and depression. STAI, State–Trait Anxiety Inventory; BDI, Beck Depression Inventory. Data from Cloitre et al. (2002b).

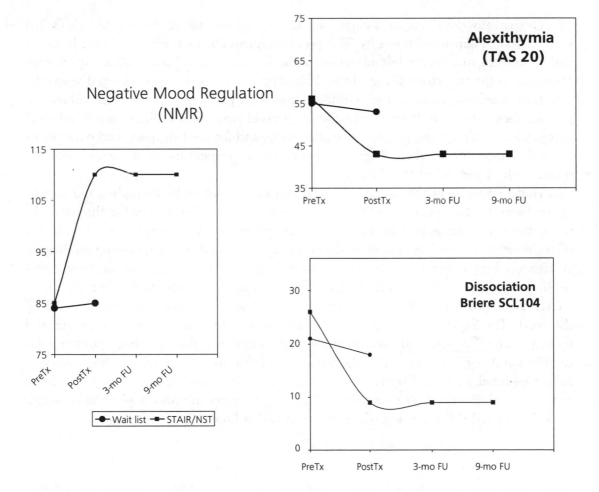

FIGURE 4.6. Improvement in emotion regulation: Negative mood regulation, alexithymia, and dissociation. NMR, Generalized Expectancy for Negative Mood Regulation Scale; TAS, Toronto Alexithymia Scale; SCL104-Diss, Symptom Checklist 104—Dissociation Subscale. Data from Cloitre et al. (2002b).

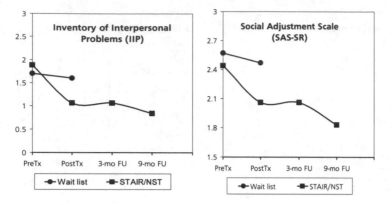

FIGURE 4.7. Reduction in interpersonal and functional impairment. Data from Cloitre et al. (2002b).

The narrative work requires going back to the past and telling about traumatic events with emotional depth and intensity. This process returns clients to their early life histories and often leads to a deeply felt awareness of the far-reaching influence these experiences have had on the trajectory of their lives. This seems more easily acknowledged when the clients have achieved some sense of distance from their past and from the more vulnerable persons they were then. From the position of present strength, the clients are able to feel compassion for the young persons they once were, and for the fear, pain, and disappointment they experienced then. They can also feel more respect for their current achievements both in and out of the therapy.

The completion of the narrative component in turn seems to strengthen the clients' appreciation for the present and their motivation to live well in it. During the narrative work, the clients grapple with the pain generated by the abuse experiences; with this effort, their emotional lives are often deepened and enriched. The experience can lead to an increased capacity for openness in emotional experiencing and greater authentic connection with others. When clients complete the narrative work, they often return to STAIR skills practice with a deeper appreciation of the emotional and social benefits of this work. The STAIR module provides the clients with tools for behaving, thinking, and feeling in more positive and competent ways, and expanding their reach for positive relationships and self-awareness. The clearest indicator that narrative work has been successfully completed, as well as its greatest benefit, is that the clients "let go" of the past in favor of the present. Recovered survivors find the present a more interesting place to be—and, with the needed skills, a place where they can feel at home.

CHAPTER 5

~

Building Emotional and Social Resources
Overview of STAIR

> Humans have the capacity for change and growth
> through the entire life span.
> —JEROME KAGAN (1980)

This chapter provides the rationale for the STAIR session topics and for their order. By conscious design, the session topics follow the human developmental trajectory in the maturation of emotional and social competencies, particularly as these competencies contribute to the growth of agency and connection with others. Agency, a sense of oneself as a source of action, originates in the ability to know what one feels and to use feelings as a guide to action. The expression of these feelings aids communication with others and, if effectively done, contributes to connection with them. Sustained connection requires the ability to express one's feelings in a way that can be understood by others and to endure certain amounts of distress in resolving conflict. It also requires the ability to balance self-interests with recognition of the interests of others. Flexibility in expectations of others, depending on their needs and the social context, allows one to have different kinds of relationships and friendships. These provide one with enriched, diverse experiences and resources for living. The skills of identifying feelings, managing and expressing emotions, enhancing assertiveness, and increasing flexibility in relationships all build on each other to create emotional and social resources.

The progression of emotional and social skills development described above is reflected in the order of the STAIR sessions. The first sessions address emotional awareness, emotion regulation, and effective emotion-guided planning and action. The first session begins with the task of identifying and labeling feeling states. Once feelings are named and their reality is affirmed, the sessions progress to the task of discriminating among feelings and communicating about them. The middle sessions introduce the critical skills of modulation of feelings and the appropriate and effective expression of these feelings to others. The second half of STAIR makes the transition to matters of interpersonal functioning—in particular, the role of emotional experiencing and expression as a central means of creating and maintaining healthy attachments. This includes developing conflict resolution skills and effectively managing power balances in relationships. The final session introduces the importance of responding flexibly to a growing range of social circumstances, individuals, and experiences. Although the growth and maintenance of self-regulation capacities constitute a lifelong endeavor, the goal of STAIR is to help the client develop core emotional and social competencies that will provide a foundation for future efforts. Below, we describe the skills that are introduced in the STAIR sessions, and we provide descriptions and rationales for the specific interventions used to develop those skills. An at-a-glance, session-by-session summary is provided in Box 5.1.

EMOTIONAL COMPETENCIES

"Emotional competencies" are the abilities to identify, monitor, manage, and express emotions for specific functional or adaptive purposes. Chapters 3 and 4 have described the developmental literature on maltreated children and empirical assessments of adult survivors of childhood abuse. The research thus far indicates that many emotional competencies, particularly those influenced by caretaker experiences, are disturbed by abuse. These include the identification and labeling of feeling states, differentiation among different emotions, appropriate danger detection, effective strategies for managing and modifying feelings, and expression of feelings in social and interpersonal contexts. We have organized emotional competencies into three core skills: (1) emotional awareness; (2) emotion regulation; and (3) emotionally engaged living, with a focus on the pursuit of valued goals.

Emotional Awareness

Emotional awareness is a prerequisite to effective emotion modulation and effective living. Whether we are aware of our feelings or not, they guide our decision making and actions. They inform others, and indeed sometimes even ourselves, about who we are. Emotions have a powerful and pervasive influence in all aspects of living. Accordingly, awareness of our feelings is a first step toward self-knowledge, self-regulation, and self-direction. Awareness of our emotions allows us to modulate them in a more purposeful, direct, and simple way than is possible when we attempt to avoid or suppress them, or when we simply experience them as a cascade of undifferentiated sensation. In addition, awareness of feelings gives us greater degrees of freedom in living. Realizing and naming what we are feeling open up options—the option to modulate a feeling, as well as the options to change it, act on it, accept it, or let it go.

BOX 5.1
Building Emotional and Social Resources:
Review of Phase I (STAIR) Sessions

Session   Content

Session 1   *The Resource of Hope—Introducing the Client to Treatment.* Treatment overview and goals; introduction to focused breathing.

Session 2   *The Resource of Feelings: Emotional Awareness.* Psychoeducation on impact of childhood abuse on emotion regulation; importance of recognizing feelings; exploration and guidance in feeling identification; practice of self-monitoring.

Session 3   *Emotion Regulation.* Psychoeducation on connections among feelings, thoughts, and behaviors; identification of strengths and weaknesses in emotion regulation; tailoring and practicing emotion coping skills; identification of pleasurable activities.

Session 4   *Emotionally Engaged Living.* Psychoeducation on acceptance of feelings/distress tolerance; assessment of pros and cons of tolerating distress; awareness of positive feelings as a guide to goal identification.

Session 5   *The Resource of Connection—Understanding Relationship Patterns.* Psychoeducation on interpersonal schemas and relationship between feelings and interpersonal goals; introduction to Interpersonal Schemas Worksheet I.

Session 6   *Changing Relationship Patterns.* Psychoeducation on role plays; identification of relevant interpersonal situations; role plays; generation of alternative schemas; introduction to Interpersonal Schemas Worksheet II.

Session 7   *Agency in Relationships.* Psychoeducation on assertiveness; discussion of alternative schemas and behavioral responses; role plays requiring assertiveness; generation of alternative schemas.

Session 8   *Flexibility in Relationships.* Psychoeducation on flexibility in interpersonal relationships; discussion of alternative schemas and behavioral responses; role plays requiring flexibility; generation of alternative schemas; discuss transition from Phase I to Phase II of treatment.

Identifying and Labeling Feeling States

The task of identifying and labeling feeling states has particular significance for abuse survivors. The social environment of an abused child is one is which the labeling of feeling is limited and, in regard to the abuse, either highly distorted or altogether absent. Because physical and sexual abuse are hidden from public view and knowledge, and are not typically topics of conversation in the social network, opportunities for correction or reanalysis of "victim blaming" or other distorted labeling is not easily available. In addition, the silence about the reality of the abuse in the home is inadvertently reinforced by the silence of the larger social environment. For the survivor, the absence of a descriptive language for a key life experience often leads to feelings of inauthenticity—and, worse, to an internalized vocabulary that is self-blaming ("You deserve what you are getting") or not synchronous with genuine feelings ("This is good for you"). As a result, childhood abuse survivors are often at a great disadvantage in coming to terms with the impact of their trauma. Feelings arising from the abuse remain inaccurately named or unnamed; moreover, the fear, anger, depression, and aggression related to the abuse are often not connected to the trauma, by the survivors or by anyone around them.

The first intervention in STAIR involves the systematic exploration of feelings—their names, their intensity, and the context in which they occur. This effort is intended to yield clarity about specific feelings, recognition of different kinds of feelings by reference to different events and experiences, and sustained awareness of the presence of feelings in daily life. The opportunity for childhood abuse survivors to name their feelings and describe their emotional experiences is vital to the process of self-discovery and ongoing self-assessment. The naming of things is the first step in each client's discovery of an authentic personal voice. The ongoing expression and organization of feelings throughout the treatment are essential to the creation of a coherent narrative of the client's personal history.

Emotion Regulation

"Emotion regulation" is defined as the capacity to modulate emotional reactions and expression. Persons who have problems in emotion regulation experience rapid and intense emotional reactions, with difficulty returning to baseline (Linehan, 1993a; van der Kolk, 1996). Such disturbance in ability to manage emotions was perhaps first discussed by Marsha Linehan as a problem that many clients bring into treatment. A psychologist, she had worked many years with clients who were chronically suicidal. She observed that many of these people experienced intense negative emotions, and that the suicide attempts were often efforts to terminate either the pain of these experiences as they were occurring in the moment, or the dread of the emotions' relentless and uncontrolled appearance in their lives. Linehan developed a program called "dialectical behavioral therapy," which was shaped by the principle that treatment should provide clients with options for how they might choose to respond to an emotion or experience, rather than being simply carried away by it (Linehan, 1993a). This principle was applied to both internal and interpersonal experiences. With this ground-breaking work, Linehan oriented therapists and research clinicians to the importance of the study and treatment of emotion management difficulties.

Basic Skills in Emotion Regulation

Difficulties in emotion regulation reflect disturbances in underlying sensory, cognitive, and behavioral systems, rather than problems with one specific type of emotional experience. The research literature has consistently identified the development of these three core coping systems across all ages—from the toddler years through adolescence into adulthood—as contributing to effective emotion management. This literature thus suggests the relevance of these systems in the treatment of clients with early-life and repeated trauma, and has provided us with a heuristic for organizing the emotion skills training. The three systems are described in this treatment as follows: (1) physical/physiological management (e.g., deep breathing, exercise); (2) cognitive strategies (e.g., self-statements, reframing of upsetting events, attentional control); and (3) behavioral management/social support (e.g., calling friends for help, talking with others about feelings).

A client's coping strategies are assessed within each system, with the goal of strengthening and elaborating these strategies. The overall goal is to create a well-integrated set of coping strategies, so that physical sensations, thoughts, and behaviors influence one another and work together toward well-modulated emotional experiences.

Modulating Negative Feelings

Fear and anger are often the emotions to which management skills are first applied. This is because fear and anger tend to be highly prevalent among trauma survivors and also create immediate and obvious problems in day-to-day functioning, particularly in monitoring personal safety (inaccurate threat perceptions) and avoiding interpersonal ruptures (anger). The applications of emotion regulation skills to other feelings, particularly shame and grief, tends to occur later in the treatment, as these feelings often first emerge when the trauma history is explored in the development of the life narrative. The emotion regulation skills described above effectively result in reduced difficulties in managing day-to-day experiences; better management of difficult feelings such as anxiety, anger, and depression; and reduction in dissociation. They also contribute, through their application during the trauma processing, to a reduction of PTSD symptoms (e.g., hyperarousal, reexperiencing).

Accepting and Modulating Positive Feelings

Although it seems counterintuitive, the experience of positive emotions can be painful to abuse survivors. Positive feelings are unfamiliar, and their unfamiliarity creates unease. Positive emotions are also threatening because they create the risk of new ways of being "out of control" or may lead to disappointment if the survivors cannot sustain the emotion. Accordingly, clients are introduced to the notion that emotion regulation includes the ability to modulate not only negative feelings, but positive ones as well. The clients are encouraged to engage in simple pleasures and to practice modulation skills to keep their feelings within bounds that are comfortable to them. The immediate consequence of introducing small pleasures is the satisfaction that the ability to confront and modulate negative feelings carries with it the reward of experiencing positive feelings as well.

However, more importantly, this exercise conveys the true meaning of emotion regulation. It refers not only to the abilities to soothe ourselves and reduce negative feeling states, but also to the abilities to raise and sustain positive feelings. It is the capacity to create an "emotional comfort zone" that is nether too intensely high nor too low, and as such allows a person to function, to learn, and to stay connected with the environment.

Emotionally Engaged Living: Toward the Pursuit of Valued Goals

For many survivors, the only alternatives to living painful and out-of-control lives are emotional avoidance, social withdrawal, limited pleasure in daily activities, and severely limited actualization of their potential. Such clients are encouraged to identify positive goals for themselves—to articulate their desires and wishes, and to consider ways in which they may realize these. Leaving the familiarity of an avoidant lifestyle requires support from the therapist and the development of several skills—making sound judgments about which goals to attempt, pacing goals, and weighing the costs and benefits of any new experience. The concept of "distress tolerance" and the skills associated with it (see Linehan, 1993b) are introduced and practiced repeatedly in the treatment. This process is intended to provide survivors with the skills necessary to control the pace of their gradual reconnection to the emotional and social world.

Distress Tolerance

Once survivors are able to identify and manage emotional reactions, they can allow themselves the experience of (well-managed) distressing feelings that serve an important purpose or goal, or are simply an inevitable aspects of certain life experiences. For example, if a client wants to get a job, a job interview is likely, and with it so is some anxiety. If a client wants to get married or have a long-term relationship, the anxious feelings associated with first meeting someone, coming to know him or her, and risking rejection are all inevitable. Interventions for distress tolerance are introduced, so that the clients can successfully achieve certain valued goals. This skill also involves weighing a goal against the likely distress it will generate, evaluating one's capacity to manage the distress, and deciding to reject or delay the goal.

Accepting Positive Feelings as Guides to Planning and Action

The clients are also introduced to the value of positive feelings in identifying valued goals. Positive feelings about certain activities, people, or projects are identified as legitimate and valuable guides in decision making. This work builds on the previous interventions in which the clients are introduced to small pleasures and practice in modulating and enjoying positive feelings. In this next step, the clients are introduced to ways to enhance quality of life by engaging in "approach behaviors" to life experiences that are positive or goals that provide intrinsic pleasure.

SOCIAL COMPETENCIES

The vast majority of survivors are motivated to come to treatment because of self-identified problems in relationships. Inevitably, problems in relationships include problems with emotions: feeling too much, feeling too little, or having a feeling poorly matched with the demands of the situation. Thus the skills developed in the first sessions are directly relevant to improving relationships. In addition, problems in relationships emerge from abuse-generated interpersonal expectations and patterns of behaviors that are not adaptive in the clients' adult worlds. Failures in the work environment, sustained conflict in intimate relationships, consistent feedback from friends about approach–avoidance patterns of relating, failures in appropriate assertiveness in the workplace or among family members, anger fits in front of their children, and fears of handing down the legacy of their abuse to their children all often have their source in abuse-related beliefs and behaviors and are all reasons for entering into treatment.

Identifying Abuse-Related Interpersonal Schemas

Chapter 2 on attachment has proposed that "interpersonal schemas" or "working models of relationships" based on experiences with important caretakers have a significant influence on the selection, character, and dynamics of later-life relationships. In STAIR, we have adapted the concept of interpersonal schemas to define and explore the negative patterns of relating that dominate clients' lives and over which they feel little control. Our research has indicated that the interpersonal schemas of abuse survivors represent "self and other" in victim–abuser patterns, where the expected contingencies for relationships, abstracted from their particulars, reflect formulations such as "To be attached means to be abused" and "Abuse is one way of attaching."

One of the central tasks in the STAIR phase of treatment is to identify abuse-related schemas and describe them as the result of a healthy impulse, attachment, which has gone wildly astray because of the malicious environmental context in which the rules for attachment were derived. Both therapists' empathy for their clients and the clients' eventual empathy for themselves are based on the understanding that schemas constitute a built-in "ambush" for abuse survivors in the form of the self-fullfilling prophecy.

Schemas have a positive function, in that they allow the anticipation of future events on the principle that "The future will be much like the past" or "The past predicts the future." People's behaviors are guided by behaviors that prepare them for *expected* rather than *possible* outcomes. Such preparations often help create the expected outcomes and close out other possibilities. This is adaptive among those who have positive expectations or live in unchanging environments. However, it leads to significant negative consequences for the survivors of childhood abuse who have left the abusive environment but still, and rather inevitably, maintain abuse-generated expectations. For example, a young woman from an abusive family who has developed the understanding that interpersonal relatedness is contingent on sexual behavior is more likely to engage in or initiate sexual activity as a way of emotionally connecting to others, whether or not she is interested in sex and whether or not her partner is actually expecting sex.

We view the identification of schemas as a critical aspect of treatment. It represents the distillation of central beliefs about self and others that provide clarity about the clients' motivations for action. The clients' behaviors become understandable to themselves and to their therapists. In addition, the source of the schemas as they derive from past experience can be explored, and the accuracy of their application to the present can be empathetically challenged. Alternative ways of thinking about self and other can be constructed.

Changing Interpersonal Schemas

A second and more difficult aspect of the treatment is to begin proposing alternative schemas—ones suggesting that the "glue" of relationships can be found in other behaviors and emotions, such as mutual respect, positive regard, and affection. This work requires moving a client from the realm of expected outcomes to that of imagined outcomes. This requires the therapist to provide guidance, suggestions, and proposals that will prompt the client to think in ways that personal history has not supported and that essentially require an act of imagination. The therapist is in some ways "reparenting" the client in the possibilities of interpersonal relationships and creating alternative "working models"—by their own relationship, as well as by explicitly proposing alternative formulations of relationships and putting them to an experiential test.

This effort is supported by each client's desire for change. The maladaptive nature of abuse-generated schemas is evident when clients' goals for themselves are disrupted by the activation of these schemas. For instance, a client may become aware that anger at a past abusive authority figure is getting in the way of forming current relationships with other authority figures. Or expectations of sexual exploitation based on sexual abuse may be creating disturbance and upheaval in current romantic relationships. The discrepancies between feelings and beliefs from the past and current goals sometimes become evident through painful real-world experiences. The treatment attempts to avoid this type of "hard-knocks" learning by using the therapy sessions as a setting in which to practice, via role plays, what clients can feel, say, and do in situations related to goal implementation. Through therapist feedback and the clients' own monitoring of feelings and statements, the clients can revise behaviors and feelings in ways that are more in accord with their identified goals, and can practice these new behaviors in sessions. A session is in essence a place to explore—to "try on" and assimilate different attitudes, behaviors, and words that match desired goals for self-expression and effective communication with others.

In STAIR, schemas are structured as simple contingency statements (i.e., "If . . . , then . . . ," or "When . . . , then . . . "). Clients find that these formulations are easy to use and effectively elicits their implicit interpersonal contingency beliefs. Typical examples include "If I do as I am told, I will be loved" or "When I ask for my needs to be met, then I am rejected." This approach allows therapists to distill clients' "core beliefs" about self and others, to provoke clients' thoughts and reactions, and to help clients develop alternative "trial schemas" for consideration (e.g., "If I don't ask for my needs to be met, then my friends will never know what I want"). This exercise is repeated from the fourth session of treatment through the trauma-processing sessions to the very end of treatment.

Linking Schemas in the Life Narrative

Schemas are the tools, and schema analysis is the strategy, for creating change in interpersonal attitudes and behaviors. Several STAIR sessions focus on identifying, proposing, and implementing alternative and more adaptive schemas. However, even when the narrative work begins, schema analysis continues. Schemas embedded in the narratives of childhood trauma are identified and compared to those that are imagined and tested daily in the present. This activity helps gauge positive changes. It also creates anchors in the implicit development of a life story. This is valuable for childhood abuse survivors, who often fear that by letting go of their past beliefs they are betraying or invalidating the reality of their trauma. It suggests that the past will be respected and recognized as part of the clients' evolving life stories and not forgotten or taken for granted, even while new schemas are elaborated in the treatment. Lastly, schemas also function across both the STAIR and NST phases of treatment to provide clients with a shorthand method for recollecting the pains of the past, without necessarily feeling those pains in depth during the recovery and change process.

Problems with Power Dynamics: Issues of Assertiveness and Control

We have observed that as survivors struggle to adopt alternative relationship roles, they often move out of victim roles and into abuser roles. This may occur in evolving relationships where an abuse survivor, in an attempt to be assertive and appropriately "in control" of events in the relationship, becomes utterly rigid and extreme. This is often related to the relative lack of variety in types of relationship templates with which a survivor is familiar. The victim–victimizer dyad is the template for relating. If the survivor has had few relationships other than the abusive ones, the client has very little room for maneuvering into new ways of relating.

We use the notion of schemas to sketch out alternative dyadic relationships that manage power in different, more egalitarian, and more mutually beneficial ways (e.g., "Having my needs recognized/recognizing those of others is a way to connect"). Because schema often effectively articulate the generalized rules with which abuse survivors have lived, schemas are quickly embraced as tools for the revision of interpersonal expectations. The new schemas are often more ideas than realities. And clients are usually stymied in their early efforts to engage in the feelings, behaviors, and language associated with dyads other than the victim–abuser pairing. For this reason, role plays in therapy sessions are critical, as are carefully selected, well-graduated exercises with others outside the treatment. These exercises provide the "real stuff" of the abstract templates, and experiential evidence of the reality of alternative ways of relating.

Flexibility in Interpersonal Functioning

The initial task in the schema work is to help clients construct and test ways of feeling, thinking, and living outside the abuse dynamic. Alternative schema generation is particularly focused on moving away from the "all-or-nothing" view of power and control that characterizes victim–victimizer dynamics, and toward a view that power and control can be shared. However, day-to-day life typically engages a person in several relationships, each with its own balance of power and control, and with a different level of intimacy and trust. The application of an egalitarian schema across all relationships would lead to poor outcomes. An insistence that a healthy diet be maintained is a reasonable and expected demand by a parent of a child—but it is not generally appropriate with a spouse (with whom decisions concerning what to eat in the household are usually shared), and certainly not with a boss who is discussing his or her favorite desserts and fondness for sweets.

Expectations for level of shared intimacy, degree of trust, and power dynamics depend on whether the relationship is with a significant other, boss or employee, parent or child, sibling or friend. The next step in STAIR moves clients toward characterizing multiple schemas that reflect different key relationships. Developing skills in these more subtle aspects of relating will facilitate the clients' ability to move fluidly and effectively in a larger social landscape. Indeed, research on interpersonal relationships has found that one of the strongest correlates of overall psychological health and life satisfaction is flexibility in interpersonal expectations and behaviors (Hill & Safran, 1994).

Schemas are effective tools for working with multiple relationship difficulties that concern abuse survivors, including repeated negative relationship patterns, pervasive difficulties in managing power and control dynamics, and problems in establishing alternative ways of approaching and relating to others. In addition, because schemas characterize both the actions and feelings in an anticipated exchange, they allow the exploration of feelings, particularly the power of feelings in derailing behaviors. In the treatment, a therapist and client develop new schemas to articulate desired interpersonal goals and ways of being. The implementation of the new schemas is often difficult, because feelings from the past conflict or compete with interpersonal goals of the present. The conflict between feelings from old schemas and the goals shaped by new schemas can be clearly brought forward to the client for examination and change. The contrast between old schemas based in an abusive past and new emerging schemas are further highlighted during NST, the second phase of treatment.

SUMMARY

Emotional and social skills are not abilities with which we are born. They are learned. The limited scope of abuse survivors' abilities does not represent personal failure or pathology, but limited opportunities. These limitations put the survivors at risk for developing problems such as anger outbursts, substance abuse, and risk avoidance. They also prevent clients from achieving what they want: having secure relationships, doing well at their jobs or careers, being good parents. For the abuse survivors, doing well in life is a mystery. STAIR provides skills that fill the gaps left by the tumult of trauma. A client completing this phase of treatment noted with relief, "It's learning things that everyone else knows." The goal of STAIR is to have the world become a little less mysterious and much more negotiable for such clients. The skills are intended to provide support for the clients to achieve important life goals and have a greater number of life choices.

CHAPTER 6

~

Working with Traumatic Memories
Overview of NST

Speaking about the [trauma] . . . provides the possibility of turning passivity into
activity. In retelling an experience, we voluntarily evoke it. Narration is thus like play
in that one can assume control over the repetition of an event which, in its occurrence,
ran counter to one's wishes. While alone at night, one may dread the vivid revival of
the experience; when telling it to others one wants to evoke it as vividly as possible.
Here is again the turning of passivity into activity: from being the helpless victim, one
becomes an effective storyteller.
      —WOLFENSTEIN, quoted by RONNIE JANOFF-BULMAN (1992, pp. 108–109)

The goals of the NST phase of treatment are to resolve PTSD symptoms through the
process of "revisiting" the traumatic memories and to put the trauma in perspective as an
experience that is part of an evolving life story. The first goal involves the process of retelling the traumatic event, with the purpose of confronting the fearful elements of the experience and dissolving the power of the memory to elicit fear. The second process involves
appraising the meaning of the traumatic experience in the context of an evolving life story.
Narratives, in both name and process, convey the message that a life story is composed of a
past, present, and future. Telling about the abuse creates and reinforces its "pastness."
Moreover, narration assumes a chronological structure that not only allows the trauma to
be located in the past, but provokes consideration of the present and imagination of a
future. The life story that begins to emerge flows from the schemas or formulations of self
and other that are anchored in time and distinguished by differences between present and
past realities. Both the repeated narration and the meaning analyses are intended to free
clients from the grip of a traumatic past, and to allow them to live in the present and imagine a future.

In this chapter, we review the rationale and history of imaginal exposure as an intervention to resolve PTSD symptoms; emerging models of the thematic nature of autobiographical memories; and the evolution and adaptation of imaginal exposure in this intervention as the heart of our narrative work. An at-a-glance, session-by-session overview of NST is provided in Box 6.1.

CONFRONTING MEMORIES: WORKING WITH FEAR

Why Revisit the Traumatic Past?

It is commonly accepted that a crucial task in resolving PTSD symptoms is the emotional processing of traumatic memories. The process we use is one of retelling or "revisiting" the past trauma. It is based on the principles of exposure therapy, particularly as developed by Edna Foa and her colleagues (see Rothbaum & Foa, 1999). Many clinicians immediately recoil when they hear the words "exposure therapy" used in treatments for trauma survivors. Therapists fear inflicting pain on their clients, or even feel themselves to be sadistic in encouraging the practice. In reality, clients experience palpable relief at having an opportunity to discuss and describe their trauma in a safe environment and in a structured and contained way. The reality is also that clients with PTSD live their memories every day, through reenactments, flashbacks, nightmares, intrusive thoughts, and images that are

---

BOX 6.1
Working with Traumatic Memories:
Review of Phase II (NST) Sessions

Session	Content
Session 9	*Introduction to NST*. Description and rationale for narrative activities; establishing commitment for narrative work; developing memory hierarchy.
Session 10	*Narrative of First Memory*. Practice with neutral memory; conducting first narrative of trauma memory; listening to tape together; exploring beliefs about self and other.
Sessions 11–15	*Narratives of Fear*. Selecting memory for narration; identifying schemas embedded in narrative and providing alternative schemas; identifying current life difficulties and implementing skills.
Sessions 12–15	*Narratives of Shame*. Same procedure as for Session 11; providing clear response of positive regard following narratives of shame; emphasizing social and personal resources that support positive appraisal.
Sessions 12–15	*Narratives of Loss*. Same procedure same as for Session 11; exploring ways of transforming loss for living in the present.
Session 16	*The Last Session*. Reviewing gains; planning next steps; addressing relapse risks; providing resources and referrals.

far more painful than the trauma-focused session work any of us has implemented. In addition, the clients' past childhood abuse experiences often profoundly dictate much of their present behavior. In reaction to the intrusion of the past into the present, clients avoid reminders of the past. They may keep relentlessly busy, abuse substances, and spurn romantic attachments. The failure of one set of avoidance strategies often begets additional avoidance strategies. The clients' experiential worlds get smaller and smaller.

Consequently, the clients' memories of the past control their lives. The intrusive, uncontrollable, and unpredictable symptoms reinforce the helplessness generated by the original trauma. At one time, the clients were subject to an ongoing reality of threat that they had no power to end or avoid. Now they are subject to the capricious and random intrusion of the memories of these events. But the reality is that the trauma is in the past, and the fear that persists is of a memory. Although the clients could not control the original traumatic events, they can have full authority over their memories. In the process of examining and exploring their memories, the clients confront them, own them, and ultimately determine their value and meaning. The process of confronting the traumatic memories reverses the relationship between the clients and their trauma. In confronting and telling about their past, the clients gain mastery over it. They move from being passive recipients of a burdensome history to becoming active agents in determining its place in their lives.

A Brief History of Exposure Therapy for PTSD

The first documented efforts in resolving PTSD through the emotional processing of traumatic memories were made by cognitive-behavioral psychologists working with combat veterans in the late 1970s and 1980s. The PTSD symptoms of fear and avoidance of situations reminiscent of the trauma were often behaviorally quite evident. The sound of a car backfiring, evoking a memory of gunfire, could elicit a startle response from a veteran. For veterans of the Vietnam War, the sound of rain and feel of humidity, reminiscent of the combat zone, could induce increased heart rate, sweating, and muscle tension. Later work with rape survivors revealed similar physiological and behavioral responses. A woman raped in an elevator, garage, or park might suffer intense hyperarousal in these settings or avoid them altogether, leading to significant restrictions in movement and travel. Effective interventions for these problems were derived from understanding this pattern of behavior as an example of a conditioned response. The sights, sounds, smells, and sensations that occurred during a traumatic event, while not necessarily intrinsically frightening, are associated so strongly with the event that their recurrence months or even years after the trauma can elicit a fear response in the absence of any real threat.

This phenomenon has been reliably observed in a series of studies where veterans with combat-related PTSD were exposed to sounds, pictures, or film clips of combat experiences. These veterans responded with strong fear reactions, as measured by affective response, blood pressure, and increased flow of epinephrine in their bloodstream, particularly as compared to similarly exposed veterans who had not developed PTSD (e.g., McFall, Marburg, Ko, & Veith, 1990; see Figure 6.1). Accordingly, treatment to resolve these useless and maladaptive reactions involved the "decoupling" of the fear response from the stimuli in a traditional behavioral manner. Via repeated exposure to the stimuli in

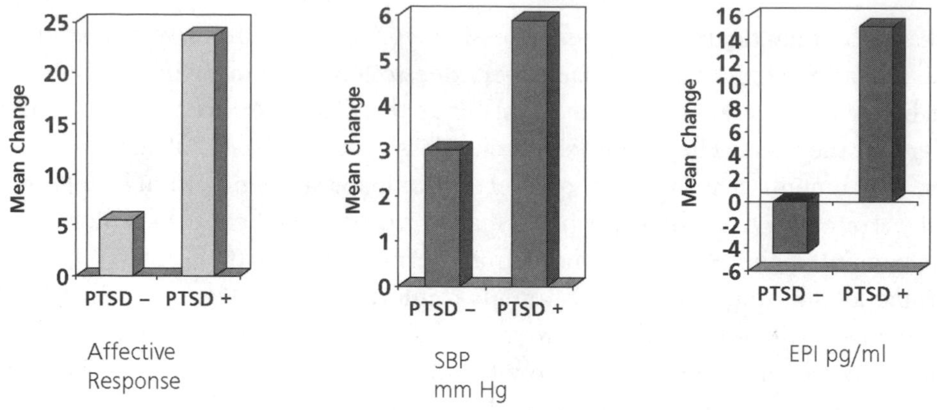

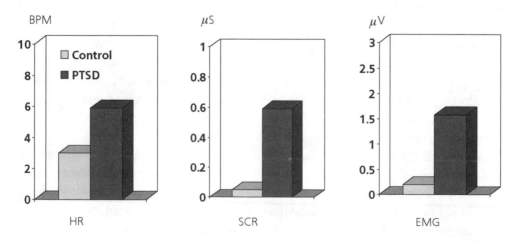

FIGURE 6.1. Conditioned fear to external cues: Psychophysiological responses to trauma-related stimuli among Vietnam combat veterans. SBP, systolic blood pressure; EPI, epinephrine. Data from McFall, Marburg, Ko, and Veith (1990).

the absence of any real threat, the clients would experience decline in the fear reaction. The stimuli, once paired rather capriciously with a real and powerful threat, now lost their potency. They became ordinary objects in the world, neutral features of the environment.

A remarkable evolution in this research occurred when it was noted that fear reactions of equivalent strength could be elicited simply through the evocation of these stimuli in memory. The physical presence of trauma-related stimuli was not necessary to elicit a fear response; the memory of these stimuli was sufficient. Increased heart rate, blood pressure, and muscle tension, all measurable aspects of a fear reaction, were induced simply by the thought of the trauma (e.g., Pitman, Orr, Forgue, de Jong, & Claiborn, 1987; see Figure 6.2). PTSD became reformulated as a disorder of memory: The feared "object," so to speak, was a memory. The process of habituation previously applied to external stimuli was adapted to mental stimuli. The rationale for the treatment was that if a therapist could

FIGURE 6.2. Fear memories: Psychophysiological responses to script-driven mental imagery of trauma. HR, heart rate; SCR, skin conductance response; EMG, electromyogram. Data from Pitman, Orr, Forgue, de Jong, and Claiborn (1987).

induce a client to bring up the image of the trauma in full and for a sufficiently long time in the context of a safe environment, the client's fearful reactions to the memory would diminish, and PTSD would resolve (see Shalev, 1997). A series of randomized, well-controlled treatment studies with veterans in the late 1980s and early 1990s, however, indicated that the intervention was only partially successful: PTSD symptoms improved but did not entirely resolve (Cooper & Clum, 1989), or veterans reported little change in subjective distress despite reduction in physiological arousal (Keane, Fairbank, Caddell, & Zimmering, 1989). In one study PTSD symptoms were not reduced, even though veterans were rated as better adjusted (Boudewyns & Hyer, 1990).

The Enduring Nature of Fear Memories

Independent of these new efforts to characterize and treat PTSD, a line of research exploring the neurobiological basis of fear responses was being conducted in animal laboratories. Joseph LeDoux and his team were among the leading scientists who determined that a relatively primitive brain structure, the amygdala, was the center of learning and unlearning of fear reactions. They were particularly interested in determining the parameters of this process. Early research tracked electroencephalographic (EEG) patterns in the amygdala during extinction of a conditioned fear response, with the expectation that the firing of the neurons related to the fear response would diminish with repeated exposure to the stimulus. In a critical study of this design, the investigators found that while there was an overall reduction in neuronal activity, the cells that had been identified as specifically related to the learned fear did not extinguish. The fear reaction as represented in the neuronal activity of the amygdala did not go away (see LeDoux, 1998).

LeDoux and his colleagues described this phenomenon as the indelibility of emotional memories. It was proposed that certain aspects of fear memories were indelibly etched into memory. The implications of these findings, translated into human functioning, suggested that traumatic memories could never be entirely freed of the overwhelming fear with which they had been encoded. This notion has been supported in a substantial number of empirical studies among both animals and humans (e.g., Bouton & Swartzentruber, 1991; Jacobs & Nadel, 1985). More recent research, taking advantage of scientific developments in protein synthesis, has attempted more sophisticated tests to determine whether established fear memories can be altered or erased (see Nader, 2003). Although there has been some success with these strategies, the initial apparent memory loss can be reversed with reminders (Fischer, Sanabenesi, Schrick, Spiess, & Radulovic, 2004) or as a result of spontaneous recovery over time (Lattal & Abel, 2004).

The idea that there are indelible aspects to traumatic memories provided an explanation for diverse observations that had been made about traumatic memories among those who suffered PTSD. If the emotional quality of traumatic memories can never be entirely extinguished, then the memories could be activated or reactivated with sufficient cueing or under circumstances of sufficient emotional power. This proposition is consistent with the observed relapse to PTSD symptoms on anniversaries of the trauma ("anniversary reactions"); delayed onset of PTSD when a survivor is presented with emotional or physical environments similar to the circumstances of the trauma; "recovered" memories that have lain dormant for years or decades; and the emergence of PTSD among elderly persons confronting chronic illness or mortality, such as World War II veterans and Holocaust survivors (see Shalev, 1997).

The enduring nature of fear memories also helps explain the limited success of the exposure therapies conducted with veterans. Certainly, some of the early difficulties were due to the newness of exposure therapy for PTSD. Since that time, however, imaginal exposure techniques for PTSD have become more refined, including the use of graded exposure controlled by the client and attention to the client's experience of safety (Foa et al., 1999a; Resick & Schnicke, 1992). Still, relapse remains high among clients with PTSD, and the residual symptomatology following pure exposure treatment indicates a need for further treatment development and conceptualization.

Toward this end, we considered the principle of extinction or habituation that was driving the scientific development of trauma therapies. "Habituation" describes a process of reduced emotional response over repeated exposures to the triggering source. To date, however, this process has been demonstrated as characteristic of only one emotion: fear. As any trauma therapist or trauma survivor can attest, fear is only one of the many emotions that generated by trauma. Others include disgust, shame, sadness, and grief. Shame is as common an emotional reaction to sexual abuse as fear. Yet clinical research has been relatively silent on the topic. Do repeated elicitations of shame-related abuse memories lead to the extinction of shame feelings? No one has ever claimed this to be the case.

Shame and grief are inevitably encountered during the recovery process, but little is understood about how these feelings are resolved. Recent investigations have begun to indicate the importance of these emotions in the recovery process. Independent of the suffering and distress caused by the presence of these disturbing emotions, shame has been identified as a risk factor for the development of PTSD, and both shame and grief have been noted to disturb the resolution of PTSD symptoms (Andrews, Brewin, Rose, & Kirk, 2000; Ehlers et al., 1998a). Perhaps the absence of focused attention on these emotions in treatments for PTSD have contributed to the observed substantial residual PTSD symptoms often observed at the end of treatment. Given their salience and potential importance, how are these emotions to be managed and resolved in treatment?

There is some evidence that imaginal exposure in the form of narratives does help resolve shame and grief (Kubany et al., 2004; Shear, Frank, Houck, & Reynolds, 2005). In consideration of these findings and with the collaboration of our clients, we devised a process of "telling" about the trauma for childhood abuse survivors. This process brought in strands of narratives related to shame and grief that were inevitably part of the experience of sexual and physical abuse.

BEYOND EXTINCTION: THE TRAUMA NARRATIVE

Imaginal exposure typically consists of repeatedly telling the story of the traumatic event, with a beginning, middle, and end. The repeated telling of the traumatic event was originally proposed as a step-by-step strategy to extinguish the fear associated with the store of trauma memories. However, it has been noted that repeated telling of the trauma also succeeds in organizing the sensory-perceptual aspects of the memory. Fragments of images and sensations, which appear intrusively without purpose or control before therapy, become organized into a coherent picture. The shards of traumatic memories "find their fit" and, like pieces of a puzzle, become an integrated and stable part of a larger picture. A study analyzing the properties of trauma narratives among rape survivors participating in exposure therapy supports this view (Foa, Molnar, & Cashman, 1995c). Comparisons between the first and last narratives indicated a reduction in the sensory characteristics of the narrative, as well as greater organization in the thoughts expressed about the trauma. Furthermore, these changes in narratives were associated with PTSD symptom reduction. The process of creating a narrative, insofar as it organizes the sensory-perceptual aspects of the memory and creates a verbally mediated interpretation of the trauma, thus appears to contribute to the reduction of PTSD symptoms independently of the process of habituation.

In addition, some clinical researchers have noted that the use of words creates another representational form of memory—one which is relatively abstract, compared to the predominantly sensory characteristics that initially constitute traumatic memory (Brewin, Dalgleish, & Joseph, 1996; Brewin, 2003). Words allow some distance from the sensory memories and engender the capacity to discuss the event without necessarily calling up the images of the event. They also drive higher-level, conceptual analyses of events, creating a system of meaning in which the sensory-perceptual memories can be interpreted and contained.

The Power of Language: Managing the Traumatic Memory

Memory has been described as consisting of two distinct forms with their own characteristics: sensory-perceptual and verbal-representational. During and immediately after a trauma, the flow of stress hormones operates on these two memory systems in contrasting ways (see McEwen, 1992). Sensory-perceptual memory functioning is heightened to such an extent that information is encoded vividly, rapidly and explosively in all sensory domains, including visual, tactile, and olfactory. Simultaneously, the memory processes involved in verbal encoding are slowed and inhibited. This disequilibrium is a component of the body's survival system when activated by the perception of bodily threat. Survival involves rapid analysis of and response to the physical environment; the processes of labeling and verbal characterization of the event are irrelevant and perhaps even detrimental to successfully meeting the demands of the moment. For some, this primitive stress-driven reaction will, as intended, enhance survival. For others, the reaction may accelerate beyond useful bounds, so that they become frozen, without the capacity for either words or action. Regardless, part of the recovery process from trauma is the recovery of the equilibrium between these two memory systems. This is a naturally occurring process. Almost everyone who has the opportunity will talk about a trauma once it is over.

The power of words and their representation in memory is quite opposite in character to that of sensory-perceptual memories. Sensory-perceptual memories make events from long ago feel as if they are happening in the moment, and can surge forward into consciousness with such vividness and dominance that all other memories fade and become inaccessible. Verbal representations of events are relatively abstract and can put distance between the recollection of an emotional event and feeling for it. Words can signify or refer to an event in a clear and direct way, but need not engage emotions. Language can therefore be a useful medium by which to diminish, modulate, or contain painful feelings.

One model of memory functioning proposes that when verbal memories develop, they automatically inhibit access to the sensory-perceptual representations of the memory (Conway & Pleydell-Pearce, 2000). Verbal representations of memories exist functionally in a hierarchical relationship to sensory-perceptual memories; that is, verbal representations organize and contain sensory-perceptual memories and modulate their expression. Moreover, verbal representations can represent synthesized information across different specific and concrete memories, and can import complex meanings to experiences. For example, a narrative, a form of verbal representation, organizes a series of memories sustained in relationship with one another by selected meanings or themes. So, for example, a person passing a bakery may catch a scent wafting in the air, which will trigger a sensory-perceptual memory of a chocolate cake with fudge icing and will make the person's mouth water. In contrast, a person sitting at a desk might write a narrative of favorite birthdays across the years and describe the presence of a favorite chocolate cake, but this experience is much less likely to elicit a flash of chocolate before a person's eyes and the accompanying mouth-watering reaction (see Figure 6.3).

These analyses suggest that beyond facilitating the internal organization of the traumatic memory, narratives can place the traumatic event in the context of other life events and in the context of an ascribed meaning that goes beyond and contains the immediate facts of the event. This process may contribute to the reduction or modulation of a variety of trauma-generated feelings, including not only fear reactions but also feelings of grief, shame, loneliness, and so on.

The therapeutic power of narrative construction to modulate multiple affects was recently demonstrated to us in the case of a man suffering from PTSD symptoms and bur-

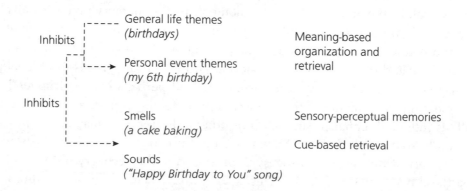

FIGURE 6.3. Functions of conceptual/contextual memory: Diagram of the relationship between verbal and sensory-perceptual images. Based on a model developed by Conway and Pleydell-Pearce (2000) and Markowitsch (1995).

densome grief that literally left him gasping for breath. The man, in his 70s, came into treatment after losing his son in the September 11, 2001, terrorist attack on the World Trade Center. He could not stop imagining his son's final moments and the particulars of his death. So frequent and extreme were these intrusive thoughts and images that when he was asked to describe his relationship with his son, he could recall nothing. It was as if the horrendous images of his son's death obscured access to any other memory about him. The situation was devastating to behold. The man had lost his son twice over: once in the World Trade Center, and now again, in his imaginal world.

The therapist began by asking this man to tell about his son as a young child, and then about his son's middle school years, his performance as a high school athlete, and his marriage to a neighborhood girl. Over time, several stories were told, and the death of his son became one of several belonging to the narrative that was his son's life. That last story was a terrible story, to be sure. But the formation of the narrative had placed the death in the context of a life lived; it was no longer simply the story of a death. When the man thought of his son, he had a narrative of how his son had lived joyfully, or another narrative about the relationship with his son and its various ups and downs. In either case, the narrative did not end with the son's death, but was continued by the creation of positive memories of the son to be handed down to his grandson. Figure 6.4 depicts the application of the model illustrated in Figure 6.3 to trauma memory in this man's case.

THE TASKS OF NST

Telling the Story

As the description provided above indicates, the primary function of narrative work for the survivor of childhood abuse is to create the story of an unfolding life, in which the trauma is only one of many events that are possible for the survivor. In Phase II of our treatment program, NST, the narrative of the traumatic event is repeated several times. It is expected that through repeated tellings, the associated fear reactions will diminish and the memory will become organized and internally coherent, so that questions about the facts of the matter (what happened and when did it happen) are answered as clearly as possible.

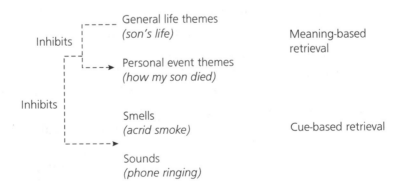

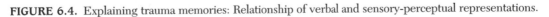

FIGURE 6.4. Explaining trauma memories: Relationship of verbal and sensory-perceptual representations.

Identifying Themes

After the trauma narrative is completed, however, the client and therapist listen to the narrative and identify interpersonal schemas within it. Because childhood abuse survivors have many particular memories, client and therapist are able to identify themes that are constant across all memories. These themes often identify the client's core beliefs about the self in the world, and are typically driven by feelings of fear, shame, and loss. Examples of such beliefs are (1) "The world is a dangerous place, and I am not competent to effectively confront or live in it" (fear); (2) "I did something to provoke this, and I did not stop it, so I am to blame" (shame); and (3) "I never had what so many take as the 'given' in a normal childhood, and I cannot ever have it" (loss and grief).

Comparing the Past and Present

The abuse-related schemas are evaluated in terms of their value and function in the present. Typically they function to bring the past into the present, via self-confirming attitudes and behaviors. These beliefs are contrasted with the alternatives that have been formulated in the first phase of treatment, and for which there is accumulating evidence of successful implementation in the client's day-to-day life. The experiential evidence for the new schemas, although limited, demonstrates that the client can have experiences different from those of the past and encourages a belief in the possibility of change. Past beliefs and feelings are validated as adaptive or inevitable, given the context of abuse from which they emerged. The experiences of the present tell a different story, however. Thus the story of the abuse and the story of the present are compared, and the beliefs belonging to each story are contrasted. Both sets of beliefs are validated by placing them in the context of time and place.

For example, a young woman who was sexually abused as a child may well have a strong feeling of incompetence. This emerges from the quite real childhood circumstances in which the client was forced to undergo sexual activity with an adult, which was beyond her competence to deal with and which she was in no position to defend herself from, escape from, or understand the meaning of. This analysis places the traumatic memory in the context of the client's childhood and creates (often for the first time) a historical or developmentally sensitive understanding of the event as an event that happened to a child. The client listens to the narrative as a story, rather than as an omnipresent memory drenched in fear and shame. This distance often provides the client with some compassion for the child in the story, who is herself. In contrast, the alternative interpersonal schema that the client has been developing in Phase I is presented as a plausible belief that can be tested and applied in her current circumstances.

This distinction between the past and the present is reiterated in all sessions. A symptom of PTSD (and a characteristic of many trauma survivors) is that time has collapsed for them. The traumatic event defines reality as it was in the past and will be in the future. Traditional narration, with its underlying chronological structure, helps clients to anchor events to moments in time and assign meaning in the context of the passing of time.

Integrating the Past and the Present

To continue with the example above, when the client feels that who she is today and who she was as a child are very different experiences of life, she may be able to take the next step in recovery—which is to accept and respect who she was. Traumatized individuals often experience themselves as in an endless state of pain (e.g., fear, shame), existing timelessly in the trauma. When the opportunity comes to distance themselves from the pain (through avoidance or "forgetting"), survivors often do so for the relief it brings. But this distancing also creates gaps and disconnections in their personal life histories, with significant negative consequences for their emotional and interpersonal functioning.

This treatment creates a context of safety that allows the survivor first to distinguish the present from the past, and then, from the safety of the present, to reconnect with her past. In the safety of the present, she does not feel like a sexually abused child, but rather has compassion for the feelings of that child. In the safety of the present, she does not relive the trauma, but simply knows that it has happened. The pain of the past is manageable, and so the feelings associated with it can be incorporated into the client's experience of the present; the events of the past can be connected to and inform those occurring today; and the traumatized self can be integrated into and enrich the experiences of the self in the present.

The client is reminded regularly of this process of integration. The therapist emphasizes the client's safety in confronting the past before the narrative work. After it is complete, the therapist guides the client in articulating ways which the past and present differ, but also they way in which the past can inform and enrich the present. Bringing the trauma forward brings the resources of wisdom—of feelings, of self-awareness, and of the facts of life and living. All of these resources can then be brought to bear on living in the present and thinking about a future.

CHAPTER 7

~

Extending the Narrative
Transforming Shame and Loss

You know, people say my writing is dark. And for me, it's quite the opposite.
It sees light in darkness and it doesn't try to distort the darkness. The essential
thing is that the seeing itself is joyful.
                    —DAVID MILCH (quoted by Mark Singer, 2005, p. 205)

The Narrative Story Telling phase of the treatment gives clients the opportunity to
develop a coherent life history with various themes that follow the thread of critical affective experiences. In addition to fear, central emotional burdens for those who have experienced sustained abuse by caretakers are shame and loss. There are, however, very few
established trauma-focused treatments that are intended to address these consequences of
abuse. Narrative work is assumed to be therapeutic in the resolution of fear through
repeated exposure to the traumatic memory and the consequent habituation/extinction of
the fear-laden response. As discussed in the previous chapter, given what is known about
emotions, there is no reason to think that feelings of shame and loss would resolve through
repeated exposure to or systematic re-experiencing of shaming or grief-eliciting memories.
Still, it became clear in our own narrative work that feelings of shame and of grief were
almost inevitably brought forth at some point in the telling of traumatic memories, and furthermore, the telling was therapeutic. We suspect that the aspects of narrative work that
make the process therapeutic are the act of constructing the narrative and the task of imbu-
ing it with meaning. Narrative work contributes to the resolution of shame and grief not
through habituation but through their transformation via the meaning the client attributes
to the trauma and through the call to action that these feelings often prompt.

NST—which includes both the telling of the story and the particular meaning analysis
that follows—is organized so that clients' understanding of who they are, because of where

they have been or what they have experienced, is no longer a source of shame or irremediable loss. Rather, it now supports the evolution of a sense of dignity and purpose. The reparative actions that transform shame and loss can begin with the simple cat of telling about the event. Narration as an act, by both its process and its content, is an "antidote" to shame and loss. Shame, which often arises from a sense of being ineffectual, is countered by the experience of agency in the creation of the story. Through telling the brutal facts of the abuse trauma, clients clearly see, often for the first time, the difficulties of their early lives and can appreciate and even marvel at their success in having survived these difficulties. The telling of the abuse story in therapy can also liberate the clients from the dark weight of secrecy that often paralyzes the capacity for self-expression. If clients can tell about the abuse, they can tell about myriad other thoughts and feelings. The stories begin spilling out; connections are made; multiple past events that have seemed to follow separate tracks come together; and important patterns are identified.

The act of narration has a similar transformative potential with experiences of loss. Narration provides a means by which a ritual for grieving and remembrance can take place. Telling about and putting words to the loss affirm that the experience has importance. Its meaning, though, is often discovered only through the process of telling the story. The loss, often initially understood rather abstractly as an "absence" of something in the life history (a loving parent, a secure home), is transformed into something with presence. This comes in the form of awareness, wisdom, or insight, and ultimately in a conscious and purposeful decision about what to make of the losses and their assigned role for life in the future.

This chapter focuses in depth on shame and loss because, despite their importance, these experiences have received relatively little attention in empirically based trauma-focused treatment formulations and interventions. Studies implementing treatments that focus on reevaluating the meaning of events associated with shame and grief have reported reduction in these feelings (e.g., Kubany et al., 2004; Shear et al., 2005). Currently, there are no reliable measures appropriate to the feelings of shame and grief that survivors of childhood abuse experience. In our own work, such changes are evaluated indirectly through reductions in depression and self-harming behaviors, and are regularly reported and recorded in the post-narrative meaning analysis. In the remainder of this chapter, we, based on our combined clinical experience of 30 years, characterize shame and loss as we have observed them in treatment and identify different thematic aspects expressed by clients in the narrative phase of the work. We present this information so that clinicians and survivors alike may have some guides in the exploration and recovery from feelings of shame and loss. Examples of NST sessions with these themes are provided in Chapters 22 and 23.

SHAME

Shame has been described as a "neglected emotion" (Allen, 1995). It is often described in contrast to other emotions (e.g., guilt, pride) and rarely as a phenomenon in and of itself, reflecting the fragmented understanding mental health practitioners and other professionals have of the topic. Yet shame is a common if not pervasive emotion associated with trauma. Shame has been reported as contributing to difficulties in adaptation across the age spectrum, from children and adolescents (Brown & Kolko, 1999; Feiring et al., 1998; Feiring, Taska, & Chen, 2002) to adults (Andrews et al., 2000; Andrews & Hunter, 1997). It has been identified as a significant predictor of PTSD independent of fear, helplessness, and horror—emotions that have been included as part of the definition of a trauma response (Brewin et al., 2000). It is also a strong predictor of slowed recovery among those childhood abuse survivors who experience adulthood trauma (Andrews et al., 2000).

In our view, shame is inextricably linked to fear, the "core" emotion resulting from trauma. Fear is a biologically hard-wired and evolutionarily ancient emotion; it alerts people to potential life threat and functions to maximize survival behaviors. Shame includes a sense of threat to survival or well-being as it relates to how individuals are perceived by others or within a community or social context. Shame arises in a threatening situation when persons feel that they have failed, that the failure is perceived by others as a sign of weakness, and that it places them at risk for ejection or rejection from the community. Often the failure is a defeat that is interpersonal in nature. Recent literature has identified strong feelings of shame among those who are raped, robbed, or sexually abused (see Andrews et al., 2000; Brewin, 2003). Those so intimately injured feel that they have failed in the essential task of self-preservation, as compared to what others might have done or as compared to what is socially expected. The beliefs associated with feelings of shame include thoughts that the persons are marked as inferior and to blame for their defeat, and ultimately rejected by others because of it. The emerging data thus seems to suggest that shame is a salient feeling among individuals injured by, rejected, and alienated from their community.

Based on our clinical experience, we have identified four different shame themes that emerge in narrative work and that are often reflected in the day-to-day functioning of survivors. These themes are "self as inferior," "self as bad," "self as annihilated," and "self as identified with the perpetrator."

Self as Inferior

Shame commonly emerges following traumas when the traumatized persons carry a sense of defeat or failure. Reactions of helplessness and powerlessness are part of the definitional landscape of a traumatic experience. In contrast, shame results from the survivors' belief that they should have done better—that they should have been able to protect themselves and did not do so. This gives rise to a sense of inferiority: "Others would not have reacted the way I did," or "Others would have escaped this circumstance, and I did not." The judgment about self is in relation to others and relative to the capacities of others for self-preservation.

In addition, shame is tied to people's capacities for self-protection as members of a social group. As noted above, shame almost always arises from victimizations that are interpersonal in nature. Individuals who have been victimized by members of their own social network feel shamed and inferior. They believe that in the social hierarchy, they are "less than" others who have not experienced this form of interpersonal defeat. Social recognition or observation of defeat by others is threatening, as it carries the identification of the defeated persons as victims, and therefore demonstrably vulnerable and at risk for further victimization. For this reason, many crime victims feel greater shame when their victimization has been witnessed by others (e.g., gang rape), and often witnesses themselves feel shame for the victims. Shame results from experiences of being "acted upon" and having no recourse or resources to avoid the victimization, escape from it, or emerge victorious.

Thus children victimized by sexual or physical abuse feel shame and inferiority because they not only *did not*, but *could not* help themselves. Feelings of shame and inferiority are further exacerbated in this as in other sexual or physical crimes, because the defeat in these events has a specific intimacy—the defeat of one's body, which leads to feelings of profound vulnerability. This is the focal point of the inferiority and shame felt by victims of physical and sexual abuse.

Crime victims often ruminate about whether they could have done anything differently to alter the outcome of the event. One purpose of replaying traumatic scenes is to determine the critical elements in the victimization. If the trauma can be attributed to unfortunate and unforeseeable circumstances, then the victims may feel that anyone would have reacted the way they did, and that the outcome does not reflect any intrinsic inferiority. They are "victims of circumstance," not victims of their own inherent weakness or vulnerability.

Childhood abuse survivors also often ruminate about the transgressions they have experienced. The fact that they were small children with limited resources, and thus were inherently vulnerable, is of little comfort. In fact, it brings their analyses of the events to the larger social environment: If they could not be expected to rely on their own resources for protection, then who should have been providing the protection? The closest members of their social world—namely, their caretakers. Yet the caretakers were also often the victimizers, and in any case they provided no protection. There is no relief from the sense of inferiority and shame. Child victims ask, "Why me?" During the years of abuse, the children often construct an answer that includes and reinforces their own sense of inferiority for the abuse: They must have deserved it.

Self as Bad

Children who are physically and/or sexually abused often believe that these events are expressions of their own intrinsic "badness." This occurs for several reasons. First, explicit statements of the children's inherent badness, inferiority, and worthlessness are frequently made by those who are inflicting the abuse. The children are identified as the cause of these events (e.g., "Look what you made me do"). This is self-evident in many cases of physical abuse, where the pain that is inflicted is often called "punishment." In cases of sexual abuse where there is little or no pain, or perhaps even pleasure, the children still understand that these activities are "bad," "dirty," or "wrong," because such activities deviate from typical, day-to-day touching experiences and because they are inevitably carried out in secrecy.

In addition, the perpetrators are aided by children's cognitive predisposition to interpret experience in a self-referential way. When bad things happen, children tend to view themselves as the source of the problem. Beatings, physical assaults, and sexual abuse convince children that they themselves are inferior or bad. Both moral and social justice are filtered through the developmentally immature, self-referential forms of cognitive processes that define childhood. A negative assessment is not circumscribed to an event (e.g., "A bad thing happened with Daddy") or designated to another actor ("Daddy did a bad thing"), but is absorbed by a child as part of his or her identity: The child *is* bad for being involved in something bad. In contrast, adult crime victims have the cognitive abilities to differentiate between internal and external causes of events, and can engage in a cognitive reevaluation that delineates the difference between events that made them feel inadequate and being inadequate persons. This type of analysis is not typical of children, and may not even be possible for younger children. Notably, even when children do recognize that the adult perpetrators are to blame, they do not necessarily excuse themselves from blame (Feiring et al., 2002; Kolko, Brown, & Berliner, 2002).

Labels of self-blame and "self as bad" stick through the years of adolescence, young adulthood, and maturity. Looking back on their childhood, adult survivors can usually see past the treachery of the self-referential logic of childhood and recognize the vulnerability of their childish minds to self-blame. This often does not help them to give up, resolve or reorganize beliefs of self-blame, however. The resistance to relinquishing these beliefs has many sources.

Self as Annihilated

Shame is associated with feeling oneself to be inferior to others and of less worth. Beyond the feeling of being "less than others" is that of being "nonexistent." These are experiences where victims feel that their very lives are of no value or regard. Brewin (2003, p. 80) reports that crime victims sometimes describe having felt that their survival was of no consequence. Prostrate bystanders at a bank robbery describe being stepped over as impediments to the goal of a successful robbery, or perhaps even being used as "human shields" to enable the robbers to escape. Brewin describes such circumstances as "encompass[ing] a total surrender of oneself and one's rights and expectations as a human being" (2003, p. 80).

This intensely disturbing state is often a chronic condition for abused children. A sense of self develops in the context of a caretaker who responds to a child's needs; soothes the child's distress; laughs when the child is funny; and engages in play, teaching, and learning. Through all of these interactions, the caretaker reflects back or "mirrors" the presence of the child, provides recognition of the child as a particular person, and acknowledges the child's agency. Physical and sexual abuse undermine these experiences. Like the robbery victims described above, abused children become objects of another's will. Parents who beat their children in fits of rage often report that their anger overwhelms them and they lose all ability to see (sometimes literally), to reason, and to control their actions. Empathy for and connection to their child has vanished, and so has the child.

Although little is known about pedophiles in general or about parents who sexually abuse their children, some research indicates that such adults do not actually see the children as persons, but rather as objects of desire—objects without any volition or emotional experience. In an unusual study of convicted pedophiles (Chaplin, Rice, & Harris, 1995), a series of pictures were developed to look like children in erotic poses and shown to the men, during which time measures of sexual arousal (i.e., erection, heart rate) were taken. The emotional states of the children were varied: One set of photos showed distressed children (crying); in the second set, children looked happy; and in the third, they had neutral expressions. The study results revealed that the levels of sexual arousal exhibited by the pedophiles were the same, regardless of the children's emotional state. These findings suggest that pedophiles experience children as sources of erotic stimulation—literally as "sexual objects"—and have little empathic connection to the children as persons in distress.

Annihilation through Self-Betrayal

If children do not exist in the eyes of their caretakers, they have difficulty existing for themselves and within themselves. Even if a child's growing identity incorporates experiences, values, and opinions obtained from outside the family, it is hard to hold on to these self-constructions while still participating in the family system. Because the sense of self is anchored in the recognition that parents or other caretakers give to their children, children are likely to compromise their moral codes to protect the family system. As a result, abused children are agents of their own annihilation through these routine acts of self-betrayal. Although they wish to tell the truth, they often find themselves lying about the conditions of their home lives; they hide their bruises and maintain the secret of abuse. Adult abuse survivors often feel shame in recollecting their childhood behaviors. They feel shame in having become accomplices in something wrong, being held captive by their circumstances, and being ineffective in escape from these circumstances. And, perhaps most damaging, they experience shame in betraying themselves and their own dignity.

Self as Identified with the Perpetrator

Rather than have no sense of self (i.e., in order to avoid annihilation), abused children will sometimes actively or purposefully participate in abusive behaviors. Some survivors report instances in which they provoked their own abuse by triggering the abusers' temper and getting (although sometimes escaping) a beating, or actively participating in or even initiating sexual activities. In much the same way that having any caretaker is better than having no caretaker, it seems to be the case that having any self, even a terribly abased self, is better than having no self. Identifying with a perpetrator's attitudes and behaviors provides self-coherence. It means that the victim can move from helplessness and passivity to active agency. The victim takes on an action plan, so that there is a capacity to act; takes on victim–abuser relational patterns, so that a relationship exists; and takes on the perpetrator's beliefs, in order to have a system of meaning.

The relationship of the victim and perpetrator is likely to have special meaning, although not necessarily in any positive sense. It has been reported that relationships among individuals who have survived the same traumatic event have a special quality. It is forged from the mutual recognition that they have experienced something beyond typical experience and beyond the power of words to describe in normal conversation or day-to-day life that sets them apart from others (e.g., Gurewitsch, 1998). A relationship of a similar nature can occur between a childhood abuse survivor and a perpetrator. These experiences have potent meaning to the victims; the events have formed their view of themselves and contributed to their self-definition. In the case of sexual abuse and sometimes in physical abuse, there is often no one else who knows about the experience, no one who was witness to the events, and no one with whom a victim has shared what happened. Recognition of a large part of the victim's identity is bound up with only one person—the perpetrator of the victimization.

A critical aspect of recovery from trauma is the disclosing and sharing of the event with a sympathetic person outside the experience. If a traumatized person is able to share and convey the reality of the experience in this way, it becomes known to a social world beyond the perpetrator. The bond between the victim and perpetrator sustained by secrecy is loosened and ultimately dissolves. The victim can become known in full to others, and then can have relationships with others in which the person's whole history and whole self are known, understood, and accepted. This work is described further in Chapter 22 (on narratives of shame).

Shame, Social Functioning, and Interpersonal Relationships

Shame burdens abuse survivors with a pervasive sense of alienation from others and diminished confidence in social interactions. They believe that "If you knew I was abused as a child, you would not connect with me." The survivors have internalized a view of themselves as "bad," "weak," "ineffective," or "defeated." These beliefs are reflected in reports of their interpersonal problems, as described earlier, with problems such as assuming blame for events they are not responsible for ("If something is wrong, it must be my fault") and being too controlling ("I am not going to let anything bad happen again"). In addition, when survivors do confront difficulties, they often exhibit a "blind spot" about calling on social support to help resolve a problem. This disinclination may be based on a general sense of being "outsiders" or not part of a particular social network or community. It may also be a result of what they have experienced and learned from their abuse situation: "Help" was not forthcoming then, and is now no longer expected. Some may believe that asking for help would expose them as the "weak" persons they fear themselves to be. In circumstances where help from others is necessary to complete a task or reach a goal, this attitude leads to failure and defeat, reinforcing the view of themselves as weak, ineffective, and critically regarded.

Survivors' negative and critical view of themselves also affects their evaluation of others. The abuse has led survivors to view certain characteristics as unacceptable—not only in themselves, but in others as well. For instance, survivors who internalize the view that vulnerability is weakness, and weakness is bad, not only view themselves with contempt but judge others in the same fashion. These survivors may prize self-confidence and self-sufficiency in others, and derogate those who show confusion, emotionality, moral uncertainty, or limited competence. The familiar mode of critical regard that is applied to the self is applied to others. The limited compassion that the survivors have for their own past experiences is now applied to others' experiences. These attitudes diminish opportunities for positive social experiences and the development of sustained interpersonal relationships.

The development of a sense of self-compassion allows such clients to live much more easily with themselves, and perhaps even with some pride and enthusiasm for themselves. In addition, a positive and more generous process of self-evaluation may lead to more generous appraisal of others. Positive changes in self-regard go hand in hand with positive changes in regard for others. The clients benefit in their relationships with others, as well as in relationship to themselves.

LOSS AND GRIEF

Childhood abuse is inevitably an experience of loss. This includes loss of protective and supportive caregivers, of a healthy sense of entitlement, and of unencumbered connectedness to others; of a child's innocent pride and easy comfort within his or her own skin; and of what the child "could have been" and the life he or she "could have had" in the absence of abuse. Identification of losses can be, at bottom, the most difficult and painful aspect of recovery. It requires clients to acknowledge that they have received less than they humanly deserved in their childhood. This can reinforce feelings of shame, because the survivors may view these losses as a reflection of their personal worthlessness. In addition, recognition of these losses can ignite feelings of grief and anger.

These losses, while very real and painful, have not been addressed in any systematic way in established trauma-focused treatments. The incorporation of themes of loss in the NST component of treatment is intended to alleviate this gap. Indeed, the use of narrative to address and resolve loss borrows directly from established rituals for mourning, which almost always include storytelling as a means of shared remembrance. This process acknowledges and confers reality to the loss. Stories about the deceased elaborate and clarify the importance of that person to the bereaved and often formulate ways of continuing to remember the person. In addition, rituals of mourning are almost always social processes that bring members of a community together. In this gathering, a network of social support is formed, reflecting the understanding that grief can be all-consuming and can paralyze the ability to function and the will to live in the present. The community cares for and protects those who grieve and keeps them emotionally and socially engaged in the present by sharing recognition of the loss and understanding of the consequent pain.

When addressing the client's losses, NST shares many functions with those observed in socially sanctioned rituals of mourning. As a witness or listener to the story, the therapist confers a social reality on the client's losses even though they are far in the past. The elaboration of the aspects of loss intrinsic to childhood abuse is an important step to understanding the past, its impact on the client's present life, and its role in the client's future. In the community of two that is the treatment, the therapist provides emotional support and care of the client as he or she recognizes and mourns these losses.

In addition, however, the therapist facilitates the transformation of grief into the purposeful selection of changes in loss-related attitudes and behaviors that have restricted the clients' ability to function and live well. There is a certain paradox in the experience of grief, in which recognition of loss can ignite energy to repair the damage and even bring forth greater effort, imagination, and determination to create meaning and value to life than would have otherwise have been the case.

Below, we have identified some common and specific loss themes that surface in client narratives. These themes are "loss of protective parental figure," "loss of childhood innocence and pleasures," "loss in interpersonal relationships," and "loss of time."

Loss of Protective Parental Figure

Children tend to accept their lot in life, for the simple reasons that they know no better and they have few other choices. Their reference points for evaluating the relative degree of life hardship are their immediate environments, particularly their families. Only through the exploration of the larger social world, via school and peer relationships in the preteen to early teen years, do abused children actually begin to realize that their home lives deviate from those of other youth. By the adolescent years, youth who have experienced abuse recognize that the goings-on in their lives differ from those of other teenagers. They recognize that their peers are *not* having the kind of experiences with which they are familiar. It may take many more years for the adult survivors to recognize that they differ from their peers not only in the *presence* of abuse, but also in the *absence* of loving care, good regard, and benign adult guidance in the world.

Exploring the reality of abuse and the context in which it was allowed to occur through the narrative work often leads survivors to painful clarity about the limited capacities and caretaking behaviors of their parents and/or parent figures. Identifying interpersonal schemas from childhood and comparing these to the ones they are forming in the present may also highlight survivors' awareness that the warmth and comfort they can now experience, or see others experience and wish for themselves, were not theirs in childhood. The persons whom they relied on for a sense of worth did not value them. Many survivors have never known "unconditional positive regard" and have never experienced a parental figure as a soothing presence. As awareness of these truths sets in, clients begin to understand on a more profound level how their most basic human rights—to be regarded with value, and with respect for their autonomy and agency—were denied them.

Loss of Childhood Innocence and Pleasures

The experience of being abused by caretakers stands in stark contrast to the innocence, safety, simplicity, and carefree ways that we, as a society, usually equate with childhood years. Even if an abused child is given the opportunity to participate in positive childhood rituals, such as playing with friends, going on first dates, or receiving honors for graduations or sports activities, the effects of trauma often pervade and overshadow the pleasure and satisfaction of these experiences. In particular, abuse by parental figures significantly decreases children's engagement with their environment and openness to others, diminishing the typical pleasures of childhood and positive memories. Such children have experiences beyond or quite different from those of their peer group. For instance, sexually abused children are prematurely forced into the world of adult sexual knowledge.

At the time of the abuse, the survivors may simply feel confused, angry, or alienated from their peers. As adults looking back on the experience, clients often feel aggrieved: They begin to see themselves as having their innocence—an attitude to life that belongs to the domain of childhood—stolen from them.

Loss in Interpersonal Relationships

The actual truth—essentially their betrayal by their parents or other trusted adults—often takes years for survivors to recognize and to accept. Intrafamilially abused teens often still cling to their attachment for and love of their parents or caretakers, even when these adults have been egregiously abusive or have repeatedly failed in parenting tasks. This connection, however, serves to maintain a template of relatedness. The affection and attachment that a child or adolescent shows to a caretaker, however unresponsive, undeserving, or implausible the caretaker may be, has an important function: It maintains the young person's capacity for human connection. The template of interpersonal schemas remains intact.

Nevertheless, specific interpersonal schemas developed in this context lead to several problems in adulthood relationships. For example, abuse survivors are more likely to choose relationships with individuals who are unreliable and unavailable—even to the point of being abusive and/or neglectful—since this is expected and accepted. In relationships where there is potential for support and caring, the clients may not be able to see or cultivate these aspects of the relationship. Clients sometimes report that while they can identify the presence of support or help others, they reject these overtures, because such giving cannot possibly match what they didn't get and still long for from parental figures. In line with this understanding, our treatment does not necessarily involve the revision or dissolution of a client's connection to an abusive caretaker. Rather, the treatment supports the growth of the client's persistent capacity for attachment. As such, it sets the goal of helping the client establish alternative interpersonal schemas and behaviors in the service of developing new and different relationships.

Loss of Time

Once clients begin experiencing fewer symptoms and improved functioning, review of their past leaves them aghast at the many years that they have not had the capacity to function well and enjoy their lives. Clients sometimes feel resentful that they will never recapture the time they have lost. They consider, for example, their teen years when they could have been studying rather than abusing drugs, or their 20s when they were too angry and hostile to establish themselves in the work world. The developing awareness of the profound and pervasive negative impact the trauma and related PTSD symptoms have had on a client's life trajectory can elicit anger and dismay. This loss, like many others related to abuse, is irreversible. However, the client does have the opportunity of the present, which, if spent in anger, will only add to the mountain of lost hours accumulated through the years. Feelings of anger, resentment, and sadness are natural parts of understanding loss. But the client and therapist need to titrate this experience so that it does not exclude the possibility of pleasure and satisfaction. Ideally, awareness of loss can contribute to an understanding of its value and effective use by the client.

A client brought this insight to her session. She reported:

"On my 30th birthday, I thought about myself as I was 10 years ago at the age of 20. I made a list of all the things that I did not have then (no education, no career training, no money, no man) and do not have now. As I made the list, though, I realized that when I turned 40 I could be doing the same thing: making a list of all the things I did not have when I was 30. I realized that it was up to me not to waste my time now—that I was free to choose what to do and how to do it. When I am 40, I want to be able to turn back and be pleased by what I did in my 30s. I put my pencil down and felt really free."

This insight is the gist of the work with all of the losses described above. In recognizing them and their consequences, the client has the opportunity to choose to live differently. Doing so makes meaning of the past, makes it "count for something," and so honors it.

SUMMARY

The guiding principle and central purpose of creating a life narrative is to transform a life viewed with fear, shame, anger, and loss into one that gives the client a sense of purpose, meaning, and dignity. It is unlikely that deeply entrenched feelings of shame and loss, and associated patterns of thoughts and behaviors, will be entirely transformed during the course of a single treatment. Given the layers of life experience that shame and loss have infiltrated, this task is more likely to be a long-term process. However, the narrative work can establish one or more templates for an improved and alternative sense of self and relationship to others, and demonstrates a process that the client learns and can use after treatment ends.

CHAPTER 8

~

Guidelines for Implementing Treatment

The paradox of structure is that it demands flexibility to be stable.
—ANONYMOUS

Treating trauma survivors poses particular challenges and rewards, over and above those encountered in standard outpatient psychotherapy. Trauma survivors have many and varied difficulties in different domains of their lives. It can be hard for a therapist—and a client—to decide exactly where to begin. Our treatment program is organized into two relatively self-contained phases, STAIR and NST, each with distinct goals. This modular approach provides flexibility in selection of treatment goals and processes. In addition, the rationale for each treatment component is clearly described in Chapters 5 and 6, and these descriptions can facilitate the process of deciding where to start and what to do. In this chapter, we address and provide guidance on potential concerns related to using a manualized treatment, deciding which clients may benefit from STAIR/NST, developing a strong therapeutic alliance, and addressing issues specific to working with childhood abuse survivors. The specific issues include: concerns related to trauma memories (seeking corroboration, confronting the abuser); client self-harming behaviors; a client's sharing the abuse history with others; the role of the couple in individual therapy; and concurrent therapy. We conclude by discussing therapist self-care.

USING A MANUALIZED TREATMENT

When we talk to clinicians in the community, many express concerns about using a manualized treatment with their clients. We understand these concerns because all of us

75

were originally trained in nonmanualized, nondirective forms of psychotherapy, and we only came to use manualized treatments after doing clinical work for several years. For this reason, we would like to address clinicians' doubts about using a manualized treatment— even one that is purported to be used flexibly, such as this one—immediately. Commonly heard concerns are as follows:

"I am a clinician, not a technician."
"If I use a manual, I will lose myself as a therapist."
"Therapy is an art, not something you can learn from a rulebook."
"My client is a unique human being, not a piece of equipment to be 'fixed' ."
"If I use a manual, I will be telling the client what to do."

STAIR/NST: A Guide, Not a Technical Manual

We know that STAIR/NST works in the format described in this book. However, the treatment has been used by all three of us in both lengthened and abbreviated forms, and has a structure and logic that is intended to provide flexibility in its implementation. Indeed, the treatment has been used in New York City for survivors of the September 11th terrorist attacks with substantial success (see Cloitre, Levitt, Davis, & Miranda, 2003). Flexibility in use of phases, types of interventions, and number of sessions, as well as flexibility in application to a variety of clients, has led to uniformly beneficial outcomes—often equal to those obtained in the more restricted conditions and client selection characteristic of a randomized controlled trial.

Flexibility in Use of Phases

This treatment contains two distinct phases. The first phase is focused on developing emotion regulation and interpersonal skills. The second is focused on processing the client's trauma history. The two-phase treatment offers flexibility. In our research, we complete the phases sequentially, with Phase II immediately following the completion of Phase I. This procedure is not unlike Judith Herman's (1992) stages of recovery, in which the therapist first ensures that the client has addressed stability, safety, and life management issues before moving on to trauma-focused work.

In clinical practice, the standard two-phase procedure, can be altered according to the needs of each client. Some clients may benefit from a repetition or lengthening of the skills-based portion of the treatment. This is particularly true of clients whose skills need further refinement, or for clients who enjoy and need only enhancement of social and emotional life skills. STAIR alone is also useful for clients who do not feel ready to address their trauma memory or whose life situation argues against their engaging in trauma processing. For example, one client was diagnosed with cancer during Phase I of treatment. The seriousness of this situation dictated focused attention to this crisis, and the Phase I component of the treatment was extended with skills training interventions directed to issues relevant to the diagnosis and treatment.

Alternatively, there may be some clients who are prepared for directly addressing their trauma memories and need only be provided with a few preparatory sessions before entering the NST phase of treatment. These may be clients who have had previous treatment that has effectively resolved life management issues, or clients who have completed a skills-based treatment and want to address some remaining trauma memories.

It is critical that the client and therapist spend time getting to know each other for between three and five sessions before engaging in the narrative work. Our research has informed us that a key factor in good outcome of narrative processing in particular is a strong therapeutic alliance, which is generally established between three and five sessions and remains stable thereafter. This period is useful for exploring the impact of the abuse history on current functioning, identifying the client's coping strategies and current life stressors, and mapping out an agreed-upon treatment plan.

Flexibility in Use of STAIR Sessions

Although the development of social skills and the development of emotional skills overlap and evolve dynamically in relationship to one another, the topics and skills addressed in STAIR are sequenced in a way that reflect the basic logic of skills development. For example, identifying feelings is a prerequisite for effectively communicating them to others, and establishing basic skills in communication is useful before attempting to resolve conflict-ridden or highly charged interpersonal problems.

The therapist can begin treatment with a session and topic that make sense for the client. For example, some clients are very aware of their feelings and have no difficulty in naming them or describing situations in which these feelings emerge and are difficult to manage. In these cases, identifying interpersonal schemas or specific problems in issues of assertiveness may be a reasonable place to begin. Our experience, however, has been that it is useful to do a quick review of feelings identification and other assumed skills before going forward. This may take only one or two sessions, but it establishes a reference point for the client's level of competence and comfort with skills that will soon be called upon. This review is likely to take as little as one session and a week of practice exercises.

Flexibility in Use of NST Sessions

The skills and planning involved in successful use of NST are not numerous or difficult. However, it will be necessary to complete the basic preparatory work for conducting narrative processing (in the first two sessions of NST, described in Chapters 19 and 20). This is as important as taking a good life history and identifying the client's "presenting problems" before initiating treatment. These sessions involve explaining the technique and rationale for the narrative work and completing the identification of memories from which the narrative work will be drawn. They are simply the nuts and bolts of the procedure, and the client must be comfortable and familiar with them in order to proceed with confidence and a sense of mastery about the task ahead. The actual material about which the client chooses to create a narrative, however, is unique to the client and selected collaboratively by therapist and client. We have identified three emotion-driven themes that are inevitably all part of a childhood abuse trauma history: narratives of fear, narratives of shame, and narratives of loss. Which theme is of most importance to the client is determined by the client's particular history, symptoms, stage of recovery, and life circumstances.

If clients are experiencing PTSD symptoms such as intrusive images and flashbacks, narration of fear-laden trauma memories is a good place to begin. However, some clients enter treatment with PTSD symptoms but feel more burdened by shame or loss. Often such feelings come to the surface as a result of recent life stressors. For example, in our work with 9/11 clients, 60% had childhood traumas; of those, many experienced a powerful depression, with the PTSD symptoms being of secondary importance. The loss of so many lives had reawakened unresolved feelings of loss, such as loss of a belief in goodness or in the possibility of a happy future. Treatment included STAIR to support symptom management, while NST focused on the telling about the losses, clarifying their meaning, and formulating activities or ways of living that honored the losses intrinsic to the clients' childhoods and to 9/11.

Flexibility in Number of Sessions

This treatment is organized into 16 sessions. It has been completed successfully in one study in 12 weeks (NST was conducted twice a week) and in another in 16 weeks (once-a-week sessions) (Cloitre et al., 2002b; Levitt, Malta, Martin, Davis, & Cloitre, in press). However, we encourage clinicians to use as many sessions as needed to address the problems that are the focus of the interventions. This can mean either extending the number of sessions to cover material at a pace appropriate for a particular client, or skipping material that is not relevant. In a recent study, clinicians flexibly applied STAIR/NST in the way described just above to clients with PTSD symptoms related to 9/11. The total number of sessions for the treatment ranged from 21 to 24, with an average of 24 sessions across all therapists and clients. Thus far, the data suggest that application of the treatment in this way produces even greater benefits than the established success rates we had already achieved. For example, the effect size for PTSD symptoms in the "lockstep" 16-session trial was an impressive 1.76, but in the flexible application the effect size was identical, indicating equal effectiveness. These data are not definitive, but they give us confidence in the benefits of adjusting the session number and content to the needs of each client.

Formal Training and Continuing Education

In this book, we have provided theory, diagnosis, treatment principles, session-by-session instruction, and numerous clinical examples to guide the clinician in a real-world application of the treatment. Still, a book, no matter how good it is, cannot replace excellent clinical training, experience, and supervision. We strongly recommend that clinicians working with childhood abuse survivors receive specialized workshop education to become informed about childhood abuse issues and about implementation of cognitive-behavioral strategies. We recommend that clinicians interested in working with this population complete at least one multiday training workshop provided by experts in PTSD related to childhood abuse or in the treatment of childhood abuse survivors. This type of training experience sets a general framework for thinking about childhood abuse, often provides hands-on experience in intervention demonstration and practice, provides a forum for asking questions relevant to a particular client or caseload, and often builds clinicians' skills and confidence to work even more effectively with childhood abuse clients.

Collaboration, not Instruction

The two-phase format of this treatment aids in building a strong therapeutic alliance. This is because the therapy requires active participation from both the therapist and the client. In STAIR, the therapist is working with the client to develop emotion regulation and interpersonal skills to reach real-life goals valued by the client. This work is collaborative with the goal of improvements in day-to-day functioning. As such improvements begin to occur, the client's trust in the therapist grows, building a strong foundation for the trauma-processing work of NST. During the NST phase, the therapist bears witness to the abuse the client has suffered. Thus the client is leading the treatment within certain guidelines offered by the therapist.

DECIDING WHICH CLIENTS MAY BENEFIT FROM STAIR/NST

Physical Abuse Survivors

When we present this treatment to therapists in the community, they often raise the question of who is appropriate for this treatment. The treatment was developed specifically for women with PTSD related to childhood sexual abuse. It quickly became apparent that most of these childhood abuse survivors had also experienced physical abuse. About 70% of women seeking treatment for sexual abuse also have a history of physical abuse— sometimes by the same person, but often by one or more additional persons (see Cloitre, 1998; Cloitre et al., 2000a). Over time, we provided treatment to women who had experienced only physical abuse, and found that they did not differ in symptom profile or clinical needs and did just as well in the treatment (Cloitre et al., 2002b).

Clients with Partial PTSD

Our current research with women who have "subsyndromal PTSD" indicate that such clients find both the STAIR and NST phases of treatment useful. It seems impractical and nonsensical to bar individuals from treatment just because they have less than a full diagnosis. Individuals with moderate levels of PTSD symptoms experience significant reductions in their symptoms following STAIR/NST (Cloitre et al., 2005). For clients who have minimal PTSD symptoms, the application of STAIR alone might be sufficient, although NST can still be implemented as a method of exploring shame- and loss-related emotions.

Clients with Significant Adult Traumas but No Childhood Traumas

As noted earlier, following 9/11, we provided STAIR/NST to adults exposed in some way to the collapse of the World Trade Center. About 60% of our clients had a history of childhood abuse. Evaluation of the treatment indicated that these clients showed significant improvement in their PTSD symptoms and also in their coping strategies, including gains in emotion regulation and in obtaining and seeking out social support and decreases in using alcohol and drugs to cope (see Cloitre, Levitt, Davis, & Miranda, 2003). The improvements in social support were especially striking, because 9/11 survivors experienced substantial deterioration of social networks (through death, building destruction, and/or job-related moves), which required them to apply coping strategies that had not been of particular importance or necessity before. The use of STAIR/NST may be relevant with clients who have recently been traumatized and are faced with the need to adapt to new environmental or social realities. We know that among these clients, the treatment provided moderate to large benefit and that those without and with a history of childhood abuse had equally good outcome.

Men

This treatment was originally developed for women, because the index trauma was sexual abuse—a form of trauma experienced approximately five times more frequently by women than by men. Through our work with 9/11 survivors, however, we found that men did just as well in the treatment as women (see Cloitre et al., 2003). Indeed, the benefits for men were greater in certain areas, particularly in reduction of aggressive behaviors and of alcohol use as a coping strategy. In reduction of PTSD, depression, and other trauma-related symptoms, men showed benefits equal to women's. Men with a history of childhood trauma tended to have more severe symptoms than men without early life trauma, but showed changes equal to or greater than those of men without abuse. These preliminary findings suggest that the treatment is applicable to men. From a clinical standpoint, we observed that the interventions and narrative process were just as relevant to men as women, and were just as well accepted and tolerated by them. It remains to be seen whether additional sessions or more refined interventions for certain symptom areas, such as aggressive behaviors or use of alcohol, would provide even greater benefits than those we observed. Nevertheless, because this treatment was developed for women with childhood sexual abuse and because the vast majority of our clients to date have been women, please note that from this point onward in the book we will use female pronouns only ("she," "her," "herself") to refer to a client in the singular.

Clients with Borderline Personality Disorder

Therapists working with clients who were abused as children often note that these clients have many characteristics of borderline personality disorder (BPD), such as emotion dysregulation and interpersonal difficulties, even if they do not meet full criteria for the disorder. These difficulties are in fact precisely the sorts of problems that several of the STAIR interventions were designed to address. Indeed, we have occasionally used this treatment with clients who met all the diagnostic criteria for BPD, and have done so with success. So the presence of a BPD diagnosis is not necessarily a reason to refer a potential client to another treatment.

Symptom Profile

As the paragraph above suggests, it is difficult to distinguish between clients who are and are not a good match for this treatment on the basis of symptoms or diagnostic criteria alone. This suggestion has been supported in a study by Heffernan and Cloitre (2000), which compared two groups of women with histories of childhood sexual abuse: women with PTSD only, and those with both PTSD and BPD. The two groups of women did not differ in severity, frequency, or number of perpetrators of their childhood sexual abuse, or in whether the perpetrators were family members or not. They also did not differ in severity and frequency of PTSD symptoms. The additional diagnosis of BPD was associated with earlier age of abuse onset and significantly higher rates of physical and verbal abuse by mothers. The group with PTSD + BPD scored higher on only one BPD symptom—feelings of being alone—and several symptom measures including anger, dissociation, anxiety, and interpersonal problems.

Identifying Motivation for Therapy

Our experience suggests two important prerequisites for determining the potential for successful treatment, regardless of the presence of BPD. These are the client's identified goals for therapy and the client's perception of the therapeutic relationship. These two issues are related. Specifically, the client's motivation and goals for the therapy must be *skills-based* rather than *relationship-based*. We have found that treatment is not effective or appropriate for clients whose treatment focus is on the relationship with the therapist rather than on learning skills guided by the therapist. In these cases, the clients' needs drift toward analysis and feelings about the relationship, and away from self-reflection and self-transformation as guided by the therapist. For example, one client who we soon realized was inappropriate for this treatment felt that the between-session exercises were the therapist's way of punishing her and trying to control her outside of sessions. The treatment quickly became primarily about the therapist–client relationship, rather than about how the client could develop skills to help her improve her life. The therapeutic relationship is critical to the success of the treatment (as we will discuss below), but this relationship supports change rather than being the primary tool or medium for it.

Assessing Treatment History

Clients who experience strong feelings of emptiness and, in conjunction, report relationships that have many ups and downs may be driven by such problems to the extent that they preclude the clients' ability to set and follow through on skills-based treatment goals.

One way to identify risk of a poor client–treatment match is to review each client's treatment history. Indicators of poor fit would include reports of difficulty in making and keeping commitments to therapy in the past, having started and terminated many treatment relationships, and stormy relationships with several previous therapists. Also of note are clients who don't seem able to view previous therapists as having both strengths and weaknesses, but only idealize or denigrate them.

Alternatively, a good record of effort in previous treatments might indicate an appropriate match, despite the presence of a full diagnosis of BPD. For example, an assessment of a 30-year-old lawyer who had been sexually abused by her grandfather yielded a diagnosis of PTSD and BPD, as well as a history of disordered eating behavior (bingeing and purging). Normally, such a client might not seem appropriate for this or any short-term treatment. However, the client had engaged in long-term psychodynamic psychotherapy for several years. She was seeking this treatment in combination with her other therapy, and her other therapist was supportive. It was clear from this woman's treatment history that she would be able to form a collaborative relationship with a therapist.

Engagement during Initial Sessions

In some cases, it is not possible to determine that a client is appropriate for STAIR/NST until the treatment has started. If the therapist starts this treatment with a client that he or she is unsure about, it is wise to pay close attention to the client's participation in the early sessions of the treatment. Does this client participate actively in sessions? Can she identify specific areas of her life she would like to work on? When she does between-session exercises, is she less focused on learning about herself and more focused on what the treatment work says about the therapeutic relationship? Clients may raise objections to some skills work or may not complete skills exercises for all kinds of reasons. However, it is notable if a client's reasoning about these behaviors concerns her reactions to the therapist rather than to the intervention.

The client with BPD who is inappropriate for STAIR/NST will also quickly require a more intense intervention and support than this treatment provides. Such clients are better off in dialectical behavior therapy (Linehan, 1993a, 1993b), which provides group and individual treatment for a sustained period of time, as well as regular phone contact for coaching.

THE THERAPEUTIC ALLIANCE

In the introductory chapters of this book, we have reviewed how caretaking environments characterized by sustained sexual, physical, and/or psychological abuse disturb the development of healthy attachment, emotion regulation skills, and interpersonal schemas (e.g., Malatesta & Haviland, 1982; Shields & Cicchetti, 1998; Shipman & Zeman, 2001). Clients bring their attachment difficulties, emotion regulation deficits, and interpersonal problems into the therapeutic relationship. The success of this treatment, and indeed of any psychotherapy, depends on the therapist's ability to build a strong alliance with the client in spite of these problems.

What Is the Therapeutic Alliance?

The foundation of a strong therapeutic alliance is unconditional positive regard (Rogers, 1951). We believe that therapists should, in general, enjoy working with their clients. It is difficult for a therapist to enjoy the work and to maintain such regard for a client he or she doesn't like. Authentic positive feelings for a client go a long way toward building an alliance. Second, the therapist must believe that he or she can help a client improve her life. Using a treatment that has empirical data supporting its efficacy, such as this one, contributes to holding and conveying that attitude.

The Importance of the Therapeutic Alliance

In a recent study, we demonstrated the importance of the therapeutic alliance to the success of this treatment (Cloitre et al., 2002b). In particular, the strength of the therapeutic alliance established during the first phase of treatment predicted successful reduction of PTSD symptoms during the treatment's second phase (Cloitre et al., 2002b). Furthermore, this relationship was mediated by participants' improved capacity to regulate negative emotions during the NST phase of the therapy. These data suggest that a strong therapeutic alliance facilitates the client's ability to manage negative emotions during trauma processing (Cloitre, Stovall-McClough, Miranda, & Chemtob, 2004). Similar results have been reported by other investigators treating clients with PTSD. In one study, Chemtob, Novaco, Hamada, and Gross (1997a) found that PTSD-related anger symptoms caused ruptures in the therapeutic relationship that directly compromised treatment outcome, including premature termination. Similarly, Tarrier et al. (1999) found that clients' feelings regarding the credibility of treatment—a contributor to the therapeutic alliance—predicted dropout from treatment.

The strength of the client–therapist relationship appears to be a critical common factor across treatment modalities, including short-term cognitive–behavioral treatment, interpersonal therapy, psychodynamic therapy, and gestalt therapy. Notably, the relationship between the therapeutic alliance and good outcome for childhood abuse survivors in STAIR/NST was twice as large as that usually observed in other treatment modalities and populations (Cloitre et al., 2005). This result suggests that the role of the therapeutic alliance in the treatment of childhood abuse survivors seems particularly important, given the interpersonal context in which their trauma occurred. Specifically, a positive alliance may serve to reverse or repair some of the interpersonal disturbances that so often undermine success in a variety of life tasks.

Threats to the Therapeutic Alliance

When managed well by the therapist and worked through, threats to the therapeutic alliance can actually improve the client–therapist relationship and the efficacy of the treatment. This can be achieved by framing threats to the therapeutic alliance as communications from the client to the therapist. Often a client's apparent difficulties with the therapist or treatment are ways of conveying fear, conflict, or a host of other problems that the client may be unable to express in other ways. If the therapist attends to alliance problems in this way, he or she may be one step closer to understanding the dynamics of their relationship.

Below, we identify four common problems in the therapeutic alliance that occur with abuse survivors. Therapists may benefit from reminding themselves about these patterns from time to time and asking themselves if these patterns are operating in any of their relationships with clients. If this is the case, or if a therapist feels vague discomfort or confusion about the nature of the therapeutic relationship, consultation with a trusted colleague can help identify and resolve these difficulties.

Breaks in Understanding

It is inevitable that there will be occasional lapses of understanding between the therapist and client. To minimize their impact, the therapist can at the beginning of treatment predict their occurrence and provide the client with guidelines about how to respond. The therapist may say something like this:

> "At some point, I am going to say or do something that upsets you, makes you angry, or makes you feel misunderstood. Although I will try my best to help you, at some point I will make a mistake. You may not even recognize my mistake at first. You may not be aware of it until you go home and think about it. When this happens, it is important that we have an opportunity to address the issue. If you are angry at me or hurt by me, come back to the next session and tell me. I want to hear about it and then make corrections about how we are proceeding!"

By warning the client that breaks in the relationship will occur, the therapist has taken away some of their power and made it more likely that the client will stay in the therapy and repair the breaks. The therapist is also showing that he or she is not afraid of breaks in relationships, that they are to be expected in the course of a relationship, and that they can be overcome. This is modeling good interpersonal skills to the client.

We have also found it helpful for the therapist to make extra efforts to reach out to the client when breaks in the relationship occur. These may include calling, rescheduling sessions, and sending letters. As we have discussed in the opening chapters, clients who were abused as children did not develop the skills to address conflict or ruptures in relationships. They tend to be easily hurt but avoidant of conflicts, and as a result, they may break off relationships when difficulties occur. The extra efforts the therapist makes reassure the client that the therapist values the relationship and believes in the client's ability to complete the treatment successfully.

Lapses in Perceived Empathy

A second issue related to the therapeutic alliance is a client's uncertainty about the therapist's ability to understand what she has been through. For some clients, this uncertainty is manifested in the question about whether the therapist is an abuse survivor him- or herself. The therapist should be aware of taking such a question too literally. Often what the client really wants to know is whether or not the therapist can help her, not the details of the therapist's abuse history. Even if the therapist is an abuse survivor, this does not make him or her necessarily able to understand the client's experience better. In some cases, rather than facilitating understanding, the therapist's own experience may cloud his or her ability to see the client clearly. Addressing the concern behind the question, the therapist might respond with a statement like this:

> "No one can really understand someone else without standing in that person's shoes. And no one's experience is exactly the same. My goal is to understand your experience as *you* have experienced it. I will listen carefully to you. In addition, I have worked with many people who have experienced childhood abuse, and I will share with you things that I have learned from them, if you think that would be helpful."

Sexualization

Sexualizing the therapeutic relationship happens often—perhaps particularly often—with clients who were sexually abused. Indeed, behaving sexually with therapists may be almost automatic for such clients. A client may wear provocative clothing to session, openly flirt with the therapist, and ask the therapist questions about his or her personal life. The therapist may react with discomfort or even with horror at finding him- or herself attracted to the client and responding to her sexual advances emotionally or flirting in response.

Many clients who act in very sexualized ways are not conscious that they are doing so; even if they recognize their behavior as such, they do not know how else to act. The therapist needs to take care to address such behavior without embarrassing or humiliating the client. A therapist may feel inclined to reprimand the client or tell her directly that her behavior is inappropriate. In actuality, the client is often merely trying to find some way to communicate or forge some connection with the therapist. The interpersonal schema at work may reflect the client's belief, based on her abuse history, that "to be attached means to be sexual." The therapist's task is to disappoint the client's expectations that this schema has generated in the client. The therapist can demonstrate in words or actions that the client is important to the therapist for reasons other than her sexual aspect, and that a sustained connection to another person need not be mediated in sexual terms.

So, for example, the therapist can explicitly note and express interest in the client's skills at her job or in her ability to compliment others. The therapist can also remark on the courage the client has shown in coming to therapy and engaging in the treatment tasks. If the client is looking for a way to connect with the therapist or to experience positive regard in the eyes of the therapist, such comments will help move the client away from sexualized behavior and help her explore other important and positive aspects of herself.

The therapist may wish to express how he or she experiences the client's sexualized behavior, but this must be done with great sensitivity. Observations such as "When you said that, I felt like you were flirting with me," or "Sometimes I feel like you are behaving toward me like you might if you wanted to date me, rather than as your therapist," or "Sometimes I feel like you ask me questions about my personal life to distract us from focusing on you" can be experienced as reprimanding or belittling by the client, who may feel "caught being bad." Rather, reactions to sexualized behavior need to be conveyed with empathy, kindness, even humor, and in a spirit of collaboration.

Ideally, this direct approach should be taken only when the therapist feels confident that the therapeutic relationship is stable and that the client feels respected and well regarded by the therapist. Under these circumstances, any sense of guilt or blame that the client experiences for the appearance of sexual expression can be quickly dissipated. The therapeutic goal is to have the client understand that sexualized modes of relating are not "bad," but also are not necessary in creating a working relationship in the treatment. This contributes to the evolution in the client's sense of self and to the development of more varied interpersonal schemas that free her from the narrow constraints of relating to others in a predominantly sexualized way. The therapist conveys to the client that she is free to be more than a sexual being, and that in the therapeutic relationship the strength of the bond comes from growth in areas beyond the appearance of sexual value.

Conflicts

The therapeutic relationship is also fertile ground for replaying the power and control conflicts that are so frequently part of victim–perpetrator schemas. For example, the client may feel victimized by the goal-directed nature of the therapy. The client may say "You are forcing me to do these exercises—what gives you the right?" Or "You are hurting me by having me think about the trauma." Alternatively, the therapist may feel placed in the victim role and abused by the client. This may be expressed in the client's anger, criticisms, and rejection of the therapist's helpful gestures ("There is nothing you can do for me," "I tried it and it did not work"). The client may begin missing sessions but call for help on weekends, may come to sessions late, or may not pay fees as agreed upon. The therapist may feel overwhelmed, incompetent, and helpless to do anything to aid the client, or may feel exploited and disrespected. If the therapist's reactions go unchecked and unexamined, they will ultimately lead to countertherapeutic behaviors that may be expressed directly to the client through verbal attacks or indirectly through rejection. It is important that a therapist in this situation closely monitor his or her feelings and behavior toward the client and work to regain empathy for the client's difficulties.

The goal of the treatment is to neutralize power/control conflicts in the therapeutic relationship. A guiding principle of treatment implementation is that the client takes the lead in setting both the pace and the goals. This philosophy of treatment, and the particular goals and pace of treatment, should be articulated in the process of the assessment and initial session work (see Chapters 9 and 10). Ideally, this structure will not so much prevent as extinguish future conflicts. The therapist may choose to reassert the agreement and remind the client that the client is in charge of the process. More importantly, it may be useful to ask the client, "What do you really want?" Often the appearance of resistance to treatment or criticism of the therapist's technique reflects clients' anxiety about going forward in the treatment and resentment about their predicament. As one client put it, clients often have this simple human desire: "I wish I did not have to do this. I wish I could be magically better." This type of question and response can break the stalemate in the conflicts of power/control and can unify the therapist and client in working toward the same goals, with adjustments as needed in the pace, process, and goals of the treatment.

SPECIAL CHALLENGES OF CHILDHOOD ABUSE TREATMENT

This section focuses on the special challenges we have encountered in working with survivors of childhood abuse while implementing this treatment. These challenges include issues focused around trauma memories (including seeking corroboration of memories and confronting the abuser); client self-harming behaviors; a client's sharing the abuse history with others; the role of the couple in individual therapy; and concurrent therapy. We review each in turn.

Truth in Memories

In the past decade, the issue of "recovered" memories has received a great deal of attention and debate (McNally, 2003). When we decided to test our treatment in a randomized clinical trial, we needed to set very specific criteria as to whom we would accept into the treatment and whom we would not. After much thought and consultation, as well as experience in working with abuse survivors, we decided to implement this treatment only with those clients who had at least one continuous memory of physical or sexual abuse. It has been our experience that individuals who report recovered memories are often highly distressed about the intrusion of such memories. The distress is related to shock at the possibility that such events could have happened, uncertainty and confusion about whether these events did happen, and the desire for corroboration. The adaptation to the experience of recovered memories requires a therapy and intervention of its own kind.

One unfortunate aspect of the debate over recovered memories is that memories of abuse tend to be presented as "all-or-nothing" phenomena. Memories are viewed as either "true and constant," or "recovered" and therefore suspect. However, in our clinical experience, most individuals reporting childhood abuse have always remembered something about what they experienced. At the same time, even those who have always remembered their abuse have had doubts or questions about some aspect of what really happened. Many of these clients find themselves wondering whether specific memories or specific details about the abuse are true.

Clients' concerns about the veridicality of their abuse memories have several sources. Many clients find that they experience an increase in memories of abuse and heightened distress when they begin trauma-focused treatment. Often such memories are not really "new" ones; they are memories that a client has always had, but that are now more accessible and present because the client is focusing on those memories. Additionally, clients sometimes report that they remember more details of their abuse experiences. They may wonder if these details are true. Lastly, some clients find that in the process of therapy, they come to a different understanding of their histories and may reframe certain experiences they had previously thought were "normal" as abusive. For example, a client reported in the initial assessment that her trauma history consisted solely of being sexually abused by her stepfather. While reviewing her history in therapy, she also reported that her mother engaged in very severe corporal punishment. In fact, the corporal punishment was so severe that the client often wore long-sleeved shirts to school in warm weather, to cover bruises on her arms. The client had not initially considered those experiences as physical abuse, but over time she came to label them as such and to view them as an important part of her abuse history that she addressed in treatment.

Many women who were abused as children and have come to treatment in adulthood have disclosed the abuse at some point, only to have their experience denied completely or invalidated. At the worst extreme, clients report having disclosed to a trusted adult when the abuse was happening, and being told that they were lying and punished for making up stories. Clients also commonly report experiences of being invalidated when sharing their abuse experiences. Clients often first try to share the abuse with friends in adolescence. Such friends, in their immaturity, are unprepared for these disclosures and may have responded by denying it, minimizing it, or just not wanting to hear about it. For example, when she was 15, one client told a friend about being sexually abused by her uncle. Her friend at first responded by wanting all the lurid details, and then stopped her from talking about it further by saying, "That is really gross. You shouldn't say those things." Another client tried to talk to her 17-year-old boyfriend about her experience of sexual abuse by her older brother. He responded by getting angry and calling her a "whore." He then tried to pressure her to have sexual intercourse with him, saying that it should be "no big deal" for her, as she had "done it all before."

Clients who have disclosed their abuse and received these types of responses may come to doubt the reality or meaning of their own experiences. Clients may find themselves wondering at times if the abuse really happened or if they did make it up—or, even if they are sure it did happen, whether they are making "too big a deal" about it. This is especially true of clients who disclosed their abuse in childhood, found its reality denied, and then continued to be abused. Such clients had to live with two realities: one of their personal reality in which they were being abused, and one of their social reality in which the abuse was denied. Minimizing or denying their experience becomes a way of coping with it in such cases.

Seeking Corroboration

By beginning trauma-focused therapy, clients are making a statement that at least some part of them believes the abuse that happened is real and worthy of serious consideration.

Some clients may begin seeking external corroboration of their abuse experiences from family members or childhood friends. Or they pore over childhood documents, pictures, letters, and school records, to see if they can find inconvertible evidence that they were abused. Clients may wish to confront their abusers and, in some cases, to pursue legal action against them.

What is the role of the therapist in such a client's search for "the truth"? There is no one accepted answer to this question, so we will give our opinion, based on our clinical and research experience with survivors. First, the therapist's job is to help the client explore what she hopes to gain from external corroboration of the abuse. Second, the therapist can help the client ponder how she will go about getting external corroboration. Third, the therapist can help the client think through the consequences of getting or not getting the corroboration she so desires.

Clients' reasons for seeking corroboration are as varied as their experiences. What many clients want is understanding from family members or friends. Clients want those individuals most important to them to recognize that these terrible experiences really happened, that they have caused them much pain and anguish, and that they have had long-term adverse effects on them. Often they have tried to talk with friends or family members about the abuse, but haven't felt understood. These clients hope that presenting some type of corroboration will be more convincing than mere words.

One woman we treated was physically abused by her mentally ill mother throughout childhood. Her father was caring, but usually physically absent: He dealt with his wife's illness by working long hours and traveling a great deal. The client and her siblings were therefore often left alone to cope with their mother's abuse. When the client reached adulthood, after her mother's death, her father and siblings talked about their mother's problems; however, they greatly minimized how abusive and chaotic the household had been. They also minimized the relationship between the abuse and our client's and her siblings' difficulties in functioning in their adult lives. This client remembered receiving medical care related to her mother's physical abuse—in particular, being taken to the emergency room for a broken arm caused by her mother's throwing her down some stairs. She wanted her medical records to show her father and siblings, so they would admit how bad her childhood was.

Her therapist asked her, "And if you get these records and show them to your father, what do you hope will happen?" The client answered, "Daddy will finally admit that my mother was a terrible mother. That she abused me and my siblings. That he never should have left us with her. That he should have protected us. He'll say he is sorry and hug me. We'll be a family again without this barrier—this ghost of my mother—between us." The therapist did not argue or debate with the client about whether or not to get the medical records or, if she got them, to show them to her family. Rather, she focused on helping the client explore how else her father and siblings might react to the medical records (e.g., with more denial) and how that might affect their future relationship.

Exploring what clients hope to achieve with corroboration is important, because often the type of corroboration clients can realistically obtain is unlikely to achieve their goals. Family members, friends, and partners who deny or minimize the clients' experiences are likely to maintain this stance even in the face of external evidence. This is because most corroboration, such as the medical records sought by the client described above, can be explained in other ways (e.g., childhood accidents). However, obtaining corroboration can be helpful to clients for other reasons. For example, one client we saw remembered having done very well in school until she started being sexually abused by her new stepfather when she was 11 years old. She obtained her school records, and they confirmed her memory: Her grades started dropping when she was 11, and her teachers noted her being more distracted in class and withdrawn, commenting on her drop in performance. Reading these report cards was very validating for the client, but was not helpful in convincing her mother, who always denied that the abuse occurred.

Confronting the Abuser

Many clients, at some point during treatment, consider confronting their abusers. This is particularly true if an abuser is a family member with whom a client still has some contact. Almost all clients wish for a confession from their abusers—the ultimate form of corroboration. Many clients imagine the day when they will confront their abusers and they will break down, confess their wrongdoing, and apologize.

The therapist's approach to the idea of confronting the abuser should be similar to the approach used with other forms of corroboration. That is, the therapist should help the client identify what she hopes to accomplish through confrontation. Many clients are seeking the ultimate confirmation to themselves that their experiences are real and true. Other clients want to prove their abuse to those who denied their experiences. Clients may also be driven by the desire for revenge: to make their abusers pay for the pain they caused, emotionally, legally, or financially. Occasionally clients may want to have adult relationships with their abusers, but feel that this is not possible until the abusers have acknowledged the abuse. We find that once clients explore what they hope to get from confronting their abusers, they often realize that the confrontation will not achieve what they hope and decide not to move forward.

For a client who wishes to move forward with confronting her abuser, a therapist can help the client think through and plan the confrontation, so that the client has the best chance of achieving her goals. The therapist can help the client plan when, where, and how she wishes to conduct the confrontation. The therapist should also explore potentially negative outcomes (e.g., denial by the perpetrator) and how she will cope with them. In rare cases, the abuser may be willing to meet with the therapist and client together. This situation sometimes occurs when the abuser has been in therapy. In such cases, the abuser's and survivor's therapists may decide that a joint meeting is most appropriate.

Mandated Reporting and Other Legal Issues

Clients also seek confrontations with their abusers for other reasons than corroboration. For example, some clients are driven by the desire to protect children from potential abuse if they believe that a perpetrator still has the opportunity to exploit other children (e.g., a priest or other spiritual leader, or a relative who may be abusing other children in a family). Situations where clients are reporting abuse by individuals who are at risk of continuing to abuse others place special ethical and legal demands on therapists. Mandated reporting statutes differ by state, but in general therapists are required to report an individual if they believe that the person is at risk of currently physically or sexually abusing children.

Clients who pursue restitution from their abusers through the legal system also pose special challenges to their therapists. If you are a therapist who has a client pursuing legal action, we strongly recommend seeking legal advice from attorneys who have dealt with such cases. Many professional organizations, such as the American Psychological Association, have contacts with attorneys who deal with these and other mental health issues. As a therapist, you may have to address issues relating to the confidentiality of your therapy records, or may face a subpoena to testify in the case. Pursuing legal action can also have direct consequences for clients' motivation to recover from the abuse. In order to receive financial compensation for the abuse, clients may have to show that the abuse was mentally damaging. This fact results in clients' needing to remain symptomatic to obtain a financial settlement. During the period when a legal process is ongoing, a therapist may choose to focus therapy on supporting the client through the process, rather than on doing trauma-focused work. The legal process in itself can be very time-consuming and stressful, and often leaves clients with few resources to focus on other areas in treatment.

Acceptance of Ambiguity

For most clients, part of the therapeutic process involves accepting that they will never receive external corroboration of their abuse or achieve certainty. They may never know for sure whether specific details of the abuse happened. The evidence for their abuse may never reach the standard of proof demanded by the legal system. Some clients will continue to have family members, partners, and friends who minimize or deny what they experienced. Ultimately, the therapeutic process is different from the legal process: The aim of therapy is not to determine truth, but to help a client understand her subjective experience, the impact of that experience on her, and the process for moving away from the past and into the future.

Client Self-Injurious Behaviors

Approximately half of the clients we have treated in STAIR/NST have a history of self-injurious behaviors such as cutting and burning. Self-injurious behaviors are common aspects of the symptom profile of abuse survivors, and clients with mild to moderate self-injurious behaviors are appropriate for and do well in STAIR/NST. A self-injurious behavior often functions as a coping strategy for emotion dysregulation—either to reduce or organize a flooding experience, or to elicit a focused feeling when a client is acutely distressed by the absence of feelings, by dissociation, or by fear of lapsing into a dissociative state (Brodsky et al., 1995). In STAIR, these behaviors often resolve and are replaced with more effective coping strategies. In addition, more positive attitudes about self and the capacity to share urges for self-injury with an empathic, nonblaming therapist contribute to recovery from this behavior. We have had no experiences of a client experiencing exacerbation in the treatment, including during the NST phase of the treatment, and we credit much of the work we do in STAIR. Moderately to very severe self-injurious behaviors (e.g., head banging, deep cutting) need to be addressed immediately, however, as they create significant and long-term health risks for an individual. Such clients are referred to other providers who specialize in the reduction and prevention of self-injury.

Sharing the Abuse History and Treatment with Others

When clients begin a trauma-focused treatment, they may also have the desire to share their abuse history and their treatment with members of their social network. This desire may be more or less appropriate, depending on the type of relationship a client has with a particular person. Clients who are abuse survivors sometimes have not yet developed good judgment about whom they can trust or whom it would benefit to share their history. A client may be inclined to tell nothing to her intimate partner, but to relay a detailed history to a passing acquaintance. Part of the therapy is to help clients learn with whom they can and cannot share their abuse histories, and what is helpful to share.

For example, one client who came to treatment was very socially withdrawn and had no real, close relationships. Her closest "friend" was the elderly woman who worked at the bakery where she bought her coffee and bagel every morning on the way to work. Each morning, the client and this woman engaged in small talk about what each was doing that day. On the day she started treatment, the client told this woman that she was going to therapy because her father had sexually abused her as a child. The elderly woman responded by saying, "In my day, one didn't talk about such things!" and walked away. This encounter was very distressing to the client, who only realized over time that her disclosure in that situation was inappropriate.

Couple Issues

A client who has an intimate partner may wish to have the partner included in the treatment. Although this treatment program was not designed to be used with couples, we routinely meet with a client and her partner if the client requests such a meeting. For those who desire couple therapy, such treatments have been developed for female partners of male veterans with combat-related PTSD (Monson, Rodriquez, & Warner, 2005; Monson, Schnurr, Stevens, & Guthrie, 2004) and may be adapted for working with couples where one member was abused as a child.

In STAIR/NST, we use the meeting to educate the client's partner about the relationship between the client's history of abuse and her current PTSD symptoms and difficulties in functioning. We find that this can be helpful for a partner who may not understand the source of the client's problems, or feels hurt by or to blame for them. For example, partner may interpret a client's avoidance of sexual intimacy as personal rejection rather than as avoidance related to a history of sexual abuse. Understanding the nature of a client's difficulties helps her partner be more supportive during the treatment. This meeting is also an opportunity to warn the client's partner that some of the client's difficulties may get worse during the treatment before improving, and that this worsening is temporary and to be expected as part of the recovery.

During this session, the therapist can also convey empathy for the partner, who may him- or herself be traumatized by the client's difficulties. Partners of abuse survivors often experience anger and sadness on behalf of the survivors, as well as anxiety about the impact of this history on their relationship. Some partners vicariously experience intrusive thoughts and other PTSD symptoms as a result of hearing about the survivor's history. It is understood that therapists sometimes feel overwhelmed by clients' experiences and may find themselves ruminating about them at unexpected times. Intimate partners of clients can be expected to experience such vicarious traumatization to an even greater degree: They share the clients' lives to a much greater extent and are not professionally trained to protect themselves. Partners may also bear the brunt of the clients' difficulties in functioning and PTSD symptoms. For example, a partner is exposed to recurring difficulties when a client has nightmares and cannot sleep, bursts out in rage, or loses her job because she cannot get out of bed and go to work. Well-functioning partners may find themselves overcompensating for such clients' deficits in functioning.

In turn, partners can contribute to the clients' difficulties and impede successful use of the therapy. Partners who are intrusive, insecure, or controlling may be threatened by the therapy, and particularly about what the clients may say about them in therapy. Although how much to share is something that always lies within a client's discretion, we discourage this particular practice as a norm. For example, in the case of a client whose partner wished to listen to tapes of sessions, we encouraged the client to describe her experiences in therapy to her partner directly, rather than indirectly sharing these through tapes. This allowed the client to preserve the confidentiality of the therapy session and to ensure that the client did not censor herself in therapy.

A therapist often does not have significant knowledge about a client's relationship with her partner until well into the treatment. It is often impossible at the beginning of treatment to judge the extent of a partner's supportiveness about the client's treatment, the partner's reaction to the client's history, and the difficulties the partner him- or herself brings to the relationship. Some clients have supportive partners; however, others tend to repeat their histories with partners who are abusive. Meeting with the partner can help inform the therapist about these issues. A meeting also gives the therapist the opportunity to refer the partner or couple to therapy if indicated.

Concurrent Treatment

Although evidence supports this therapy's effectiveness for addressing the problems faced by child abuse survivors, it is not always all that a client needs. Some may need, or may come to STAIR/NST already using, other forms of treatment (e.g., medication, couple therapy, or supportive therapy), particularly if they are in life circumstances of chronic stress. Consequently, we routinely worked with clients who were in other forms of treatment. For research purposes, we asked that clients not make changes in their other treatments (e.g., medication dosage or frequency of therapy sessions) during the length of the research protocol (3 months). We asked this to ensure the validity of the research protocol. However, this requirement is obviously not necessary in routine clinical practice.

Our clinical experience suggests that, given certain prerequisites (such as the agreement of all involved), STAIR/NST can be successfully conducted concurrently with other forms of individual or group therapy or with medication management. Providing STAIR/NST to a client who is already in a long-term treatment arrangement can be very helpful to the client. A typical example is the client who has been in long-term psychodynamic psychotherapy with a trusted provider and has an excellent relationship with this provider. This client may at some point want to do some more directed, skills-based, and trauma-focused work. A therapist who has been trained psychodynamically and is nondirective may see the value in such work for the client, but may not be comfortable with doing it or may not wish to do it. The client may benefit from pursuing the treatment in this book concurrently with another provider, while continuing with her long-term psychodynamic psychotherapy.

Concurrent therapy can only be successful if the client's present therapist is supportive of the concurrent treatment and feels he or she can work together with another therapist. Occasionally a client appears to be seeking concurrent treatment, but is actually unhappy with her present therapy and is exploring other options. If that is the case, it is recommended that the therapist not begin with this client until she has made a determination about whether or not to continue with her present therapist. When the present therapist is supportive and the client pursues concurrent treatment, it is essential to maintain open communication among all of the client's mental health providers. Such communication ensures that all providers have the information they need to treat the client most effectively, and it prevents the client from creating conflicts between providers.

THERAPIST SELF-CARE

> The effects of trauma are catching, and the listener is always in danger of empathically resonating with the victim and thus converging emotionally within the same traumatic envelope. . . . As Euripides said several thousand years ago, "where there are two, one cannot be wretched and one not."
> —SANDRA L. BLOOM AND MICHAEL REICHERT (1998, p. 145)

Psychotherapy involves "complex demands, human costs, constant risk, and often limited resources" (Pope & Vasquez, 1998, p. 1). Treating clients who were abused as children is particularly challenging for two reasons. First, the clients bring their difficulties in attachment, emotion regulation, and interpersonal relating into the therapeutic relationship. Second, the therapist is consistently confronted with hearing about some of the most vile behaviors human beings can inflict on one another. These are events that most people choose to avoid or distance themselves from, but the therapist who treats traumatized clients cannot engage in avoidance. Thus cultivating self-care is essential for the trauma therapist.

Working with traumatized individuals can leave a therapist feeling disillusioned, alone, or frightened. Several authors have explained these types of reactions as an effect of secondary exposure or vicarious traumatization (Baker, 2003; Courtois, 1993; Kottler, 1998; McCann & Pearlman, 1990a, 1990b; Pearlman & Saakvitne, 1995; Pope & Vasquez, 2005; Ruzek, 1993). Such traumatization is evident when therapists caring for survivors of crime, sexual abuse, natural disaster, or combat develop a posttraumatic-like reaction from hearing about the traumatic incidents and seeing its effect on their clients. Many therapists who work with trauma survivors talk about being surprised by the intensity of their reactions after vicarious exposure to traumatic material. It is not uncommon to hear descriptions of becoming hypervigilant and anxious, or of experiencing sleep difficulties and feelings of anger about the injustices clients have described. Some describe functional difficulties, such as withdrawing socially from their peers. Some therapists have noted that people whom they typically depend on for support are sometimes unable to understand the difficulties involved in working with traumatized clients.

We will not review all the principles of good self-care here; rather, we refer our readers to other authors who have written extensively on the subject (see Appendix A) . Psychotherapists in training may wish to refer to a brief summary article on this topic (see Koenen, 1998). However, we would like to put forward a few principles we espouse in relation to self-care.

The first is the importance of seeking consultation with other trauma therapists. Throughout our work on this treatment, we have sought out other professionals' advice and wisdom about the challenges of working with trauma survivors, and this has led to simple but effective revisions in our interventions. We have learned to be attentive to our appointment schedules. It is good practice to avoid clustering multiple appointments together, and to give ourselves time to relax, debrief with others, or take a walk in between client meetings. We have also learned to balance our caseloads. A full-time practice requires diversity; not all clients should be trauma survivors. In any given set of trauma clients, it is advisable to avoid the intensive processing of trauma memories with many of them at the same time.

We have also come to value maintaining a healthy lifestyle through diet, exercise, and enjoyable activities. One of the most important self-care practices is to monitor and appreciate our limitations. As therapists, we all have many demands on our time. If we begin to feel overwhelmed while treating our clients, it is time to make some adjustments so that we can be more emotionally available to our clients. Finally, we have come to realize that the social support we receive from other professionals in the field is essential. Many excellent books and websites provide further information on this subject, and they are included in Appendix A.

CHAPTER 9

~

Assessment of Client and Match
for Treatment

Not all responses to a traumatic event fall within the orbit of PTSD, and many factors besides PTSD are relevent to establishing a treatment plan . . . and must be adequately assessed if treatment is to show maximum benefit.

—JOHN MARCH (1999, p. 200)

OVERVIEW

The primary goal of this chapter is to provide guidelines for assessing trauma clients and for considering whether clients' needs are a match for the STAIR/NST treatment. The assessment should touch on these six domains: trauma history, PTSD symptoms, emotion regulation problems, interpersonal difficulties, harmful or risky behaviors, and resilience or coping strategies. In this chapter, we discuss how to assess each domain, and we recommend measures that can be used by clinicians interested in performing a more structured assessment. We then provide guidelines for assessing whether a client is appropriate for this treatment. Finally, we talk about giving feedback and treatment recommendations to the client after assessment has been completed. We begin below by discussing some important general guidelines for assessing trauma clients.

THE "A, B, C, D, AND E" OF TRAUMA ASSESSMENT

A: Actively Support the Client

Some therapists, depending on their theoretical orientation, might generally assume a neutral stance with their clients. Although this approach may be appropriate in certain situations, many trauma clients react negatively to a clinician's neutral response to their abuse history. Trauma clients have often avoided sharing their histories because of shame or fears of rejection. For such clients, the assessment session may be the first time they have acknowledged their abuse histories. Others may have shared their histories previously but have had them denied or refuted. These clients are especially sensitive to a therapist's response and will quickly interpret neutrality as denial, condemnation, or rejection. Openly supportive statements that acknowledge a client's difficulties can go a long way in building an alliance with the client. For example, a therapist might say, "Thank you for trusting me enough to share that experience with me," "That must have been very frightening/upsetting," or "I appreciate your difficulty in telling about these events."

B: Behavioral Descriptions, Not Value Judgments

The cardinal principle of trauma assessment is to ask questions that describe abusive behaviors, rather than asking a client to evaluate whether or not she has been abused. For example, a therapist assessing for physical abuse might ask the client, "When you were a child or adolescent, did a parent or someone who took care of you ever do something on purpose to you that gave your bruises or scratches, broke bones or teeth, or made you bleed?" rather than "When you were a child, were you ever physically abused?" The second question asks the client to make a value judgment about her experience and to define it as abuse.

Although clients may have experienced what trauma research typically defines as abuse, they may not view it in those terms. For example, Maria, a 37-year-old Puerto Rican woman, at first reported being sexually abused by her father but denied experiencing physical abuse. However, in response to the first question above, she answered affirmatively and went on to describe how her mother regularly punished her by making her kneel with bare knees on gravel for hours at a time. After Maria had done this for a while, her knees would start bleeding. She would not be allowed to get up to go to the bathroom and would sometimes wet herself. Maria did not view this as physical abuse because she defined such abuse solely as physical beating, which her parents did not engage in.

C: Contain the Client's Narrative

Some clients come to treatment overwhelmed by memories of abuse. These memories intrude on their work, their sleep, and their relationships. The therapist may find that such clients can't seem to stop talking about their abuse history once they begin. Rather than avoiding the therapist's questions, they will talk about their abuse experiences in great detail. The therapist needs to help such a client contain her narratives of abuse. Letting her go into too much detail in the first assessment session may lead her to feel overly or unexpectedly vulnerable, and may thus make her less likely to return to treatment. In addition, the therapist may decide not to work with the client. If the client reveals a great deal of personal information and the therapist decides the client is not appropriate for his or her practice or program, the client can easily feel rejected, taking the therapist's decision personally.

An effective way to contain the client is to describe explicitly the task at hand. The therapist might say something like this: "Now I am going to ask you some questions about some difficult experiences you may have had in childhood. I am not going to ask you to go into detail at this time, but just collect some general information about things you have been through." If the client's narrative becomes overly detailed or extended, the therapist might say, "I am going to stop you from going into more detail here. I appreciate the difficulties of telling your history. But there are still many aspects of this consultation remaining, and I am hoping to help pace us through it all. Telling all of your history is not necessary right now, and can be very tiring and painful. Is this all right with you?" Keeping an opening for the client to respond is key, as the client may have been slowly working toward disclosing a critical part of her history. This inquiry may help her move forward.

D: Don't Avoid

Traumatic events such as child abuse are difficult to talk about. Even therapists find it difficult to ask clients questions about their abuse experiences, for fear of upsetting them or even upsetting themselves. One of the principles of trauma therapy is that clients' avoidance of memories, feelings, and thoughts related to their traumatic experiences has played a role in maintaining their symptoms. Therapists must therefore be careful not to avoid asking about traumatic experiences or to subtly redirect clients who are taking about such experiences.

This advice may seem contradictory to our last recommendation regarding containing a client. A therapist must perform a delicate balancing act in terms of containing a client without promoting avoidance. Clients are often very sensitive to therapists' reaction to their abuse disclosure, and may take redirection from a therapist as a message that the therapist can't manage hearing about their abuse. Countering this expectation is an another reason why we recommend being openly supportive of a client's disclosure rather than maintaining a neutral stance. When containing a client, we use direct language and explain why we are not going into more details about the abuse at this time. We also state explicitly that we will go into more detail later.

E: Expect More

Whatever a client reveals in this session, a therapist can be fairly confident that she has held back some experiences. Usually clients seem to hold back their "worst" experiences. For some clients, these will concern their most brutal abuse episodes; for others, these will be their most shaming or grief-provoking experiences. A client will reveal more about herself as she comes to know and trust her therapist better.

These five guidelines should be kept in mind from the first contact with the client and throughout the assessment process.

FIRST TELEPHONE CONTACT

The first contact between the therapist and the potential client will often take place on the telephone. For some therapists, this contact may merely involve getting the client's name and contact information and setting up the initial assessment session. Others may also choose to obtain information about why the client is seeking treatment. If a therapist's practice is primarily trauma-focused, questions concerning current problems and abuse history will help determine the appropriateness of this type of treatment. It is sometimes evident that the primary focus of treatment will not at first be past trauma if there are current significant life-threatening behaviors or other disturbances, such as sustained substance abuse, eating disorders, self-injury, or initial reactions/working through of recovered memories (see Chapter 8 for discussions of the last two issues). If the therapist does not specialize in these problems or have consultation available for these types of treatment, a referral, kindly and reassuringly provided, will save the abuse survivor time and frustration.

ASSESSMENT SESSION

The assessment session will most often be the first time a client and therapist have met in person. It is a time to gather systematic information about whether or not the client is appropriate for the treatment. It is also the first opportunity to start building the therapeutic alliance.

"What brings you to treatment now?" is the most important question to be asked and answered in the assessment session. This question begins the process of building the therapeutic relationship by demonstrating that the therapist cares about the client's concerns and reasons for being there. The client's answer to this question will provide preliminary information about her goals and hopes in coming to treatment. The client's answer to this question will also give the therapist information about the client's level of insight into the relationship between her abuse history and current difficulties. The answers we have heard to this question are varied. In response to the question "What brings you to treatment now?", clients have said the following:

> "I have never been able to get past a first date with a man. If anything remotely sexual happens—like he tries to kiss me or even just hold my hand—I freeze. Last weekend, at my friend's wedding, I met a man I like. He has asked me out, and I don't want to blow this chance. I need to find out what is wrong with me."—Susan, a single, heterosexual, 35-year-old Jamaican woman and successful architect

> "I visited my parents at Passover for the first time in years. Since getting back to New York, I have been completely blocked in doing my art. I can't concentrate, get frustrated, and lash out at my studio-mates. I thought it would pass, but it hasn't."—Rachel, a single, lesbian, 50-year-old unemployed Jewish artist

"I find myself losing my temper with James [her 3-month-old son] all the time. It's all I can do to stop myself from hitting him, so I end up screaming at him instead. If he starts crying and doesn't stop right away, I feel overwhelmed and helpless and like a terrible mother. I know what I am supposed to do, but my feelings just get in the way."—Jane, a 30-year-old European American married woman

"I used to be able to keep going no matter what. I just kept busy all the time, worked hard, went to the gym, went out with friends, took active vacations, traveled. I just can't do it any more. I can't keep going. I don't know what to do."—Maria, a 40-year-old Latina advertising executive

"I am here because my husband says he can't take it any more. If I don't change, he will leave. He is tired of my irritability, my yelling, my distance, and my lack of interest in sex. I don't want to lose him!"—Kashana, a 35-year-old African American married woman

As indicated in the examples above, clients will not always state their abuse histories as the reason they are coming into treatment, even though they are aware that the service or therapist they are calling specializes in trauma treatment. Rather, clients tend to focus on the problems that are currently causing them difficulty. While they recognize that they have been abused, they don't necessarily connect their history with present problems. Clients typically do not come into a consultation and state, "I am coming for treatment because I have PTSD symptoms related to being sexually abused as a child." Rather, clinicians need to obtain information on clients' abuse and trauma histories through careful assessment.

Many clinicians in nonresearch settings find it helpful to use standardized assessment measures. Such instruments can help assure a therapist that he or she is covering all the domains of assessment thoroughly. We have found this especially important with regard to a client's trauma history, as often a clinician will remember to ask about certain types of traumatic experience (e.g., abuse) and forget others (e.g., sudden, unexpected death of a close friend or relative). Conducting a complete assessment is essential for treatment planning, as the more information the therapist has in the beginning, the more effective he or she can be in connecting the interventions to the client's specific difficulties. Below, we cover the six domains we believe are important to assess. For most of these domains, Appendix B provides specific self-report and therapist-administered instruments we have used in our assessments, as well as references for these instruments.

SIX DOMAINS OF ASSESSMENT

Trauma History

Before obtaining the client's trauma history, the therapist can say something like this:

"Now that I know why you are coming to treatment at this time, I would like to go back and ask you some questions about your childhood. In order to make sure I

gather all the information I need to help you, I have a list of questions I ask everyone who comes to see me. Some of these questions may seem very personal or
difficult to answer. You don't have to answer anything you don't want to. Please
also feel free to stop me at any time if you want to ask me something or need a
break. OK?"

The therapist can begin eliciting the client's history by asking the client some background questions about where she grew up, with whom she lived, whether she had siblings, and so forth. The therapist can then move to asking the client about specific abuse
experiences. How the clinician introduces this topic will depend on whether he or she is
using a specific assessment instrument or is conducting an entirely open-ended interview.
In either case, the therapist should remind the client that she should feel free to decline to
answer any questions she does not wish to answer.

Therapists who are inexperienced in assessing abuse and trauma histories should
receive training and supervision in how to conduct a trauma assessment. Using structured
interviews designed to assess histories of child abuse can be very helpful, particularly for
therapists with less experience in this area. Such interviews have been designed to give
specific wording on how to ask about different forms of abuse. As we have stated previously, questions about abuse experience should be worded behaviorally. We give some
examples of such wording below, following descriptions of the specific types of abuse
(these descriptions are based on those of Briere, 1992).

Sexual Abuse

Sexual abuse includes activities by a parent or caretaker such as fondling a child's genitals,
penetration, incest, rape, sodomy, indecent exposure, and exploitation through prostitu-
tion or the production of pornographic materials. Sexual abuse can also occur between
peers or siblings if a substantial age difference exists between the victim and perpetrator
or if the sexual activity is performed without the victim's consent.

> *Sample question*: "When you were a child, did a parent, family member, or some-
> one else in charge of your care ever touch or fondle you in a sexual way?"

Physical Abuse

Physical abuse can range from minor bruises to severe fractures or death as a result of
punching, beating, kicking, biting, shaking, throwing, stabbing, choking, hitting (with a
hand, stick, strap, or other object), burning, or otherwise harming a child. Such injury is
considered abuse, regardless of whether the caretaker intended to hurt the child.

> *Sample question*: "When you were a child or adolescent, did a parent or caretaker—
> such as a grandparent, other adult relative, or babysitter—ever do something on
> purpose to you (for example, hit or punch or cut you or push you down) that gave
> your bruises or scratches, broke bones or teeth, or made you bleed?"

Emotional Abuse

Both sexual and physical abuse of children often co-occur with emotional abuse and neglect. Emotional abuse is a pattern of behavior that impairs a child's emotional development or sense of self-worth.

> *Sample question*: "When you were a child did a parent or caretaker say things repeatedly to you like 'You will never amount to anything'?"

Emotional abuse may also include constant criticism, threats, or rejection, as well as withholding love, support, or guidance.

> *Sample question*: "When you were a child, did a parent or caretaker ever threaten to hurt or kill either you or someone (a friend) or something (a pet) you cared about?"

Neglect

Neglect involves the failure of a child's caretaker to meet the child's basic needs. Neglect may be physical, medical, educational, or psychological.

> *Example question*: "When you were a child, were you ever not properly fed or clothed by your parent or caretaker?"

When the therapist has completed the assessment of the client's abuse history, we recommend taking a few moments to check in with the client and ask how she feels before moving on to assess other traumatic experiences.

Revictimization History and Other Traumatic Experiences

One of the most profound consequences of childhood victimization is subsequent, repeated victimization in the form of rape, physical assault, and domestic violence (Browne & Finkelhor, 1986; Polusny & Follette, 1995). Women with childhood sexual abuse are acutely aware of these problems, which are often among their most pressing reasons for seeking treatment. Trauma assessment therefore includes reviewing clients' adulthood as well as childhood trauma histories. We have found using a measure designed to screen for a wide range of traumatic experiences to be helpful in assessing clients' victimization histories and other traumatic experiences. Many of these screening measures have been designed for clients to fill out themselves, but they can also be used to guide a clinical interview (See Appendix B).

PTSD Symptoms

There are many books and articles on the assessment of PTSD (see especially Wilson & Keane, 2004). Therefore, we do not go into detail about this here, but only review the diagnosis briefly with respect to women who have been abused as children. We recommend that therapists use a structured clinical interview to make a diagnosis of PTSD (see Appendix B).

Definition of a Traumatic Event

The diagnosis of PTSD as defined by DSM-IV-TR (American Psychiatric Association, 2000, p. 467) requires exposure to an event involving a "threat to the physical integrity" of oneself or others, and the subjective response of "fear, helplessness, or horror" in relation to that event. PTSD is characterized by three clusters of symptoms.

Reexperiencing Symptoms

The first symptom cluster involves reexperiencing, which consists of intrusive memories, thoughts, and feelings related to the trauma. To meet criteria for a diagnosis of PTSD, clients must have at least one reexperiencing symptom. Clients may express that they can't stop thinking about the abuse, or that thoughts or images of the abuse come into their minds without warning. They may describe having nightmares about the abuse (or nightmares that evoke emotions similar to those they experienced when being abused). At the extreme, clients may have flashbacks, in which they actually feel like the abuse is happening again. Such flashbacks are sometimes so real that they can be misdiagnosed by clinicians unfamiliar with PTSD as psychotic symptoms. For example, one of our clients who was very severely physically and emotionally abused by her mother reported to her psychiatrist that she was "hearing voices" that insulted her and told her to punish herself. During our assessment of this client, we discovered that the "voices" were actually flashbacks of her mother yelling at her. The client knew that such voices were not real, but when these flashbacks occurred, she felt as if she was a child and the abuse was happening again.

Avoidance and Numbing Symptoms

The second cluster of PTSD symptoms involves avoidance and numbing. To meet criteria for a diagnosis of PTSD, clients must have three such symptoms. Avoidance symptoms consist of clients' avoiding thoughts, feelings, places, or persons that remind them of the traumatic experiences. Such symptoms are challenging to assess in women who experienced childhood abuse, because often avoidance began early in life and has become such a part of the clients' ways of being in the world that they are not even conscious of it. For example, a 47-year-old client who was sexually abused was very socially withdrawn. She had never had an intimate relationship, had few friends, and supported herself financially by editing scientific publications (which she could do from home). Her social withdrawal started in adolescence as a way of avoiding sexual attention from males, because such attention reminded her of the abuse and made her extremely anxious. At 47 years old, this client had been socially withdrawn for over 30 years. She had structured her entire professional and personal life to avoid being around people, particularly men. She did not even fully recognize how her avoidance had shaped her life.

"Numbing" refers to the tendency of individuals with PTSD to experience restrictions in their emotional experiences. Some researchers argue that rather than being emotionally "numb," individuals with PTSD are hyperreactive to negative triggers (particularly those related to the traumatic events), and therefore need more intense positive stimulation to experience positive emotions (Litz & Gray, 2002). Women who have PTSD related to abuse may describe feeling at times "numb" or "dead inside" or "nothing" or "like a zombie." They may report difficulty feeling love or joy, as well as anger or sadness. They describe being confused because things that produce emotion in other people (e.g., a daughter's wedding) have no impact on them. Numbing appears to be the counterpart of hyperarousal (Litz, Schlenger, Weathers, Fairbank, & LaVange, 1997). That is, numbing may result from the depletion of emotional resources. Thus numbing is a component of the emotion dysregulation that is characteristic of women with abuse histories. Such women tend to cycle between feeling overwhelmed by emotion and feeling "nothing."

Hyperarousal

The third cluster of PTSD symptoms involves hyperarousal. This cluster includes symptoms that overlap with other psychiatric disorders, such as trouble concentrating (major depression), irritability and outbursts of anger (generalized anxiety disorder), and difficulty sleeping (major depression). The one symptom in this cluster that is unique to PTSD is exaggerated startle response. The classic example of this symptom is a Vietnam combat veteran who falls to the ground when he hears a car backfire.

Which Trauma to Assess?

Most assessments of PTSD include asking how much each symptom bothers the individual and how often the person has the symptom. One challenge in assessing PTSD related to child abuse is that such clients have often experienced multiple traumatic events. Typically, a trauma clinician focuses on the "worst" experience of child abuse, as determined by the client. This is not necessarily the event the *therapist* views as most distressing or difficult, but the one that troubles the client the most at this time.

Another challenge in PTSD assessment is that many interview instruments attempt to specify whether specific symptoms only started after the traumatic event. This is difficult for women with chronic abuse histories, because often the abuse began early in life and they do not remember what they were like before the abuse occurred. In these cases, it is only possible and certainly sufficient to link the clients' PTSD symptoms (particularly reexperiencing symptoms) to particular events.

Emotion Regulation Problems

Emotion regulation is the ability to modulate powerful affective states. As noted above, clients with a history of child abuse find themselves fluctuating between two emotional extremes: either being overwhelmed by their feelings, or feeling nothing or "numb." Clients report that these extreme states often occur unpredictably. They also may find that they get upset unexpectedly over minor things, have trouble letting go of upsetting things, and have difficulty calming themselves down. As a result, such clients are also often "emotion-phobic." That is, they avoid feeling anything because of their fear of being overwhelmed and unable to cope with their feelings. All of these problems reflect emotion regulation difficulties.

The therapist may begin the assessment of emotion regulation by saying something like this:

> "Some people who experience abuse have difficulty managing their feelings. Sometimes they may feel nothing, numb, or empty. At other times, for seemingly no reason, they may be overwhelmed by feeling too much. At these points, they not even know what they feel—only that they are 'upset.' Does this sound familiar to you?"

The therapist may then go on to assess which emotions are most difficult for the client and how they are handled. Common problems include severe anxiety, depression, and (most particularly) anger.

Another component of emotion regulation difficulties is a lack of distress tolerance—that is, an inability to sit with difficult feelings and not be overwhelmed by them. When clients are faced with overwhelming emotions, they often experience them as intolerable and will do almost anything to make the feelings stop. Such attempts may include self-harming behaviors, such as suicide attempts, substance abuse, and aggression against the self, and are believed to reflect maladaptive efforts to manage or terminate high-distress experiences or situations.

The assessment of emotion regulation is a relatively new area of research focus and instrument development. In Appendix B, we list some instruments we have used in our research. However, therapists should be aware that new and more refined instruments are being developed.

Interpersonal Problems and Role Dysfunction

As mentioned previously, many clients cite interpersonal problems as their primary reasons for seeking treatment. Therapists can get a sense of clients' interpersonal difficulties by asking about their social support network; whether they have close friends; and whether they are in or have ever been in an intimate relationship, and, if so, what those relationships have been like.

Depression and Anger

Problems with emotion regulation and mood often lead to interpersonal problems among those with histories of childhood abuse. Several studies have found that depression and anger, rather than PTSD symptoms, are the predominant correlates of the interpersonal and role dysfunction reported by women with abuse histories (e.g., Beckham et al., 1996; Chemtob et al., 1997a; Chemtob, Novaco, Hamada, Gross, & Smith, 1997b). A therapist can query whether a client has noticed that she gets depressed or angry, and whether these feelings seem to interfere with her relationships or functioning at home, at work, or in social life. The therapist may ask (in regard to depression), "Do you cancel social events or call in sick because you are feeling too down to go out?", or (in regard to anger), "Do you ever find that when you are angry, you do or say things that you later regret?"

Types of Interpersonal Problems

An assessment of the types of interpersonal problems experienced by women with abuse histories revealed that, compared to women who had never been abused, those with abuse histories reported significantly more problems in being both too submissive and too controlling, greater difficulty in being assertive, and more problems in taking on too much responsibility in situations for which they might not be responsible (Cloitre & Koenen, 2001; Cloitre et al., 1997). These data suggest that women with abuse histories have significant difficulties centering around issues of power and control in relationships. A therapist can gently inquire whether a client feels she has these sorts of difficulties, with queries such as "Do you find yourself having difficulties standing up for yourself or afraid of conflict?" or "Do your friends ever say that you are argumentative or need to have your own way?"

Measures identifying common interpersonal problems that childhood abuse survivors experience, including those related to negative emotional states, are provided in Appendix B. These forms can be given directly to clients to complete or simply to review. Alternatively, the therapist can use them as a basis for further queries. Often, when clients complete or review the items on these measures, they are surprised but pleased that the emotional and interpersonal difficulties they experience are identified on these sheets. Some clients have commented that they are relieved that their experiences are known and understood, and that other survivors share the same problems.

Harmful/Risky Behaviors and Comorbidity

The assessment of harmful or risky behaviors is something that has been addressed in detail by other authors (e.g., Linehan, 1993a, 1993b; Miller, 1994), and so it is not discussed in detail here or included in Appendix B. The present discussion is limited to the task of identifying clients who are well matched for the interventions in STAIR/NST. Such clients are those whose primary presenting problems are emotion dysregulation, interpersonal difficulties, and PTSD symptoms. Clients whose primary presenting problems demand immediate attention—such as imminent suicidality, alcohol or drug dependence, severely disordered eating behaviors (such as regular bingeing and purging), or severe dissociation that meets criteria for a dissociative disorder diagnosis—should be directed to treatments that immediately address these issues. These clients often need more intensive treatments, such as inpatient or residential treatment or detoxification.

Self-harming or risky behaviors are strongly associated with a history of child abuse, and therefore should be assessed in clients presenting with such a history. Clients who have these difficulties may be appropriate candidates for STAIR/NST at a later time, when they are stabilized and are no longer a threat to themselves or others. We have had several clients who engaged in STAIR/NST after successfully completing an inpatient or residential treatment program for one of the above-mentioned problems.

Resilience and Coping Strategies

The topics of resilience and coping among women with histories of child abuse are receiving growing attention (Grossman, Cook, Kepkep, & Koenen, 1999; Harvey, 1996; Harvey, Liang, Harney, & Koenen, 2003; Lam & Grossman, 1997; McGloin & Widom, 2001). We view clients who were abused as children and are now seeking treatment to be resilient. Such clients must have had some coping strategies that were effective and have enabled them to survive. Our interest in resilience is reflected in our assessments, which attempt to gather information about the clients' resilient domains of functioning and successful coping strategies. Such information can help therapists tailor interventions to best utilize clients' resources and strengths.

A therapist may begin to engage a client in talking about her strengths by asking how she coped when the abuse was going on: "How did you manage to function?" The therapist can then guide the client toward evaluating those strategies and whether they continue to work in the present. Another way of talking about the client's strengths is to ask the client directly what she thinks they are. However, many clients have trouble identifying anything positive about themselves. If this is the case, the therapist might have the client talk about what her boss, best friend, neighbor, or boyfriend might say are her best qualities. The therapist might gain information on the client's strengths by talking about her intellectual or social interests or activities, such as drawing, reading, church/temple work, or volunteer work.

Measures of resilience and positive coping are provided in Appendix B. The assessment of resilience and positive coping is an area under development, so our list is not meant to be exhaustive.

MATCH BETWEEN CLIENTS' NEEDS AND TREATMENT INTERVENTIONS

Match for Treatment

If you are a therapist considering using this treatment, a simple rule of thumb is to ask yourself whether the client's primary presenting problems are emotion regulation difficulties and interpersonal problems that appear to be connected to a history of child abuse. If the answer is yes, and if the client is not at imminent risk from self-harming behaviors, then it is appropriate to consider using this treatment with the client. Therapists may wish to use only the STAIR module to address these difficulties, and to use the module or particular sessions as often as needed. If the client also has significant PTSD symptoms, then the addition of the NST module is appropriate.

Clients who have used STAIR/NST successfully almost inevitably have comorbid anxiety disorders and major depression. They may meet criteria for an Axis II Cluster A personality disorder, such as dependent or avoidant personality disorder. They may also engage in some disordered eating behaviors (such as some restrictive eating, over-exercising, or bingeing and purging) and/or in substance abuse. As noted in Chapter 8, the treatment has even been successful with clients who have borderline symptoms if they are not imminently suicidal or self-harming.

Readiness for Treatment

If the client's presenting problems indicate that the treatment is appropriate for her, the therapist should consider whether the client is motivated and has the time and other practical resources to participate. STAIR/NST requires a commitment of 12 weeks and additional time to complete between-session exercises. The trauma-processing work during NST in particular requires sustained and unbroken effort for a minimum of 4 weeks. Clients obtain the greatest benefit with the least possible distress when this work is conducted in a sustained fashion. The treatment as a whole requires not only a time commitment, but a commitment to use available emotional and social resources to complete the work. During STAIR/NST, clients are asked to confront not only their abuse histories, but also parts of themselves and their lives they have avoided for years. Clients who enter into this treatment must therefore be motivated to make changes in their lives and to commit the practical and emotional resources it demands.

Clients who cannot attend treatment regularly—say, because of personal or professional demands or generally chaotic lives—are likely to obtain less benefit from this treatment. For instance, clients who travel a great deal on business and will miss sessions for weeks will not obtain maximum benefit. Such clients can be provided with supportive or other forms of therapy until they are able to attend treatment regularly.

It is also common that clients come to treatment in the middle of a personal or family crisis, such as when a parent is terminally ill. Such crises seem to trigger unresolved abuse histories or exacerbate PTSD and other trauma-related symptoms. However, some clients in such situations may not be able to commit to an intensive, trauma-focused treatment. They may benefit from a less directive, more supportive form of therapy until the crisis resolves.

It is difficult to predict ahead of time which clients will be able to commit to the treatment. Therapists will have to think through these situations on a case-by-case basis. Some clients are able to overcome great odds to commit to the treatment. One client we treated was an impoverished single mother, who worked full-time while raising four children. She was also in recovery from alcoholism and regularly attended Alcoholics Anonymous (AA). Despite these barriers to treatment, she never missed a session and regularly completed between-session exercises. This success was partly the result of good planning. Early in treatment, the client and therapist thought very practically about how to arrange her schedule to maximize her ability to complete the therapy. The client made backup arrangements for child care with friends, and got up 30 minutes earlier in the morning to complete her exercises. She was also fortunate enough to have a supportive supervisor at work who allowed her to attend her AA meetings during the day. Thus this client was able to activate her social supports in order to commit to treatment, in spite of having few financial resources and large family responsibilities. We encourage therapists to work with clients to help them identify barriers to treatment and address those barriers before they become a problem.

FEEDBACK

When the therapist has completed the assessment, the therapist should summarize to the client what his or her understanding is of the client's presenting problems and how those fit with STAIR/NST.

A Sample Case

Annie was a 35-year-old divorced woman with three school-age children. She worked as an administrative assistant for an official in a local government agency. Her husband had left her when her children were very young, and she had since been preoccupied with supporting her family and raising her children. She reported a history of sexual abuse by her father from ages 7 to 10, and physical abuse by her mother throughout childhood (*trauma history*). She called our clinic after she saw an advertisement for our treatment in a local newspaper. She came to treatment when she reached her 35th birthday.

In Annie's initial session, she reported that she was an alcoholic and had been sober for 3 years. She was actively involved in AA (*history of harmful behavior [substance use] but not current*). She reported that since she stopped drinking she had became increasingly anxious (*emotion regulation problems*), and nightmares of the abuse had become more frequent (*PTSD symptoms: reexperiencing*). She reported frequently having thoughts and images of the abuse come into her head when she was at work. She had difficulty concentrating and was easily startled (*PTSD symptoms: hyperarousal*).

Annie reported that she had coped with her symptoms by keeping very busy. She had been at her current job for 7 years and had a good record (*resilience and coping strategies*). She stated that her agency was currently offering a training program for employees who wished to move from administration to management. She had wanted her boss to nominate her as a candidate for the program, but had been too anxious to ask him (*emotion regulation and interpersonal problems*). Her work experience revealed a consistent pattern of good employment but unassertiveness. She appeared to have a record as an excellent employee, but had never built on that to request any sort of advancement for herself (*role dysfunction*).

Annie reported several close friendships with members of AA (*social supports, resilience*) but she had not had an intimate relationship since her husband left her, and wasn't sure she could ever love anyone in that way again (*interpersonal problems*). She struggled to be a good parent to her children, but frequently found herself caught between being overly indulgent because she felt guilty about not being more available to them and being overly controlling and strict (*role dysfunction*). She reported that sometimes she lost her temper and found herself screaming at them. She reported impulses to hit her children, but had never done so (*emotion regulation problems*). If she found herself particularly enraged, she would lock herself in the bathroom until she calmed down. She reported suicidal thoughts, but had never attempted suicide and reported no plans or intention to attempt suicide. She reported a tendency to overeat when she was anxious or depressed, but denied bingeing or purging (*risky behaviors not a priority*).

Interpreting the Assessment Findings

If Annie was imminently suicidal, self-injurious, or currently substance-dependent, she would have been inappropriate for this treatment. If this had been the case, the therapist would have given Annie the reasons for needing to be provided with an alternative treatment, and would have referred her to a treatment program focusing on her suicidality, self-harm, and/or substance abuse. Often we encourage clients to return to us for treatment after they have addressed problems such as substance dependence.

Annie was a client who was clearly appropriate for STAIR/NST. She presented with PTSD symptoms (intrusive thoughts, images, nightmares) related to her childhood abuse history. She also reported emotion regulation difficulties that were affecting her interpersonal relationships (anxiety, lack of assertiveness on the job, role dysfunction with her children). Annie's substance dependence was under control, and she did not report any other self-injurious behaviors that would have taken priority at this time.

Therapist Feedback

After completing and evaluating the assessment information, the therapist informed Annie that her problems were appropriate for STAIR/NST treatment. In speaking about how STAIR/NST would help Annie, the therapist focused on three specific issues: her nightmares and intrusive memories of the abuse; her difficulty with being assertive at work in asking for advancement; and her distress over her parenting. The therapist spoke with Annie about how part of the treatment would focus on how to manage her feelings in interpersonal situations to achieve goals she had identified. The therapist suggested that Annie might choose speaking with her boss about his nominating her as a candidate for the training program as an initial goal to focus on. The therapist also spoke about how the trauma-focused work in the second part of the treatment would help reduce her nightmares and intrusive thoughts about her abuse history. Thus the therapist was able to tie the specific problems Annie was currently experiencing to the interventions used in STAIR/NST.

SUMMARY

This chapter has focused on orienting therapists to how we assess clients and consider the match between clients' needs and STAIR/NST. We have discussed how to talk to clients about their trauma histories. We have reviewed the six domains of assessment: trauma history, PTSD symptoms, emotion regulation problems, interpersonal difficulties, harmful or risky behaviors, and resilience or coping strategies. (In Appendix B of this book, we offer some suggestions for assessment measures.) In the next section of this chapter, we have outlined guidelines for determining whether a client is appropriate for this treatment. Finally, we have talked about giving feedback to the client after assessment has been completed.

PHASE I

~

Skills Training in Affective
and Interpersonal Regulation
(STAIR)

Building Resources

CHAPTER 10

~

SESSION 1
The Resource of Hope
Introducing the Client to Treatment

> The very making of an appointment with a total stranger
> to deal with the greatest intimacies and vulnerabilities of
> one's life is an act of profound faith.
> —DIANA FOSHA (2000, p. 5)

OVERVIEW

By the time a trauma client comes to therapy, she has often reached the limits of her capacity to function. She is likely to be feeling substantially demoralized and defeated. Visiting a professional is often an act of desperation. Still, by coming to therapy, the client is clinging to some vestige of hope. The therapist's primary task is to sustain and strengthen this hope. Hope emerges from a sense of being understood and a belief in the possibility of change. Thus the first of the therapist's tasks is to listen carefully to the client and reflect back an accurate and empathic understanding of the client's symptoms and life circumstances. In addition, the therapist must then propose a treatment plan that addresses these problems, and, in a collaborative process with the client, must come to a shared understanding about the goals of the therapy and the means by which these goals will be reached. Box 10.1 outlines the theme and curriculum for Session 1 of treatment.

REVIEW CLIENT'S EVALUATION EXPERIENCE, ABUSE HISTORY, AND SYMPTOMS

The therapist begins by inquiring about the client's experience of the evaluation process. This will provide an understanding of the client's emotional state and potential concerns about the treatment. If the evaluation has been completed by someone other than the ther-

115

BOX 10.1
Theme and Curriculum for Session 1:
The Resource of Hope—Introducing the Client to Treatment

THEME

By the time a trauma client comes to therapy, she has often reached the limits of her capacity to function. Still, by coming to therapy, the client is standing on some island of hope. The therapist's primary task is to sustain and strengthen this hope. Hope emerges from a sense of being understood and a belief in the possibility of change. Thus the first of the therapist's tasks is to listen carefully to the client and reflect back an accurate and empathic understanding of the client's symptoms and life circumstances. In addition, the therapist must then propose a treatment plan that addresses these problems, and, in collaboration with the client, must come to an agreement about the goals of the therapy and the means by which these goals will be reached. The therapist will also give the client "something to go home with by beginning skills training in a mind–body exercise (focused breathing).

PLANNING AND PREPARATION

Review client's evaluation materials, particularly abuse history, symptoms, and coping skills. Bring handouts on treatment rationale and focused breathing (Handouts 10.1 and 10.2).

AGENDA

- Review client's evaluation experience, history, and symptoms.
- Establish the therapeutic contract.
- Provide overview of treatment plan.
- Explain Phase I goals: Emotion regulation and interpersonal skills development.
- Explain Phase II goals: PTSD symptom reduction and creation of life narrative.
- Review rationale and benefits of a two-phase treatment.
- Provide a coping skill: Focused breathing.
- Provide rationale for between session exercises.
- Assign between-session work:
  - Practice focused breathing twice a day.

SESSION HANDOUTS

Handout 10.1. Treatment Overview: About STAIR/NST
Handout 10.2. Instructions for Focused Breathing

apist, it will be important to acknowledge that the therapist has become acquainted with the evaluation materials and presenting problems. If the evaluation has been completed by the therapist, it is still useful to summarize the material from the evaluation, including abuse history, symptoms and presenting problems. This will serve multiple purposes, including verifying that the information the therapist has is correct and providing the client an opportunity to add anything further that feels important for the therapist to know.

The therapist is actively working here, conveying that he or she has made an effort to know about the client and also that the therapist is not overwhelmed by the material. At the same time, the therapist is careful not to overwhelm the client by confronting her with too stark a summary of her abuse experience. Thus the therapist may often pause to make room for the client to confirm, clarify, or add information, conveying an expectation of collaboration. This may take 10–30 minutes, depending on the complexity of the client's abuse history and/or her inclination to elaborate.

Possible Challenges

Some clients may be reactive to hearing their abuse history summarized. The clinician should be alert for this and address it with the client as necessary. For example, it may trigger symptoms in the client, leading her to feel overwhelmed already before the treatment has even begun. The therapist should "normalize" this, explaining to the client that it is natural for talking about the abuse to trigger symptoms at first, but that this will become manageable as the therapy proceeds.

ESTABLISH THE THERAPEUTIC CONTRACT

The initial and perhaps unarticulated agreement when the client walks through the door is that the client has come to therapy for help and the therapist has agreed to help her. How this will take place is the next immediate question, and the answer to it needs to be clearly discussed and negotiated.

Certain parameters guide this process when a therapist plans to implement an empirically based treatment like STAIR/NST. In this situation, the therapist begins with the proposal that the results of the assessment—particularly the client's identified PTSD symptoms, problems with emotion management, and difficulties with relationships—indicate that STAIR/NST is a good match to her needs. The therapist can express confidence in this approach and say something like this:

> "The treatment was developed specifically for women with problems very similar to yours. The therapists who developed it relied heavily on the input and feedback of abuse survivors who came to treatment and had the same problems and issues for which you are now seeking help. We also know that this treatment works to resolve the problems you have mentioned. It has been systematically evaluated with several dozens of women similar to you over the last 10 years and has been

found to be effective. Clients have also reported that the treatment process itself was, although sometimes difficult, a positive experience and worth the effort."

If the client is concerned that the treatment may be too rigid or structured, and will not take into account her individual needs, the therapist can reassure her. As described in Chapter 8, the treatment has built-in flexibility. The therapist can say something like this:

"The therapy has become flexible enough over time to be tailored to each individual's needs without compromising effectiveness. For example, the application of fewer or more sessions—as well as the emphasis on some types of skills training over others, based on your needs—in no way compromises the effectiveness of the treatment. In fact, application of the treatment in this way is known to provide even greater benefits. So I look forward to working with you on determining how to tailor this treatment so that it will really be effective for you."

The initial proposal of this structured program is most often met with cautious enthusiasm. Clients are typically relieved to hear that their problems are not unusual, are well known to professionals, and (most importantly) have been the focus of sensitive and considered thought and treatment development. The therapist can then proceed to review the treatment rationale and specific interventions. As described below, the therapist should engage in a dialogue with the client to make sure that each aspect described is matched to the client's specific needs in a way that is understandable and relevant to her. Number of sessions, length of treatment, and areas of concentration for skills training should be discussed and planned.

Reminders about the Therapeutic Alliance

The therapeutic alliance is a working partnership between the therapist and the client, and it is an integral if not critical part of an effective treatment. In particular, therapy settings "pull" for power dynamics, owing to the therapist's perceived position of authority. The power balance between therapist and client can be delicate to negotiate, given the client's experiences of misused authority.

On the one hand, the therapist is in the position of an "expert" or an authority figure, as he or she has skills that are intended to help guide the client in reaching desired goals. This role is legitimate and has positive value for the client. The therapist's knowledge and capacity to implement the treatment provide much-needed structure for the task at hand. It also provides the client with a sense of safety and security, which is a prerequisite for effective treatment.

On the other hand, the client's reaction to authority figures, because of her abuse experience, is likely to include feelings of fear, hostility, and suspicion toward the therapist. The client may feel herself to be disregarded and controlled by the therapist and ineffectual in managing herself in this setting. To counteract this obviously negative interpersonal dynamic, the therapist must make clear that his or her role as an "expert" is in the service of the client's needs and desired recovery. The interventions, their use, and their timing follow the pace and experience of the client. The treatment has been developed to be flexible for this very reason. Given the client's background, she is likely to have had little opportunity to be attended to, taken seriously, and truly seen and heard. The clinician's attitude of receptivity and responsiveness to her experience is a therapeutic intervention in its own right.

Ideally, agreement about the therapy goals and means will be readily established between therapist and client, and therapy will proceed. Therapist and client will remain attuned to each as they work toward these goals, one adapting technique and the other accepting guidance along the way. The support of the therapist will empower the client and affirm her value in the effort. The client in turn will appreciate the therapist's expertise as an instrument of support, rather than as a negation of her needs or experience.

PROVIDE OVERVIEW OF TREATMENT PLAN

The therapist explains that this is a two-phase treatment, which usually consists of 16 hour-long, weekly sessions. The first phase will focus on learning skills for living more effectively with specific emphasis on emotion management problems and interpersonal difficulties. In the second phase, sessions will focus on the emotional processing of the client's traumatic experiences, as well as continued work on enhancing life skills. Handout 10.1 can be used to provide the client with an overview of the STAIR/NST treatment. (Note that this and other client handouts are grouped together at the ends of treatment chapters, for ease of reproduction.)

EXPLAIN GOALS OF PHASE I (STAIR)

Emotion Regulation Skills Development

The therapist explains that one main goal of the first phase is to help the client develop emotional awareness and provide skills to modulate negative feelings and tolerate distress. The client may benefit from learning that many women who were abused as children have difficulty knowing what they are feeling and/or managing their feelings. Some people feel overwhelmed by their feelings, while others may have learned to cope by not feeling anything at all. The therapist should stop and ask the client about her experience with this. It may help to give examples, such as "Some women are never able to feel anger, while others don't feel able to manage their anger at all, so that they 'blow up.' "

The therapist explains that one goal of the treatment will be to learn together how the client can experience her feelings without becoming overwhelmed. This will first involve the client's becoming more aware of her feelings and what triggers them. People abused as children may have difficulty experiencing and labeling feelings because their feelings were mislabeled or disregarded. Again, the therapist should give examples and elicit examples from the client.

To get an initial sense of how others responded to the client's feelings when she was a child (this subject is pursued in more detail in Session 2), the therapist should engage the client in discussion. If the client does not spontaneously respond to what the therapist is describing, inviting her to do so with comments such as "Does this strike a chord anywhere for you?" may help.

Interpersonal Skills Development

A second goal of this phase is for the client to learn how to improve interpersonal skills by using interpersonal goals rather than feeling states to guide her interactions. The therapist and client will also talk about how she can use these skills in her relationships—specifically, to manage certain emotions that can at times interfere with or overshadow her relationship goals. The therapist should ask the patient about difficulties she experiences in interpersonal relationships, prompting with examples and questions as necessary—for instance, "Some women who were abused as children have difficulty in being assertive or let people take advantage of them. Is this familiar to you?" or "Are there certain feelings you have problems expressing to people? What makes it difficult?" The client's answers should give her interpersonal style and problem areas. These topics are taken up again in more detail in later sessions.

Selection of Specific Coping Skills

Finally, the therapist tells the client that she will have the opportunity to learn a number of skills and emotion management strategies, and that she will select from a "menu" of coping strategy options what works best for her. The results of the Generalized Expectancy for Negative Mood Regulation-Scale (see Appendix B) to assess the client's relative strengths in cognitive, behavioral, and social support strategies for managing current distress. This information will be used at a later point in treatment to select coping strategies that address the client's current problems.

EXPLAIN GOALS OF PHASE II (NST)

The therapist explains that in the second phase of treatment, the client will tell about her abuse experience(s) repeatedly, in order to identify and explore the feelings that go with the experience(s). One important goal of this work is for the client to be able to think about the trauma, or encounter reminders or triggers of it, without experiencing her particular symptoms at the intensity she does now.

Review of PTSD Assessment Results

The therapist provides an overview of the symptoms that constitute the diagnosis of PTSD, and explains how the client's symptoms fit into the diagnosis. PTSD is described as a syndrome that can develop after a person has been exposed to a traumatic event, such as childhood abuse, rape, combat, being in a plane crash, or witnessing a murder. Often PTSD develops soon after the trauma; however, it can begin at any time after the event. Using the client's self-reported PTSD symptoms (obtained from evaluation materials), the therapist and client together review the three PTSD symptom clusters (i.e., reexperiencing, avoidance and numbing, and hyperarousal); determine which of these symptoms the client reported in the assessment; and clarify her understanding of what the symptoms are and how they fit into each category.

Narrative Work for the Purpose of Decreasing Fear and PTSD Symptoms

The client's current symptoms (nightmares, flashbacks, anxiety, etc.) indicate that there is "unfinished business" related to the past trauma. The therapist notes that some people try to cope with this by avoiding traumatic memories, which is understandable but ultimately does not work. Other people cannot avoid their memories at all and feel overwhelmed by them. And some people experience both of these elements at different times. The aim of the treatment is to help the client process the memories of her abuse in such a way that she attains more control *over* them, rather than being controlled *by* them. The therapist can tell the client something like this:

> "The goal will be to help you make meaningful connections between your feelings and your experiences in a safe and supportive environment. Staying with these memories rather than running away from them can be very distressing at first, but over time it will help decrease the anxiety and fear that are associated with them. This process is called 'deconditioning' or 'habituation.' "

Narrative Work for the Purpose of Organizing Traumatic Memories

A second goal of the narrative work is to help the client to assimilate and integrate her experiences. Some clients find the following analogy helpful: The mind can be viewed as a kind of file cabinet in which a person's experiences are organized and stored, helping the person to make sense of them and put them in their right place. So, for example, children might have a file for "birthday parties," where they store memories of particular parties, plus their accumulating knowledge about what one brings to a party, what to expect at a party, and so forth. But where does a child file and organize the experience of abuse? Typically, the abuse experience is not labeled and discussed. Thus the feelings and memories continue to interfere with life in the present, frequently in the form of PTSD. The symptoms reflect the unorganized and unassimilated feelings associated with the trauma. Part of the goal of processing abuse experience(s) is for the client to be able to organize these distressing feelings and memories and find a place for them.

Narrative Work for the Purpose of Developing a Life History

During the narrative phase of the treatment, the conclusion of each telling (or a series of tellings) will involve a review of the client's perceptions of herself and her life circumstances, including her relationship with those who abused her. These will be directly compared to the beliefs she holds about herself now and to her perceptions of her current circumstances and relationships. Some perceptions of self and patterns of relating will be identical to those of the past. These will be reviewed for their current positive value to the client, and will be either accepted and reinforced or identified as perceptions that may be due for revision. There will also be observations about the way in which the client has changed, and changed for the better. Client and therapist will identify the positive and more adaptive beliefs about herself that have developed during Phase I, as well as the internal and external resources for life functioning that have accumulated. The comparison of current self and past self often highlights the positive changes the client is making, which are easy to lose sight of during the change process. This type of contrasting activity also places an emotional distance between the client's past and present. Narrative analysis organizes experience as a story with a beginning, middle, and end. The sense of time this process instills reinforces the idea that the trauma is in the past and therefore cannot hurt the client. Lastly, narrative analysis will yield some understanding of how the past has influenced the present but need not continue to do so. With this awareness, the client may begin to exercise choices about who she will be and what she will do.

REVIEW RATIONALE AND BENEFITS OF A TWO-PHASE TREATMENT

There are several reasons for organizing treatment into two phases, each with its own specific goals. The immediate goal of the therapy is to help the client improve functioning and reduce suffering in day-to-day life as quickly as possible. The first phase of treatment, STAIR, is intended to address this goal. This initial phase of work also allows a period of time for the therapist and client to get to know each other. The client has time to become comfortable with the therapist and satisfy herself that the therapist is someone she trusts enough to engage in a process that involves experiencing painful feelings. In a complementary fashion, the therapist will develop a good working knowledge of the client's strengths and vulnerabilities, which will help the therapist guide the client in titrating the emotional intensity of the narrative work. During this time, the client will develop better skills in emotion regulation, which she can use during the more emotionally intense narrative work. The development of emotional and interpersonal resources will also build the client's self-esteem and provide her with greater awareness of her strengths, so that thinking about the past will be, if not less painful, at least less frightening.

Lastly, both therapist and client should review for themselves the number of times they believe it might be useful to cycle through the STAIR component of the treatment. Repeated use of STAIR can be reinforcing for some clients, particularly for those who suffer more from difficulties with daily life functioning than from PTSD symptoms.

PROVIDE A COPING SKILL: FOCUSED BREATHING

An important and final task of the first session is to provide the client with the beginning of emotion regulation skills instruction. This gives the client "something to go home with." It is intended to boost the client's hope that the treatment will improve her functioning in day-to-day life. It also demonstrates the engagement of both body and mind that is typical of emotion regulation activities, and it is an example of the collaborative process between client and therapist that skills acquisition involves.

Rationale and Overview of Focused Breathing

The therapist begins by explaining the rationale for focused breathing to the client:

> "One technique for dealing with distressing feeling states involves decreasing your physiological arousal through focused breathing. When people are in an aroused state, they tend to breathe from their chests and breathe more quickly. This can actually increase symptoms of anxiety, including dizziness, breathlessness, and even disorientation. The aim of this exercise is to slow down your breathing and decrease the amount of oxygen you take in, which will lead to a decrease in anxiety. In addition, the exercise has a meditational component intended to help you reduce disorganized thinking and thought flooding by focusing on a single sensation and single task—namely, breathing. Focused breathing can be used to manage states of irritation or anger, and as a meditative tool for feeling calm and grounded. It is also an exercise that highlights the relationship between the mind and the body. By clearing the mind of all thoughts, and by directing your concentration toward regular breathing, you will experience the influence of mind over body. In a complementary fashion, the relaxation of the body that comes from regular breathing will also reduce your flow of undirected thoughts, completing the circle so that you can experience the influence of the body over the mind."

The therapist should emphasize that experiences of the body and mind are highly interrelated. Focused breathing is an exercise that will help the client connect and integrate experiences of the body and mind in a healthful way.

Instructions to Therapist for Teaching Focused Breathing

1. *Assess baseline.* Observe the client as she breathes in her usual way. Have her pay attention to her rate of breathing and whether she breathes from her chest or diaphragm.

2. *Teach technique.* Model breathing from your diaphragm, placing one hand on your chest and the other on your stomach, and have the client imitate this. Explain that when she is breathing from the diaphragm, only the stomach hand should move up and down, while the chest remains still. It can help to invite the client to think of how a baby sleeps—how only the lower abdomen moves up and down. Or she might imagine her stomach as a balloon, filling with air and expanding as she inhales, then letting out the air and shrinking as she exhales.

3. *Slow down rate of breathing.* Instruct the client to take in enough air to fill the space under the diaphragm, then gradually let it out slowly. Sometimes breathing through the nose is easier because it is a smaller opening, which will help to control the rate of exhalation. Instruct the client to pause briefly after exhaling before inhaling again. Some clients will tend to hold their breath too long at first; explain that the pause should come after *exhaling*, and use imagery to convey the desired movement and flow. For example, the ebb and flow of an ocean wave is a helpful image for some. The image of climbing up a slide (inhaling) and then sliding down (exhaling), and briefly pausing at the bottom before climbing up again, has also been helpful.

4. *Meditational component.* In order to help the client slow her thoughts and focus attention on breathing, instruct the client to count her breaths as she inhales, and think "Relax," "Calm," or some similar thought as she exhales. She should continue counting until she gets to 10, and then go back to 1. Explain, "It is perfectly natural for other thoughts to come into your mind. Try not to get angry or frustrated; just allow the thoughts to pass through your mind and bring your attention back to counting as often as you need to." Some people find it helpful to concentrate mostly on the physical sensation of their breathing, others on the counting or "Relax" statement. Still others will have other ways of focusing that come most naturally to them. Encourage the client to do what works best for her.

PROVIDE RATIONALE FOR BETWEEN-SESSION EXERCISES

The therapist should provide the client with take-home exercises, which incorporate the skills that are taught during treatment. There are several reasons for doing this. The first is that the assignments will provide the client and therapist with important data on the client's real-life experiences that can be used in session to inform interventions. The therapist can use examples from the homework when introducing new information or skills. Another reason for between-session assignments is that they enable the client to practice skills learned in the session in the context of her real life. Generalizing what is learned in session to real life is one of the fundamental principles of this therapy. A further reason is that this is a relatively brief treatment that asks clients to learn a large number of skills in a short period of time. The only way for clients to accomplish these tasks is to practice on their own.

The therapist then gives the client the focused breathing handout (Handout 10.2) for use between sessions. She should be instructed her to put aside some time each day where she will be undisturbed and comfortable, and to practice the technique for at least 5 minutes twice a day. The therapist emphasizes that her skill will increase with practice, and that only then will it be available to her as a coping device when she is anxious.

ASSIGN BETWEEN-SESSION EXERCISES

The client is instructed to practice breathing retraining twice a day for at least 5 minutes each time.

Treatment Overview: About STAIR/NST

RATIONALE FOR THE TREATMENT

This treatment was specifically designed for adults with a history of childhood abuse who suffer from posttraumatic stress disorder (PTSD) symptoms and experience difficulties in functioning due to problems with emotion management and interpersonal relationships. The first phase of treatment directly addresses current relationship and emotion management problems. Phase I of treatment will also prepare you to work effectively in the more emotionally intense Phase II, which involves discussion and analysis of painful memories of childhood trauma. People often try to cope with traumatic memories by avoiding them. This is understandable, but ultimately it does not work, and the memories return in unpredictable and uncontrollable ways. The goal of Phase II is to organize your memories of trauma and resolve your feelings about them, so that you control the memories rather than the memories' controlling you. In addition, the process of describing your past is a means by which you will be able to identify beliefs about yourself and patterns of relating that might have been adaptive in abuse circumstances, but no longer are adaptive and need to be changed. The skills training from Phase I will help you leave behind old patterns of functioning and develop interpersonal behaviors and emotion management strategies that are consistent with your current life goals.

OVERVIEW OF THE TREATMENT

This is a two-phase treatment. In the first phase, called Skills Training in Affective and Interpersonal Regulation (STAIR), 1-hour sessions will take place once a week for 8 weeks (unless you and your therapist decide that a different number or spacing of sessions would be appropriate). This phase will focus on learning skills for dealing with distressing feelings and for improving interpersonal situations. In the second phase, called Narrative Story Telling (NST), 1-hour sessions will also be held once a week, also for 8 weeks (again, unless you and your therapist decide differently). These sessions will consist of emotional processing of your traumatic experiences, as well as continued work toward improving your day-to-day life.

Phase I: STAIR

The first goal of Phase I is to develop emotional awareness and build skills for handling negative feelings and managing distress. A second goal of this phase is to learn how to improve your interpersonal skills by learning how patterns you learned in early relationships continue to guide your current relationships. Time will also be spent on how to use emotion regulation skills in relationships—specifically, how to manage certain emotions that can at times interfere with or overshadow your relationship goals.

(continued)

Phase II: NST

In Phase II, you will engage in the emotional processing of your abuse experiences by repeated narration of the events of your early life. The goal will be to help you make meaningful connections between your feelings and your experiences in a safe and supportive environment. Staying with these memories rather than running away from them can be very distressing at first, but over time it will help decrease the anxiety and fear that are associated with them. In addition, this process will allow you to identify the ways in which the present is different from the past, freeing you to behave and think differently. It will also provide you with a life narrative, which will allow you to take a long view of your life and see your trauma as only one of many possible experiences that you may have.

Instructions for Focused Breathing

In one way or another, the body is involved.
—DIANA FOSHA

RATIONALE

One technique for dealing with distressing feeling states involves decreasing your physiological arousal through focused breathing. The aim of this exercise is to slow down your breathing and decrease anxiety, breathlessness, and disorientation. In addition, the exercise has a meditational component intended to reduce disorganized thinking or thought flooding by focusing on a single sensation and single task—namely, breathing. Focused breathing can be used to manage states of irritation or anger, and as a meditative tool for feeling calm and grounded. It is also an exercise that highlights the relationship between the mind and the body. By clearing the mind of all thoughts and by directing concentration towards regular breathing, you will experience the influence of mind over body. The relaxation of the body that comes from regular breathing will also reduce the flow of undirected thoughts, completing the circle so that you can experience the influence of body over mind. The body and mind are highly interrelated, and focused breathing is an exercise that will help you experience the connectedness and integrity of the body and mind in a positive and healthy way. The ability to engage in focused breathing in a meditational fashion is difficult and takes practice. So do not be discouraged; practice regularly and with patience, and your skill will develop over time.

PROCEDURE FOR DIAPHRAGMATIC BREATHING

Getting Started

Place one hand on your chest and the other on your stomach. Take a slow, deep breath, and pay attention to which hand moves. When you are breathing from your diaphragm, only the hand on the stomach should move up and down, with little movement coming from the chest. It can help to think of how babies sleep—how their stomachs quietly move up and down. Or you might imagine your stomach as a balloon, filling with air and expanding as you inhale, then letting out the air and shrinking as you exhale.

Slow Down Your Rate of Breathing

Take in enough air to fill the space under the diaphragm, then let it out slowly. Sometimes breathing out through the nose is easier because it is a smaller opening, which will help to control the rate of exhalation. Pause briefly after exhaling before inhaling again. Some people tend to hold their breath too long at first; the pause should come after *exhaling*. Imagery can be helpful in maintaining a slow and steady rhythm. For example, a wave is a helpful image for some. The image of climbing up a slide (inhaling) and then sliding down (exhaling), and briefly pausing at the bottom before climbing up again, may also be helpful.

(continued)

Meditational Component

In order to help slow your thoughts and focus your attention on breathing, count your breaths as you inhale, and think "Relax," "Calm," or some similar thought as you exhale. Continue counting your breaths until you get to 10, and then start over at 1. It is perfectly natural for other thoughts to come into your mind. Try not to get angry or frustrated; just allow the thoughts to pass through your mind, and bring your attention back to counting as often as you need to. Some people find it helpful to concentrate mostly on the physical sensation of their breathing, others on the counting or "Relax" statement. Experiment with different methods, and do whatever works best for you.

Practice

Practice is essential to develop this skill, so that it becomes something you can use to decrease distress in stressful situations. You should practice the technique in a comfortable, quiet place where you will not be disturbed. Take a few seconds to relax, and then practice the breathing exercise for at least 5 minutes. This should be done at least twice a day. When you are beginning to learn this skill, it is best not to practice when you are already distressed. The idea is that if you practice the breathing when you are in a calm state, it will become a habit that you can then call upon when you are distressed. As you become more skilled at it, you may begin practicing using it in mildly distressing situations, such as when you are feeling impatient while waiting in a line.

CHAPTER 11

~

SESSION 2

The Resource of Feeling
Emotional Awareness

Reality is when something is happening to you and you know it and can say
it and when you say it other people understand what you mean and
believe you.
—ANDREA DWORKIN, quoted by CATHARINE A. MACKINNON (2005, p. 13)

OVERVIEW

Identifying and naming feelings may seem to be a simple activity. But, in fact, many abuse
survivors have not had sufficient opportunity to do this. Feelings are a critical resource for
living. Feelings provide information about potential threats in our environment, guide
our decision-making processes, and motivate our actions. They also contribute to self-
knowledge, as when they inform our preferences (likes and dislikes), and they powerfully
communicate to others our intentions and beliefs. Developmentally, awareness of feelings
often grows in tandem with naming. Naming heightens our awareness of a feeling, provides a vehicle for its expression, and clarifies its meaning and potential purpose. Through
naming, a feeling becomes real.

Chronic childhood abuse often leads to pervasive and long-term impairment in a survivor's ability to identify and name feelings (this impairment is called "alexithymia"). The
ability to identify and name feelings facilitates emotional awareness, organizes emotional
experiences, and supports effective decision making and actions. The survivor's difficulty
with identifying and naming feelings creates disturbances in all of these experiences; perhaps most devastatingly, it undermines the survivor's confidence in the accuracy of her
feelings and perceptions, and in the authority of her actions.

BOX 11.1
Theme and Curriculum for Session 2: Emotional Awareness—
The Resource of Feelings and the Power of Naming

THEME

Identifying and naming feelings may seem to be a simple activity. But, in fact, many abuse survivors have not had sufficient opportunity to do this. In this session, the therapist helps the client enhance her ability to identify and label her feelings, their sources, and associated thoughts and actions. In addition, the therapist helps create a sense of safety in the client's experiencing and naming of feelings, provides clarification of different kinds of feelings, and furnishes support for their expression and felt reality.

PLANNING AND PREPARATION

Review client's evaluation materials related to difficulties with emotion regulation. Bring copies of Self-Monitoring of Feelings Form (Handout 11.2) and other handouts. Prepare examples for Self-Monitoring of Feelings Form.

AGENDA

- Begin with emotional check-in and review of between-session exercises.
- Introduce concept of emotion regulation.
- Explore and identify client's emotion regulation difficulties.
- Introduce session goal: Awareness and monitoring of feelings.
- Provide rationale for monitoring and understanding feelings: Effective living.
- Use elements of emotion to name feelings.
- Discuss discrimination among different kinds of feelings.
- Practice with Self-Monitoring of Feelings Form.
- Assign regular practice in monitoring feelings.
- Summarize the goals of the session and between session exercises:
  - Practice focused breathing twice a day.
  - Complete Self-Monitoring of Feelings Form once a day.

SESSION HANDOUTS

Handout 11.1. The Impact of Childhood Abuse on Emotion Regulation
Handout 11.2. Self-Monitoring of Feelings Form
Handout 11.3. List of Words You Can Use to Describe a Feeling
Handout 11.4. Feelings Wheel

In this session, the therapist helps the client find words to describe her feelings, understand their sources, and become aware of the thoughts and actions associated with them. These skills are learned through instruction and repeated practice in self-monitoring of feelings. At the same time and of equal importance, the therapist helps create a sense of safety in the client's experiencing and naming of feelings, provides clarification of different kinds of feelings, and furnishes support for their expression and felt reality.

Conscious awareness of feelings is a first and vital step in self-discovery. It is intended to give the survivor confidence in her visceral experience of emotion. This liberation in emotional experiencing is intended to create new resources, give the client renewed energy, and contribute to her experience of a real and authentic self. Box 11.1 outlines the theme and curriculum for Session 2 of treatment.

BEGIN WITH EMOTIONAL CHECK-IN AND REVIEW OF BETWEEN-SESSION EXERCISES

This session and all that follow begin with an inquiry about the client's reaction to the previous session and any difficulties she may have had implementing the between-session tasks. Clients may have questions that need answering before they can comfortably go on with the current session. If a client reports significant difficulties with the skills work from the previous session (in this case, focused breathing), the therapist and client should plan to reserve time at the end of the session for extra practice.

In this particular session, a client may have second thoughts or concerns about the treatment plan. The goals and means to reach treatment goals must be relevant to the client and also must be adapted to the client's sensibilities, and so any concerns she has should be addressed. In addition, what the client has to say at the opening of the session is a demonstration of or exercise in the expression of feelings—her preferences, her sense of collaboration, and her fears about the coming weeks of work. The session thus begins with an experience of the central goal of the session: practice in identifying and expressing feelings.

INTRODUCE CONCEPT OF EMOTION REGULATION

"Emotion regulation" encompasses the ability to identify, label, modulate, and effectively express feelings. All these aspects of emotion regulation are addressed in this and the next several sessions. The therapist should convey the meaning of the concept and explore the client's experiences with all these aspects of emotion regulation. The therapist should keep in mind, however, that the skills work for this particular session focuses only on the prerequisite to all other aspects of emotion regulation: emotional awareness. This is learned through self-monitoring of feelings, which gives the client practice in the specific skills of identifying and labeling feelings.

The therapist now introduces the notions that (1) emotional awareness and expression are skills that are learned; (2) childhood abuse is an experience in which a child's feelings are often ignored or mislabeled, and this experience is in itself is a "learning experience," albeit a negative one; and (3) negative or maladaptive habits of self-monitoring and expression can be unlearned and changed for more adaptive functioning. These ideas can be more meaningfully discussed and reinforced in the context of the client's own history and experiences. Handout 11.1 can be used to provide the client with a summary of these ideas.

EXPLORE AND IDENTIFY CLIENT'S DIFFICULTIES WITH EMOTION REGULATION

To begin the process, the therapist can first engage the client in describing any difficulties in managing feelings she is aware of and/or would like to change. In our experiences, two simple questions yield a great deal of information and discussion: "How were feelings handled in your family as you were growing up?" and "How have your traumatic experiences affected the way you feel?" These questions will provide specific information relevant to the client's needs.

The therapist then pursues an open-ended discussion of how trauma has affected the client's feelings and ability to manage them. Not all clients have the same difficulties. For example, a client may have no difficulty labeling her feelings, but may respond poorly to them or not know what to do with them. Some clients may need help primarily in being able to attenuate states of intense emotion, while others may need a lot of work to help them access any feelings at all.

Discuss How Feelings Were Managed in the Family

Because the childhood experiences of an abuse survivor have a strong influence on her beliefs and management of feelings, queries into family history can be very enlightening. The client can tell about ways in which caregivers responded to her feelings in the past. For example, were her feelings considered important? Were they ignored? Were they mislabeled (e.g., the client was told, "You're fine, stop crying" when upset)? Did expression of emotion result in negative reactions from caregivers (e.g., "I'll give you something to cry about")? In addition, the client can discuss how caregivers handled their own emotions. For example, did they sweep things under the rug, drink, or express frightening, out-of-control anger?

The therapist can note where appropriate that parental guidance shapes learning via role modeling, some of which may not have been ideal or effective. In addition, the client will probably have developed ways of coping—some of which are adaptive, but others of which take a toll on the client's current well-being. The client and therapist should explore and identify which emotional "coping styles" are problematic for the client now.

Discuss How Abuse Has Influenced Feelings

The discussion described above often facilitates the client's ability to describe how the abuse has influenced her "habits" of emotional awareness and expression, and which of these habits the client wants to work on to change. Common responses to the question "How have your traumatic experiences affected the way you feel?" are listed below and can be used by the therapist to guide this discussion.

Confusion

Abuse survivors frequently comment that the most common feeling they have, even years after the abuse, is confusion. "Confusion," while not exactly a feeling, accurately represents something about our clients' state of affairs. The secrecy and denial typical in families of abused children have made this particular type of trauma "the problem with no name." If the problem did not have a name for decades, it is not a surprise that the feelings associated with it have no names either. Words have the power to organize experience. With few labels for their experience, abuse survivors often do not know what they felt as children and do not know exactly what they feel now, or how to link their childhood and adult feelings to the abuse events.

Chronic Fear, Hypervigilance, and Dread

The burden of managing the trauma (which in itself is a threat to the child's physical and psychic well-being), and the frequent absence of support or intervention about the abuse, often create a chronic sense of anxiety, hypervigilance in monitoring for potential assaults, and a sense of dread and hopelessness about the future.

Emotions as a Roller-Coaster Experience

It is also not unusual for clients to experience alternating acute states of overwhelming emotions and numbing—in effect, to experience an emotional "roller coaster." In response to these overwhelming emotions, some abuse survivors learn to "shut down" altogether to protect themselves from the acute reactions of the repeated trauma, as well as the chronic fear and anxiety.

Keeping a Distance from Emotions

Abuse survivors often like to keep a distance from intense emotions. As one client who had been beaten regularly during childhood put it, "I have been on the wrong end of the stick many times, and I know the damage that anger can do to a body and soul." Abuse survivors, by virtue of their own experience as victims, are intimately familiar with the painful and damaging consequences of intense and out-of-control emotions. Many of them shy away from experiencing intense emotions, because experience has taught them that intense emotions are linked to negative outcomes. One of the goals of therapy is to demonstrate to such clients that this is not always the case and less likely than they think.

Therapist's Attitude: Respecting the Client and Her Experience

Two important attitudes to convey in this discussion concern a client's feelings about herself and about her family of origin. It is important to acknowledge that the coping strategies of the past that create difficulty in her life now were almost certainly the coping strategies that were the best she could do in her given situation, and sometimes were the necessary and only adaptive responses available. In addition, many clients have conflictual bonds to their abusers and may feel the need to defend their behaviors during their childhood. For example, a client with alcoholic parents may say, "They did not know what they were doing. If they hadn't been drinking, they would not have done any of these things." The therapist should respond in a way that respects this need, and in language that does not imply judgment—for example, "Your parents, for whatever reason, were not able to/ did not help you to cope with difficult feelings."

INTRODUCE SESSION GOAL: AWARENESS AND MONITORING OF FEELINGS

The therapist should now explain that this session revolves around the introduction and use of the deceptively simple Self-Monitoring of Feelings Form (Handout 11.2). This sheet provides a strategy for systematically identifying feelings, their intensity, situational triggers, and associated thoughts and behavioral responses. It is essentially a telegraphic diary of the client's emotional life and is used throughout the STAIR module.

The completion of this monitoring form over several weeks, and the development of the skills described above, are intended to accomplish the therapeutic goal of enhancing the client's emotional awareness. Practice in using the Self-Monitoring of Feelings Form facilitates the labeling of feelings and their links to specific events, clarifies differences between feelings, and identifies the contexts in which they happen. Lastly, the therapist can point out that the final column of the sheet, which asks the client to attend to her behavioral reactions to each trigger and emotion, provides information about how the client responds to difficult emotions, and so lays the groundwork for later efforts in building coping skills.

Value of Self-Monitoring for the Client

The therapist should explain that the client will be asked to make daily entries between sessions. As the task is repeated over several weeks, the therapist and client can identify the range and pattern of emotions the client experiences. The therapist can provide some examples of how this form has been useful to other clients. For example, some clients discover over weeks of diary keeping that they are really almost always angry at a sister, or almost always anxious during sex. Other clients learn that feeling angry is really a cover for disappointment. Still others come into each session with nothing written down and report that they have no feelings. Learning about the client's emotional style is one aspect of the client's journey of self-discovery. It may also provide some evidence of the type of emotional reaction the client may have during the emotionally demanding processing of the trauma during the second phase of treatment.

Therapist's Attitude

The therapist should understand that beyond the immediate value of self-exploration, self-monitoring also provides the client with an experience in which someone (the therapist) is taking an active interest in the client's feelings—what she feels, how much she is feeling it, and when she feels it. This may be a relatively novel experience for abuse survivors, whose feelings have often been ignored, or who themselves believe that their feelings are irrelevant or too threatening, dangerous, or ugly to be given attention. The simple act of working together and attending to a client's emotional life ideally allows the client to have her feelings validated or feel more "real" by virtue of being named and shared.

PROVIDE RATIONALE FOR SELF-MONITORING AND UNDERSTANDING FEELINGS: EFFECTIVE LIVING

Clients need to be presented with a rationale for why they should take the time to monitor and understand their feelings. Discussion about feelings may elicit distress, and some clients at this point may reconsider their desire to come into contact with their feelings, their need to change, and their commitment to the therapy. A supportive reminder that they have chosen this task is helpful. So is exploration of the value of accurate and well-modulated emotional experiencing. Some reasons clients have given for self-monitoring their feelings are as follows:

> "My danger sensor is smashed, and I can't tell what is safe and what is threatening."
> "I never know what I am feeling. A friend asks 'Are you happy?' and I don't know!"
> "I feel nothing. And then a small thing happens, and I can't get out of bed."
> "I can't trust my feelings, so I try not to feel anything."
> "I just feel angry all the time."

Rehabilitation of the Arousal/Threat System

One of the primary reasons clients should take the time to monitor and understand their feelings is that accurate perceptions of and reactions to our emotions contribute to adaptive living. Emotions provide us with information and help guide our decisions and behaviors. This is especially pertinent for a client who requires assistance in understanding what situations to approach or avoid. One of the clients quoted above reported that she had been beaten in such an indiscriminate fashion and experienced a series of such unexpected assaults that she felt as if her "danger sensor" was smashed, and she'd lost all capability of distinguishing situations in which she was safe from those that might be an immediate threat to her well-being. Rather incongruously, she was chronically hypervigilant and fearful of going outdoors, but on those rare occasions when she elected to go out, she thought nothing of a stroll though a poorly lit park at night. She had been raped in broad daylight and as a child had been assaulted for no apparent reason. The world of safety–threat cues did not apply. Her threat detection system was badly out of kilter. Persons with a history of sexual abuse are more prone to being victimized repeatedly and will greatly benefit from being able to interpret emotional cues accurately. One goal of this treatment is to rehabilitate the emotional threat system that has been disturbed by abuse. Regular review of the Self-Monitoring of Feelings Form to identify feelings of threat (or their absence) is a first step in this process.

Enhanced Confidence in Using Feelings to Guide Decisions and Actions

Many abuse survivors have little confidence in their emotional perceptions, and thus are stymied or suffer severe indecision because they do not trust their emotional experiences as an accurate source of information. Part of the goal in this series of interventions is to build confidence in the accuracy of emotional experiences, so that they become a resource for the survivor in simplifying daily life. Building and strengthening emotion regulation skills is difficult. Thus the therapist will benefit from explaining the evolution of the client's progress through treatment from developing the ability to identify and label emotions, to gaining the skills necessary to regulate them.

Enhanced Engagement in Living and the Possibility of Pleasure and Happiness

Awareness of feelings can help the client make decisions not only to live more safely, but also to live with greater satisfaction, both about herself and about her relationships with others. Once the client feels relatively safe, she can turn her attention to experiencing positive feelings and identifying positive life goals. Awareness of positive feelings, and of when, where, and with whom they occur, can lead to greater clarity about the survivor's desires and wishes for her work life and relationships. It can lead to the pursuit of personal goals that are intrinsically pleasurable or satisfying to the client, such as sports or dance. Lastly, the client's ability to "follow her feelings" can ignite a sense of creativity and self-appreciation that may never have been experienced or may have been lost a long time ago. It is often worthwhile to note that approaching pleasure and positive experiences can be frightening to a survivor, for fear of disappointment or of simply being overwhelmed with sensation or arousal. One of the treatment goals will be to help such a survivor modulate her feelings and manage her distress, particularly in the pursuit of valued positive life goals.

USE ELEMENTS OF EMOTION TO NAME FEELINGS

Some people have difficulty in naming feelings. For these clients, labeling a sensation or physical reaction is a useful first step. Clients are usually able to identify experiences of acute sensations or rapid changes in their physical state, such as trembling hands, rapid breathing, or a hot face. The next step is to identify the associated thoughts and behaviors and make an inference to an emotional label. For example, rapid breathing and the thought "He's a jerk" may describe anger. Therapist and client can review models of emotion that break down emotional experiencing into three channels or modes: physical sensations, thoughts, and behaviors. The client can be asked to become more aware of bodily sensations and changes in these sensations as an entry point to connecting to feelings. Awareness of bodily sensations can be followed by questioning or observing associated thoughts and behavior. All of these elements combined ultimately contribute to the experience of an emotion (see Box 11.2).

The causal relationships among thoughts, feelings, and behaviors are multidirectional; change in any one of these can cause change in any other. We begin this exercise with physical sensations, because many clients do not have experience with linking these sensations to their thoughts and behaviors. Given that most emotions are linked to specific types of physiological changes, an effort to compose a list of commonly experienced physiological changes is worthwhile. The therapist and client can generate such a list, including such phenomena as alterations in heart rate, amount of sweating, muscle tension, and so on. This can be followed by the names of emotions that are typically paired with specific bodily changes. For example, an increase in heartbeat may reflect a myriad of emotions, such as the approach of a potential mugger or the presence of a romantic partner. Rapid breathing can be a sign of either anger or extraordinary happiness. Once these are noted, the client can then begin to link her own physiological

---

BOX 11.2
The Three Channels of Elements in an Emotion

Physiological Change: One or more noticeable bodily changes/sensations.
  ➤ Extremely sweaty hands. Heart racing.

Cognitive Interpretation: How you understand the physiological change.
  ➤ "I am nervous because I have a job interview."

Behavior: The action you choose to take.
  ➤ Abandon the interview site, or utilize a relaxation technique and bolster up my courage.

BOX 11.3
Sample Feeling Identification Scenarios

SCENARIO 1

You notice that your heart is racing and that your palms have suddenly become very sweaty. The you notice that there is a car coming toward you at you at 50 miles per hour, and you are only halfway across the street. How do you think you would feel?

SCENARIO 2

You notice that your heart is racing and that your palms have suddenly become very sweaty. You have just seen someone you are romantically interested in approaching you. How do you think you would feel?

---

changes with emotion labels based on inference from her thoughts and behaviors. The client can move from a sensation to an interpretation of the sensation by reference to her associated thoughts and behaviors.

Essentially, an emotion is the recognition and interpretation of a change in bodily state, which can be triggered by behaviors or thoughts. The therapist and client should examine methods of how to recognize these changes and distinguish their meanings. To illustrate this point, the therapist may present a diverse array of examples (Box 11.3). The therapist can also utilize the model depicted in Figure 11.1 to elucidate how the three types of elements interact in the dynamic process of emotional experience.

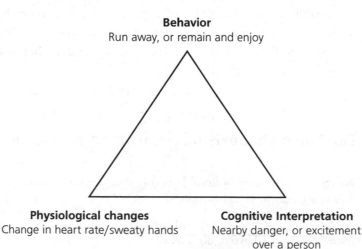

Behavior
Run away, or remain and enjoy

Physiological changes
Change in heart rate/sweaty hands

Cognitive Interpretation
Nearby danger, or excitement
over a person

FIGURE 11.1. A model of how physiological changes, thoughts, and behaviors interrelate in emotional experience.

DISCUSS DISCRIMINATION
AMONG DIFFERENT KINDS OF FEELINGS

Some people with PTSD are chronically anxious and frequently become flooded with sensations. Anxiety per se can be adaptive, but when it is chronic and excessive, it floods a person's ability to differentiate feeling states. In addition, some abuse survivors have not been encouraged to explore the wide range of feelings that can be expressed and understood. This restricted knowledge of feelings limits their self-awareness and their evaluation of and communication with others.

There are several different methods for enhancing a client's capacity for discriminating feelings and expanding an emotional vocabulary. First, we have found it helpful if the therapist provides the client with a list of feeling words (see Handout 11.3, the List of Words You Can Use to Describe a Feeling). The client can immerse herself in the luxury of a rich set of feeling words and consider which are appropriate descriptors of her current experience or are typical of her.

The Feelings Wheel (Handout 11.4) provides the opportunity for the client to identify a single emotion and follow the radial depiction of related emotions, or those that may result from this original emotion, given certain circumstances. During this exercise, the client may become more aware of the variety of emotions that exist and their complex relationship to one another. The therapist can point out that more than one feeling can be involved in an emotional experience. For example, sadness and anger may go together, as may demoralization and anxiety. In addition, contrasting or opposing emotions can occur together, such as hatred and pity or love and fear. The client can provide examples of times when these emotions have been combined and how she handled herself in these circumstances.

PRACTICE WITH SELF-MONITORING OF FEELINGS FORM

The goal of this intervention is to impart several simple and individually tailored methods for the client to be able to adequately identify and label feeling states and to understand how such interpretations affect behavioral actions. The best way for the client to learn all this, however, is simply to work through the Self-Monitoring of Feelings Form with the therapist. In Box 11.4, we describe a case example of self-monitoring, and then describe how this client and her therapist discussed the use of this form in session. Example 11.1 shows how this client completed the form.

This case demonstrates how self-monitoring provides a structure and process that helps the client develop clarity and insight about the presence and diversity of her feelings, about the fact that certain feelings predominate in her daily life, and about the presence of a pattern or typical mode of reaction to them. The ultimate goal of the treatment is for a client to have the freedom and ability to experience emotions with greater awareness (and less intensity, if she wishes), and to engage in a broader range of behavioral reactions than those depicted in this scenario.

BOX 11.4
Case Example: Self-Monitoring of Feelings

Janet had been physically and sexually abused by her father, as well as physically abused by several other caretakers throughout her childhood. Although she was able to hold a job and had achieved a relative degree of success there, she had a problem with binge eating and had few friends. When the therapist introduced the Self-Monitoring of Feelings Form to her, along with the Feelings Wheel, she was intrigued by the number of words one could use to describe a feeling.

IDENTIFYING A SITUATION AND FEELINGS

The first situation Janet described, when asked to identify a time when she'd had strong feelings, was a conflict with her son. She said she'd felt "upset" when he did not clean his room after she had asked him to. With the help of the feelings Wheel and some prompting of "What else did you feel?", she was able to identify more *specific feelings*—shame, sadness, and anger (see Example 11.1). In addition, it was helpful for the therapist to ask her how her *body* felt, so that she could identify some of the *physical connections* to her emotions. For example, her fists were clenched, she was flushed, she had a headache, and she was breathing quickly. After the feelings were labeled, the therapist discussed with her how it is possible to have *more than one feeling at a time*, and noted that although this may be confusing occasionally, it is not unusual.

IDENTIFYING INTENSITY OF FEELINGS

Together, the therapist and Janet numbered the intensity of each feeling she'd had on a scale of 1 to 10, where 10 was the most she could ever imagine feeling something (e.g., so angry she could explode, so sad she wanted to die) and 1 was the least. By labeling the intensity, Janet began to develop perspective on the degree of emotions she was experiencing in various situations, rather than having all of her feelings blend into one big, unmanageable, and scary knot.

IDENTIFYING THOUGHTS

The next step, and one of the hardest, was for Janet and her therapist to figure out the thoughts that went along with her emotions. Since Janet had never tried to link her thoughts to her feelings before, the therapist had to help her out with suggestions of things she might have been thinking. In discussing the situation at home, they noticed that Janet felt responsible for her son's behavior; when he failed to do something, she felt like a failure too. So her shame and sadness were coming from thoughts like "I'm a bad mother," and "If he loved me, he would do what I say." Her anger was connected to thoughts of "He doesn't respect me, and he knows he can take advantage of me."

(continued)

BOX 11.4 *(continued)*

IDENTIFYING RESPONSES

Eventually Janet and the therapist would work on replacing this kind of thinking with more positive and less self-blaming thoughts, but for now they just tried to identify what she did in response to the feelings. To make herself feel better, Janet ate a whole bag of candy.

DEVELOPING SELF-AWARENESS

Once she had learned how to monitor her feelings in session, Janet was able to complete the self-monitoring sheets over the course of the following week. When she came to the next session, she said to the therapist, "I was going to tell you I'd had a good week, but when I looked back at my worksheets I realized I'd felt bad almost every day!"

In looking at the sheets together, Janet and the therapist not only noticed when and where she was feeling bad; they also noticed that whenever she had strong feelings, she either went on an eating binge, immersed herself in her work, or went to sleep for a long time. Basically, all of her coping responses for strong emotion involved escape tactics. One of the first therapeutic tasks became helping Janet find additional coping responses for managing her feelings.

Note. Case prepared for this book by Tamar Gordon.

Feeling	Intensity (0–10)	Trigger	Thoughts	Response/coping strategy
Anger	10	Son didn't clean room after I told him to.	He doesn't respect me, and he knows he can take advantage of me.	Eating a whole bag of candy.
Shame	10	Same.	I'm a bad mother.	Same.
Sadness	7	Same.	If he loved me, he would do what I say.	Same.

EXAMPLE 11.1. Self-Monitoring of Feelings Form: Case Example of Janet.

Typical examples of emotions that generally appear in self-monitoring exercises are feelings of sadness, anxiety, or anger. Yet there will be situations where clients will only be able to write that they felt "overwhelmed" or "upset." In these instances, the therapist can provide positive feedback regarding their ability to identify these states, and work with them to identify and label more completely the specific emotion(s) involved. For example, the therapist can pose questions such as "Were you crying?", "Did your muscles feel tense?", or "What other physical sensations were you aware of?" in order to tease out specific emotions.

ASSIGN REGULAR PRACTICE
WITH SELF-MONITORING OF FEELINGS FORM

The client will complete the Self-Monitoring of Feelings Form at least once per day until the next session. The form will indicate situations the client faced that raised strong feelings, and will also provide data on the client's coping strategies. The therapist and client will benefit from reviewing the form at the beginning of the next session. That way, any practical difficulties or misunderstandings regarding the use of the form, such as what information goes in which column, can be addressed. If necessary, the therapist and client can complete the Self-Monitoring of Feelings Form together (e.g., if the client has not completed the work during the week, or if there are aspects of the experience that are unclear to the client).

Once the client has become more adept at completing these assignments, the therapist can emphasize the utility of this form in providing important data for the therapeutic sessions and allowing the therapist a window into her experiences. The therapist should also stress the importance of recording the details as soon as possible after the moment: "This will provide the two of us with the most helpful data."

SUMMARIZE THE GOALS OF THE SESSION
AND PLAN BETWEEN-SESSION EXERCISES

In the first few sessions, it is worthwhile to review the key ideas and goals at the end of each session, as many clients will be unfamiliar with these concepts and may be feeling anxious and somewhat distracted.

In summary, in this session, the therapist has discussed with the client how her experience of abuse impaired her ability to identify and understand her feelings. The client and therapist have worked together to identify the client's emotion regulation difficulties. The three channels of emotion have been reviewed: physiological, cognitive, and behavioral. The therapist and client have practiced having the client use elements in one channel— physiological—to help her identify the other elements of a specific emotion (e.g., anger).

In order to help the client identify her feelings, the rationale for and process of self-monitoring feelings have been reviewed. The therapist and client have filled out Handout

11.2, the Self-Monitoring of Feelings Form, together. The therapist has also reviewed two other emotion identification tools with the client: Handout 11.3, the List of Words You Can Use to Describe a Feeling, and Handout 11.4, the Feelings Wheel.

Finally, the therapist has presented the rationale for between-session work and assigned self-monitoring for the client to complete between sessions. The therapist should provide the client with several copies of the Self-Monitoring of Feelings Form (Handout 11.2), and with a copy of each of the other forms (Handouts 11.1, 11.3, and 11.4) for the client's review.

The Impact of Childhood Abuse on Emotion Regulation

For many people, abuse experiences have a powerful impact on emotional functioning in adulthood. Good parenting provides children with emotion regulation skills, which include the ability to identify feelings, understand their sources, and manage them for optimal functioning. Sexual or physical abuse elicits a range of powerful and confusing feelings. Often childhood abuse survivors have been raised in a family context where caregivers—whether or not they are the abusers—offer poor soothing during times of distress and poor guidance in modulating feelings. Many abuse survivors feel overwhelmed by their emotions or, in contrast, feel numb and unable to experience many or all emotions.

TYPES OF EMOTION REGULATION DIFFICULTIES

Difficulties in emotion regulation vary by person and sometimes by situation. Some people have trouble labeling and identifying their feelings. They may feel either "bad" or "okay," and have little sense of differences between their emotions (e.g., anxiety vs. sadness). Other people lack an understanding of what triggers their feelings. It may seem that their emotions randomly come "out of the blue" and make no sense. Many people can learn to recognize a "triggering situation," but will have more difficulty knowing what to do with the intense feelings that emerge. Such feelings may be experienced as overwhelming or even dangerous, and people often feel ill equipped to handle them.

THE ROLES OF FEELINGS

Learning how to modulate and attend to feelings is a critical skill, because feelings once managed, serve important roles in effective living. One role of emotions is to serve as guides for action. For example, a feeling of fear should guide us to leave an unsafe situation and take steps to ensure safety. Anxiety can be adaptive, but when chronic and excessive, it floods the ability to differentiate feeling states. It causes people to overreact to situations, or to underreact because they are trying so hard not to overreact.

Feelings also contribute to effectively communicating how one feels and what one needs from others. Some people who have PTSD or have experienced sustained childhood trauma are chronically anxious, angry, or sad, or are so numbed that they cannot use this kind of information. By working on attending to your feelings and modulating them, you will be able to make better use of information from your feelings and to express them more effectively.

Lastly, feelings can be used to inform you about your preferences (likes and dislikes) and to help guide you in the selection of valued life goals. Awareness of feelings includes awareness of positive feelings and, in combination with emotion modulation skills, can enhance your experience of life, your creativity, and your appreciation of yourself.

(continued)

SELF-MONITORING OF FEELINGS

One way to begin learning how to identify feeling states and their triggers is to monitor your feelings in different situations. Using the Self-Monitoring of Feelings Form, you will practice labeling your feelings and identifying the situations and thoughts that trigger those feelings. With your therapist, you will review your completed copies of this form to increase your skills in identifying feelings and their triggers and to build your awareness of the patterns in your feelings. The completed copies of the form will also serve as important data for developing new coping strategies.

Self-Monitoring of Feelings Form

Feeling	Intensity (0–10)	Trigger	Thoughts	Response/coping strategy

List of Words You Can Use to Describe a Feeling

Affectionate	Glad	Relaxed
Afraid	Gloomy	Relieved
Amused	Grateful	Resentful
Angry	Great	Resigned
Annoyed	Guilty	Sad
Anxious	Happy	Safe
Apathetic	Hateful	Satisfied
Apprehensive	Helpless	Secure
Ashamed	Hopeless	Sexy
Bitter	Horrified	Shy
Bored	Hostile	Silly
Calm	Impatient	Strong
Capable	Inadequate	Stubborn
Cheerful	Inhibited	Stuck
Comfortable	Irritated	Supportive
Competent	Isolated	Sympathetic
Concerned	Jealous	Tearful
Confident	Joyful	Tender
Confused	Lonely	Terrified
Contemptuous	Loved	Threatened
Controlled	Loving	Thrilled
Curious	Loyal	Touchy
Defeated	Manipulated	Trapped
Dejected	Manipulative	Troubled
Delighted	Melancholy	Unappreciated
Depressed	Miserable	Uncertain
Desirable	Misunderstood	Understood
Despairing	Muddled	Uneasy
Desperate	Needy	Unfulfilled
Determine	Nervous	Unimportant
Devastated	Numb	Unloved
Disappointed	Out of control	Upset
Discouraged	Outraged	Uptight
Disgusted	Overwhelmed	Used
Disillusioned	Panicky	Useless
Distrustful	Passionate	Victimized
Embarrassed	Peaceful	Violated
Enraged	Pessimistic	Vulnerable
Excited	Pleased	Withdrawn
Frantic	Powerful	Wonderful
Frightened	Prejudiced	Worn out
Frustrated	Pressured	Worried
Fulfilled	Proud	Worthwhile
Furious	Provoked	Wronged
Generous	Put down	Yearning

Feelings Wheel

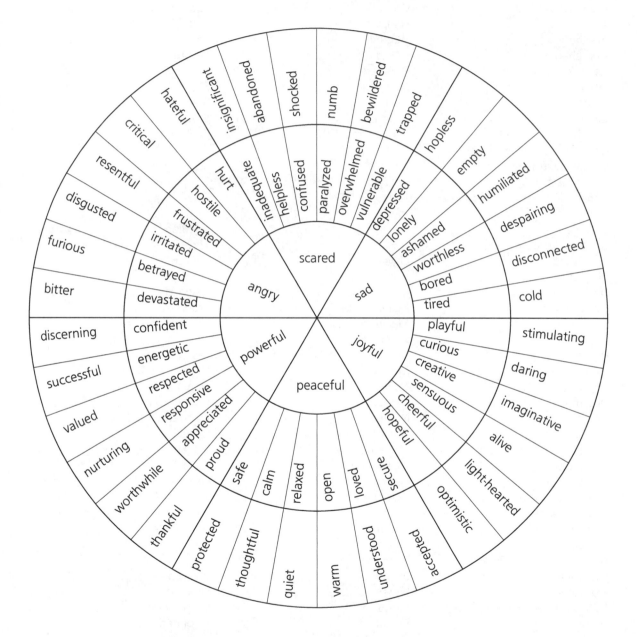

CHAPTER 12

~

SESSION 3
Emotion Regulation

The art of soothing ourselves is a fundamental life skill.
—DANIEL GOLEMAN (1995, p. 57)

OVERVIEW

Clients who have been abused as children appear both to experience more negative feelings and to have more difficulty modulating feelings than those who have not experienced the trauma of childhood abuse. Often such clients will vacillate between being overwhelmed by distress and feeling nothing or numb. Clients often attempt to cope with overwhelming feelings via strategies that make them feel better in the short run, but are ultimately self-destructive. These include using drugs or alcohol to cope and engaging in other self-injurious behaviors (e.g., cutting or bingeing and purging). Session 2 has focused on helping clients know what they are feeling by learning to name and describe them. This exercise allows the clients to experience greater emotional awareness in daily life. The primary goal of Session 3 is to help clients develop and strengthen skills that will enable them to modulate feelings without resorting to self-destructive behaviors. Doing this will enhance their competence and confidence in the process of exploring emotion-laden experiences.

This session focuses on the concept of emotion regulation, with an emphasis on strengthening capacities for self-soothing. The emotion regulation skills proposed here build on Session 2's organization of emotional responses into three channels or modes of experiencing (physiological, cognitive, and behavioral), and exercises are selected to strengthen regulation skills within each channel. The client is also made aware that she can slow down the movement from one mode of experiencing to another, particularly the transition from arousal (physiological) to action (behavior). This is an experience with

149

BOX 12.1
Theme and Curriculum for Session 3: Emotion Regulation

THEME

Individuals learn emotion regulation early in life in the context of relationships with caregivers. Clients who were abused as children often have caregivers who cannot regulate their own negative feelings. Such caregivers may lash out in rage or use alcohol or drugs to make themselves feel better. Thus clients may never have learned positive and effective emotion modulation strategies. Instead, such clients go to extreme measures to avoid difficult feelings (e.g., social withdrawal or substance abuse). Understanding such behaviors as ineffective attempts at emotion regulation is a first step in learning new, positive, and effective strategies to cope with feelings.

PLANNING AND PREPARATION

Review emotion regulation self-report measures to identify patterns that can guide your work with the client. Bring extra copies of the Self-Monitoring of Feelings Form (Handout 11.2). Prepare several examples of emotion regulation strategies for each element of emotion.

AGENDA

- Begin with emotional check-in and review of between-session exercises.
- Elaborate on the concept of emotion regulation.
- Identify and discuss problematic emotions.
- Discuss dissociation (as relevant).
- Identify and evaluate client's current emotion regulation skills.
- Identify and practice adaptive emotion regulation strategies.
- Help client "slow down" in moving from feelings to thoughts and actions.
- Introduce positive emotions and plan pleasurable activities.
- Review misconceptions about emotion regulation work (as necessary).
- Summarize the goals of the session.
- Assign between-session exercises:
    - Complete Self-Monitoring of Feelings Form once a day.
    - Practice focused breathing twice a day.
    - Identify three coping strategies and practice each once a week.
    - Schedule one pleasurable activity per week.

SESSION HANDOUTS

Handout 12.1. Examples of Emotion Regulation Skills for the Three Channels of Emotional Responding
Handout 12.2. Suggestions for Pleasurable Activities: Regulation of Positive Feelings
Additional copies of Handout 11.2. Self-Monitoring of Feelings Form

which traumatized individuals who have PTSD or live in a chronic "crisis state" tend to be unfamiliar. Lastly, the client is introduced to the practice of experiencing positive emotions. For some survivors, strong emotions of any kind can be frightening, even those that are positive. A rationale for the functional value of positive emotions is given, as well as assurances that emotion regulation skills apply to managing positive as well as negative emotions. Box 12.1 outlines the theme and curriculum for Session 3 of treatment.

BEGIN WITH EMOTIONAL CHECK-IN AND REVIEW OF BETWEEN-SESSION WORK

The therapist should begin by reviewing the client's Self-Monitoring of Feelings Forms and inquiring about the client's progress in using focused breathing. The client's self-monitoring can provide useful examples of emotion modulation difficulties that the therapist can highlight throughout this session. If the client did not do the self-monitoring, the therapist should take a few moments to review the rationale for between session work and to fill out the form, using at least two examples.

ELABORATE ON THE CONCEPT OF EMOTION REGULATION

The first step in this session is for the therapist and client to continue discussing the concept of emotion regulation. "Emotion regulation" refers to the responses that individuals develop to help them create an emotional "comfort zone" that is neither too intensely high nor too low, and that as such allows them to function, to learn, and to stay connected with the environment. A prerequisite to effective emotion regulation is the capacity to be aware of and to monitor one's feelings—skills introduced in Session 2. While "emotion regulation" functionally refers to the capacity to manage feelings, it also importantly implies the necessity of a certain degree of emotional awareness. Moreover, emotion regulation is linked to enhanced life engagement, as it directly contributes to improved functioning in interpersonal relationships, parenting activities, and work effort.

Emotion regulation includes our abilities to soothe ourselves and to reduce intense emotional states of all kinds, including fear, anger and sadness. It also includes the ability to raise and sustain feelings that facilitate effective and positive engagement in life. This might include finding humor in a difficult situation, being curious about how things work, feeling yearning to spend time with loved ones, or being satisfied with a job well done.

The therapist should emphasize that emotion regulation includes both reducing overwhelming or negative emotions and increasing positive ones. A well-modulated emotional state varies from person to person and from one circumstance to another. The ideally modulated emotional state is one in which the person is "comfortable in her own skin" and effectively and appropriately engages in her environment, with the people in it, and in the tasks she is pursuing.

Review the Development in Childhood of Emotion Regulation

Before proceeding to skills work on emotion regulation, the therapist should have a detailed discussion about the normative course of development of emotion regulation. We have found that understanding how emotion regulation develops helps clients feel less "crazy" and understand why they behave the way they do. In addition, emphasizing that emotion regulation skills are learned behaviors encourages the clients to learn new, more positive, and more effective ways of managing their moods. The developmental perspective also helps clients avoid feeling discouraged by emphasizing that emotion regulation develops over years in childhood, and that the clients should expect learning new strategies to take some time.

Provide Examples of the Normative Process of Learning Emotion Regulation

Throughout development, a child learns strategies to regulate emotions in two primary ways: through caretakers' responses to the child's moods, and through modeling or observing caretakers' management of their own moods. Abused children often have parents who have deficits in both areas. Such parents are unable to respond or ineffective in responding to their children's needs, and also—sometimes because of their own trauma histories—are unable to cope with their own emotions in a positive and effective way. It is often helpful to provide examples to illustrate to clients how emotion regulation strategies develop in the context of normative child–caretaker relationships. Such examples can easily be linked to the skills clients are learning in the therapy.

The therapist can describe the following (or a similar) scenario. Consider a situation in which a 4-year-old child who is climbing a jungle gym in the playground slips and falls. The child starts crying. What does the child's caretaker do? The caretaker runs to the child and helps the child get up. He or she asks the child, "Did you hurt yourself? Where does it hurt?", and inspects the child for physical injury. Finding no real damage but realizing that the child has a scraped knee and was scared by the fall, the caretaker might say while holding and comforting the child, "I know, I know, it's scary to fall like that. I know your knee hurts. But I'm here; it will be okay." The caretaker might rinse out the scrape with some water. Once the child calms down, the caretaker might ask, "Do you want to climb the jungle gym again?" If the child is hesitant, the caretaker might say, "Do you want me to help you climb?" Then the caretaker might stand behind the child so that the child feels safe while climbing.

This scenario provides an illustration of a caretaker acting as an external regulator of the child's emotional experience. The caretaker's guidance also acts as instruction to the child, who, by this example, will learn how to manage his or her own distress over time. This example includes the prerequisite presence of emotional awareness in the caretaker for the child. The caretaker is aware of the child's feelings and reactions, and provides labels for them ("It's scary to fall like that" and "I know your knee hurts"). The caretaker also signals acceptance of the child's expression of these feelings by naming and thus verbally "echoing" them, rather than ignoring or censoring them. The caretaker monitors the child's emotions from the first instant after the fall, as he or she holds the child (bodily soothing and comforting), evaluates the situation and takes action ("It's not too serious; let's rinse the scrape out"), and finally guides the child back to and monitors any hesitation ("Do you want me to help you climb?"). By encouraging the child to climb on the jungle gym again, the caretaker facilitates reengagement in a pleasurable activity and the resolution of any remaining fear by helping the child confront rather than avoid the source of the misadventure.

A child's capacity for emotion modulation grows out of such experiences. Over time, the child internalizes lessons in managing distress. Children learn various strategies to soothe themselves: physiological strategies to create body comfort (e.g., focused breathing, stretching); cognitive strategies (e.g., telling themselves it is going to be all right, planning solutions); and behavioral strategies (implementing an action plan, confronting rather than avoiding). Finally, the example above illustrates the presence of strong emotional support, suggesting that requests for help will be met and so encouraging a final behavioral strategy: recruitment of social support. The caretaker is giving the child a message that "If you are upset, someone will listen to you and help you feel better." By asking if the child needs help, the caretaker is also teaching the child, "If you need help, let someone who cares about you know." And by standing behind the child while he or she climbs, the caretaker is teaching the child recruitment of social support: "You can rely on others to give you help if you ask for it."

Discuss the Impact of Abuse on Development of Emotion Regulation Behaviors

How might this example be different for a child whose caretakers are abusive? We can envision a number of scenarios in response to that question. The therapist can provide examples as relevant to the client's own personal experiences in childhood. Often the current patterns of emotion management that the client reports have parallels to those she experienced and observed in her caretaking environment. A couple of common scenarios are described below.

For example, an abused child is often also neglected. In that case, there may not be a caretaker around at all in the playground example. Another possibility is that the child's caretaker, even if present, may respond angrily to the child and say, "Stop being a baby. You are fine. Stop crying." The caretaker is thus not acknowledging the child's feelings and not helping the child identify these feelings. If the child actually runs to such a caretaker, the caretaker may push the child away. Or the caretaker may dismiss the child due to being incapacitated from depression or substance use. Yet another maladaptive response by the caretaker may be hitting or punishing the child who is crying in this example. The child then learns that his or her feelings are not important and that when they are expressed, they will bring negative responses from others.

Abuse survivors often have not developed the ability to recognize their feelings, avoid certain feelings altogether, or engage in self-destructive behaviors when feelings seem overwhelming or unavoidable. Such clients often do not understand why they behave the way they do and cannot see a connection between their feelings and behaviors. When clients begin to see that many of their behaviors are learned responses from childhood, they begin to feel "sane" and develop some compassion for themselves.

Discuss the Impact of Emotion Regulation Problems on Parenting Skills (as Relevant)

Another area to explore with clients is their own behavior as caretakers. Clients who have been abused as children are at higher risk of abusing their own children. Although most abuse survivors do not abuse their children, they often worry about behaving toward their children in ways that their parents behaved toward them. They often struggle with the question of how best to parent their children. They do not want to repeat their own parents' mistakes, but do not know how to behave differently. When their children are distressed and crying, clients may feel overwhelmed and helpless. When their children are angry, clients may feel vulnerable and victimized. Rather than helping their children learn to regulate their own feelings, clients who were abused as children find themselves reliving their own histories through their role as parents.

The therapist can provide a case example from our work (or his or her own) about such a situation. A client named Judy had parents who belittled and made fun of her whenever she cried. Her earliest memory of this dated from when she was 5 years old. Judy was an overweight child and would often be teased at school about this. One day, walking home from kindergarten, some older boys followed her, teased her for being overweight, and laughed when she tried to run away. She arrived home in tears. Her mother's response was to say angrily, "Look at Judy; she's such a baby. Boo-hoo-hoo." When Judy cried more, her mother threatened punishment: "If you don't stop crying, I will give you something to cry about." As a result, Judy learned quickly not to cry or to show when she was hurt, afraid, or vulnerable in any way. She learned this so thoroughly that she developed a very "thick skin" and had difficulty recognizing any feelings of vulnerability in herself. She also developed little tolerance for vulnerability in others. She had internalized her mother's punitive coping style and now inflicted it on those around her, including her daughter. When her daughter cried, she found herself getting angry and wanting to yell at her.

When viewed in the context of her developmental history, Judy's response to her daughter was not surprising. Judy was merely repeating what she learned from her own parents and applying the same rules to her daughter that she applied to herself. By learning in therapy how children develop emotion modulation skills, Judy became able to understand herself and her behavior better. As she learned to recognize her own feelings, she was able to identify how her daughter's behavior triggered her own history. She was then better equipped to differentiate her daughter's feelings from her own feelings and history. By understanding that emotion modulation skills are something learned, Judy became empowered to respond to her daughter in a way that would teach her emotional modulation skills, rather than feeling victimized and overwhelmed in the face of her daughter's behavior.

IDENTIFY AND DISCUSS CLIENT'S PROBLEMATIC EMOTIONS

The therapist can begin by reviewing the completed Self-Monitoring of Feelings Form with the client, noting which feelings seem to be problematic, and identifying any patterns. Are there feelings that seem to emerge repeatedly (anxiety, anger, depression)? Are there situations that typically trigger these feelings? And how does the client typically cope with her feelings? Some clients may have difficulty with this process because they are not used to considering/naming their feelings, and because their coping strategies are not intentional but occur automatically.

The therapist can talk with the client about each example on the sheet and help her more clearly and fully consider the questions above. Listed below are negative emotions that are often chronically experienced by survivors. The therapist can select for discussion those emotions with which the client is particularly burdened. The information below provides a starting point for discussing these feelings. It includes information about the adaptive functional roles emotions play, how trauma conspires to create dysregulation of these emotions, and what can be done to bring these feelings "back in line" or into synchrony with the client's goals of adaptive and healthy functioning. The aims here are to help the client understand (1) why she feels the way she does, so that she becomes less confused and overwhelmed by her feelings; (2) that these feelings have an important and possibly beneficial presence in her life; and (3) that a focused goal of the treatment will be to have the client learn to master and modulate her feelings. In the descriptions below, we have identified the coping strategies that we have found a "good match" for modulating the particular emotions, and that we use in this treatment. All of these strategies are described in this chapter and later chapters on STAIR sessions.

Anxiety

Anxiety is a state of arousal that signals danger. It is common among trauma survivors because it is typically generated by experiences that are unpredictable, uncontrollable, or unfamiliar—the very characteristics of a trauma. Anxiety has an adaptive function, which is to ensure readiness for coping with an unidentified danger. It informs us to stop what we are doing, in order to attend and plan for response to an imminent danger. This experience of "heightened alert" occurs chronically and without evident purpose among trauma survivors. This may be because there are multiple, unidentified traumatic reminders in the environment that trigger anxiety, or because the trauma has caused the survivors to psychologically and biologically adapt to and persist at an anxious set point.

The state of chronic "anxious apprehension" is exhausting. It has been described as having one's feet simultaneously on both the gas and brake pedals of a car: The individual is aroused and ready to go, but resisting the initiation of action. When the physiological arousal initiated by anxiety is used toward some action (e.g., fight or flight), the arousal is hardly noticed; indeed, the arousal and the action flow as one. If no action is or can be taken, however, the arousal "idles" and continues uncomfortably until it (and the individual) is exhausted. Accordingly, it is easy to see why effective modulation of anxiety involves the physiological reduction of arousal (e.g., focused breathing), the evaluation of thoughts ("I am safe here"), and the selection of behaviors that integrate arousal and movement. Indeed, one of the most important and long-term goals of the treatment is the perfect antidote to anxiety—that is, to replace feelings of helplessness and uncertainty with competence and confidence.

Anger

Anger is a feeling that typically occurs among people both with and without trauma histories, and it is a justified response to abuse. Anger is adaptive when it prepares us for active coping (fight), invigorates and sustains our actions, and fuels a healthy sense of power. However, anger becomes problematic when it is misdirected toward people or situations *unrelated* to the trauma, or expressed as violence toward self (e.g., self-injury) or others (e.g., physical assault). Additionally, the intensity of anger, even when it is warranted, can do harm to important relationships or interfere with valued support from others. Misplaced or intense anger, particularly when it leads to destructive behaviors, can have long-term negative social and legal consequences.

In order to use anger effectively, its presence must be recognized, modulated, and appropriately directed. Anger management strategies often include the combined recognition and delay of its expression (counting to 10, leaving the situation); reduction of its intensity (focused breathing, exercising, going for a run); appraisal of the outcome of expressing the anger ("What will be the result of this action? Is it consistent with my goals?"); and appraisal of the accuracy of the source of the anger ("At whom am I angry? What in this situation has made me angry?") Skills in the ability to discriminate between feelings and goals, particularly interpersonal goals, are the topics of several sessions (Sessions 6–8).

Depression

In contrast to anxiety, which is a state of high negative emotion, depression is a state of low negative emotion. It is a sustained state of absence of pleasure and excitement, and of disengagement from the world. Whereas anxiety is a state of heightened readiness to respond, depression is a state of giving up the attempt to cope. It is associated with the view that nothing can be done and no effective action can be taken. Despite their contrasting characteristics, many people experience both anxiety and depression in alternating fashion. A person may become highly anxious in anticipation of a feared or threatening event, but may then give up in depression or become depressed when the outcome of the event is negative.

Depression typically results from experiences of failure or loss. It is not surprising that depression is so often associated with chronic abuse by caretakers. Survivors of such abuse often reason that it happened because they deserved it—that they failed in some way, or even that they failed to protect themselves, regardless of the reason for the abuse. In addition, sexual or physical abuse is essentially a form of loss. Those abused by caretakers have been psychologically abandoned and have experienced several losses, including loss of safety, security, and love. Repeated, inescapable physical or sexual abuse also contributes to a sense of loss of mastery and control. Abuse survivors have often experienced situations where they could not control their circumstances or create other circumstances where they could feel safe, be free from suffering, or obtain important nurturance or human warmth and connection.

Several activities in this treatment are intended to counter depression. The client is prompted to recognize that her early circumstances—which more than justified her depression—no longer apply to her current situation. The client now has the opportunity to experience mastery of her environment, and to seek safety and human connection. The reality of this proposal is demonstrated in the treatment through the creation of experiences of safety, mastery, and pleasure. This includes the active role playing in sessions of alternative experiences; revision of interpersonal schemas; intentional efforts at experiencing pleasure; and the provision of energy, nurturance and support in the therapeutic alliance. General mastery is demonstrated through growing emotional and social competence. Mastery of symptoms and of the client's trauma history in particular result from the successful completion of narrative work.

DISCUSS DISSOCIATION (AS RELEVANT)

Dissociation should be introduced in this session for those clients who experience it. Therapist and client will be familiar with the client's tendencies to dissociate as a result of the evaluation. For clients who experience dissociation, a discussion of its nature and function can be provided as follows.

"Dissociation" is an experience in which a person is cognitively and emotionally removed from the current environment. Dissociation is not a feeling, but rather an automatic response to overwhelming feeling. It is a protective response in which the individual "escapes" from the pain or intensity of an emotion that is unbearable. Dissociation is most frequently a response to fear, anxiety, or acute nonspecific distress. It is a reaction that is fairly unique to traumatic situations—uncontrollable, unavoidable, and threatening circumstances from which physical escape is not possible.

Dissociation may be seen by the clinician and experienced by the client as an emotional "shutting down" where the client shifts from a feeling state into an affectless one. In the cognitive dimension, a client may lose touch with a sense of being present in the "here and now"; she may perceive herself as either somewhere else or "nowhere." Dissociation has a protective function but also has a substantial cost, in that the individual loses touch with present reality, which can put her in greater danger or can delay a response that would be effective in the moment but will have little value later. Most important, dissociation is often reported as a distressing experience in and of itself and can be deeply disturbing and disorienting.

The intervention for dissociation is essentially prevention. The ability to effectively modulate feelings will reduce the risk and the need for dissociation. Although dissociation may have been the only possible coping response for the client during her childhood abuse, her life circumstances have changed, and it is likely that other forms of emotion management will now be more effective. In addition, in the absence of the opportunity to learn other strategies, the client may have become overreliant on dissociation, so that it is now a response of habit rather than necessity. The emotions that tend to "trigger" dissociation, as well as particular individuals and situations that tend to provoke it, can be identified and tracked with the Self-Monitoring of Feelings Form. The strengthening of modulation capacities, particularly in regard to "triggering" emotions, should then reduce dissociative responses.

IDENTIFY AND EVALUATE CLIENT'S CURRENT EMOTION REGULATION SKILLS

Review Negative Mood Regulation Assessment

The next step is to have the client identify her own emotion modulation strategies. Before this session, the therapist should review the client's results on the Generalized Expectancy for Negative Mood Regulation (NMR) Scale or other self-report measures of emotion modulation. Thus the client can be given information about her relative strengths and weaknesses in physiological strategies, cognitive strategies, behavioral/social support strategies, or any other forms of emotion modulation relevant to the client. The therapist and client can use their selected measure as a basis for continuing to build on skills already present and to identify areas of vulnerability. If scores on cognitive strategies such as self-talk are relatively strong, the client can be made aware that she has a skill in this domain and can explore ways in which such strategies can be applied more often and in more varied situations. In a similar fashion, if a client does not have or is not using emotion regulation skills in other areas of emotional responding (physiological or behavioral), these potential resources can be brought to the client's attention as a first step in developing skills in these areas.

Review the Self-Monitoring of Feelings Form

The Self-Monitoring of Feelings Form should also be used as a source of information about the client's typical emotion management strategies. The therapist can talk with the client about each example on the sheet and help her identify how she responds to each identified feeling. Some clients may have difficulty with this process because their coping strategies are not intentional, but automatic and unconscious.

Elicit Examples of Modulation Strategies

If a client has difficulty coming up with examples, it is sometimes helpful to ask, "What do you do to make yourself feel better when you feel bad?" The therapist can then work with the client to make a list of the different things she does to make herself feel better. These activities are the ways she attempts to regulate her emotions. Once the client provides a few examples, the therapist can start from the beginning and help her evaluate the strategies used. This process can be facilitated by asking, "Did doing X make you feel better?" If the client did feel better, the therapist can move on to evaluate the broader consequences of the strategy. How long did the client feel better? Were there any negative consequences to this strategy? Evidence from the client's life can be used to determine whether this is a useful, effective strategy for regulating emotions.

Identify Specific Strategies for Each Channel of Emotional Responding

The therapist and client can use examples from the Self-Monitoring of Feelings Form to identify the three channels of emotion responding for each example. This process will facilitate understanding the client's primary ways of coping with negative feelings. The therapist should work with the client to connect her coping strategies to the three channels of emotional responding reviewed in Session 2 (see Handout 12.1). For example, the client's response to a work difficulty can be broken down into the three channels. The client is unjustly criticized by a coworker in a large meeting. Her heart starts beating faster, she gets shaky, and she finds herself sweating and breathing quickly (physiological); she becomes self-critical and catastrophizes (cognitive); then she shuts down and withdraws, saying nothing for the rest of the meeting (behavioral).

Identify Timing of Strategies

Identifying and evaluating the client's emotion modulation strategies should also involve investigating *when* the client uses the strategies. Many clients are very avoidant in coping with their emotions. As a result, rather than engaging in emotion modulation strategies when they first start feeling distressed, they wait until they are completely overwhelmed and they have no choice but to deal with their feelings. By learning to identify what they are feeling when they start having the feeling, such clients can learn to use coping strategies before being overwhelmed. For example, a client may be feeling anxious after having a very difficult day at work. If she recognizes that she is feeling anxious, she can decide to do something after work that will make her feel better. For example, she may call a good friend and ask her to go for coffee, or go for a walk in the park. If the client does not recognize that she is feeling anxious, or if she ignores or discounts her feelings, she may choose to do something that doesn't make her feel better and, in fact, may make her feel worse. Identifying feelings while they are still at relatively low intensities helps the client manage them successfully.

IDENTIFY AND PRACTICE
ADAPTIVE EMOTION REGULATION STRATEGIES

The next component of the session is to help clients develop new emotion regulation strategies. Interventions can be targeted at any one channel, with the expectation that they will have an impact on the other channels as well. Clients will differ in terms of the channel in which it is easiest for them to intervene; it is best to begin where clients are most skilled and then help them develop skills in other channels. It is very important to make clear to clients that these and other affect modulation skills are *not* designed to cover over or avoid feelings, but to improve the clients' ability to manage emotions in a more positive and effective way. Below, we review examples of coping strategies for each channel of emotional responding. Obviously, most strategies target more than one channel. Several strategies are listed under each element. A therapist and client can select the ones that work best for the particular client and add any that come to their attention. Both flexibility and practice in application are key ingredients to improved coping.

Physiological Strategies

Many different techniques are effective in targeting the physiological channel of emotion. These include focused breathing, progressive muscle relaxation, self-hypnosis, and mindfulness-based techniques such as meditation. Because each of these techniques has been described in detail by other authors, we do not go into more detail here. However, a key aspect to all of these modulation strategies is that they must be practiced regularly and in nonstressful circumstances. One of the most common problem clients have in learning body-based regulation exercises is that clients tend to implement them only under stress. This is a difficult circumstance in which to learn. The clients are burdened with simultaneously trying to remember how a skill works while managing their overwhelming feelings. Skills need to be practiced regularly and in relatively relaxed and quiet conditions, so that they become ingrained and automatic behavior patterns that require little effort to initiate under stress. In a triggering situation, a client should only have one task: managing her distress. The skills are intended to be resources that can be immediately recruited and automatically initiated.

We have included a list of references in Appendix A for therapists and clients interested in expanding their repertoire of strategies in this area. This is also a good time to review with clients their practice of focused breathing and any difficulties that have come up since it was introduced.

Cognitive Strategies

Cognitive strategies provide significant methods for coping with distress. Of particular relevance is the stress reaction that results from thoughts relating to the trauma experience. Since reminders of their traumatic experiences cannot be completely controlled by clients, methods for confronting the feelings and thoughts associated with these events will be beneficial for preventing the clients from feeling overwhelmed when they are presented with a reminder. Previous authors have written in detail about cognitive strategies (Burns, 1999; Resick & Schnick, 1996).

Attention Shifting

One cognitive strategy we use with clients is attention shifting. That is, when clients recognize they are having a trauma-related thought, they acknowledge it and then make the decision to shift their attention to something else. For many clients, this works best if the attention shifting involves a change in activity as well. For example, a client has an intrusive thought while she is in her office writing a report for work. She is taught to acknowledge the thought to herself and then get up and take a moment to water her office plants. She is not avoiding the thought, because she is acknowledging it, but she is choosing to shift her attention away from that thought. Examples of activities that can be used to shift attention include cleaning the house, calling a friend, planning a vacation, recalling pleasant past events, and counting backward by sevens.

Positive Self-Statements

An additional cognitive strategy we commonly use with clients is to create a list of positive self-statements that can be used to counter negative cognitions. For example, a client who is very self-critical may generate a counterstatement such as "I am doing the best I can." Material from the client's self-monitoring sheets should be used to determine areas of negative self-talk that could be countered with more helpful statements. For example, many clients report fearful cognitions about experiencing and expressing feelings. A client may report cognitions such as these:

> "If I let myself get angry, I will lose control and become abusive."
> "If I show my true feelings, my partner will think I am weak and will not love me."
> "Crying is pathetic."
> "It doesn't matter what I feel. No one cares."

Once such cognitions are identified, the client can generate examples of positive self-statements such as these:

> "It is okay to feel angry. It is what I do with my anger that is important."
> "I can manage my anger in a positive, effective way."
> "Expressing my feelings is courageous."
> "By expressing my feelings, I enable my partner to be more supportive of me."

Each client will compose a list of positive self-statements that directly counter the negative thoughts surfacing both within and outside therapy. For example, if a client receives a bad test grade, instead of resorting to the opinion that she is inherently unintelligent, an alternate self-statement can resemble the following: "It is too bad that I didn't do well this time. I will have to study harder next time and get a better grade, just like I have done before." Every time a negative thought enters her mind, the client is instructed to generate a positive counterstatement. A virtual reservoir of positive statements will increase the probability of positive—or at least less catastrophic—reinterpretations of events. This will enable clients to stem more extreme negative reactions.

Positive Imagery

Another cognitive strategy is to use positive imagery. Such work has proven useful in effecting positive emotional states. This method requires the evocation of specific memories or images that induce positive (nonhurtful or, preferably, pleasure-producing) thoughts or feelings. These images are to be as detailed as possible so that each detail can serve as a retrieval cue, thereby increasing the ease with which these images are recalled. During times of distress, clients are to summon these images in order to combat the negative effects of invading thoughts or circumstances and to induce more positive emotional states.

All of these techniques can help clients stop negative thoughts from spiraling into fully distressing reminders of their trauma. In order to do this, clients first must learn to identify the thoughts that accompany their feelings. This can be done through use of the Self-Monitoring of Feelings Form. Once this goal is accomplished, clients may then proceed to practice various techniques for addressing these thoughts.

Behavioral Strategies

Behavioral emotion modulation strategies are the easiest for clients to identify, because they include anything people do in everyday life to make themselves feel better. Such strategies may include calling a friend, watching a movie, preparing for a meeting, going for a run, taking a bath, or making a favorite food.

Time Out

"Time out" in STAIR means leaving the environment that is creating the emotional disturbance for a set period of time. This is not to be used as an avoidance strategy, but as a modulation strategy. This means that the client's intention is to return to the setting or goal once her feelings have returned to baseline or have settled to a level that allows her to reengage effectively. In some cases, time out lasts for only a few minutes; in other cases, it may last for days or weeks. High-distress reactions often occur unexpectedly, and taking time out occurs relatively immediately upon exposure to a trigger. For these circumstances, the client can prepare herself with particular sentences or behaviors to use on an as-needed basis. Clients may rely on phrases such as "I can't continue this conversation any longer, but why don't we plan to resume later?" when they feel their anger or anxiety rising. If a reaction is very intense (say, a strong anger reaction) and the words that will spill out will be negative or hurtful, the client can do a short time out from the conversation (by counting to 10) or a longer one (by simply keeping quiet and listening). If a client is beyond words and moving into aggressive action, the client needs to be ready simply to leave the room or location. The potential embarrassment of such abrupt behavior is far less than that which follows letting loose with a verbal tirade or getting into a fight.

Replacement Behaviors

Clients often find themselves engaging in old, ingrained emotion modulation strategies automatically and in a fixed, repeated pattern. Such patterns are hard to break, and the drive to move into such an action is nearly unstoppable. These actions include reaching for a drink or a pill, cutting, bingeing on food, or engaging in unconsidered and/or unsafe sex. These strategies are often successful in their aim, which is rapid emotional relief. This success reinforces the pattern. Still, a client pays a high price in both the short- and long-term consequences of such strategies. One method of breaking such a behavioral habit is to replace it with another "action pattern" that can be speedily introduced, has the same end result (reduced arousal), but does not cause the collateral damage. Rather than engaging in compulsive behaviors, the client can engage in other activities that have their own fixed action pattern. These may include cleaning the house, running the jogging circuit several times, returning items that have been on loan, mowing the lawn, washing the car, jumping rope, or going to the gym.

HELP CLIENT "SLOW DOWN" IN MOVING FROM FEELINGS TO THOUGHTS AND ACTIONS

As described in Session 2 (see Chapter 11), awareness of feelings creates options. If a client realizes that "this is what anger feels like," the awareness creates a space between the feeling and the need to act. In that space the client can observe the feeling and can choose to modulate it, act on it, or let it go. The analysis of emotions as occurring in three distinct channels can be used to reinforce this idea. The physiological arousal of anxiety, fear, or anger need not lead directly or automatically to actions or even to specific thoughts. Those who have been abused or exposed to repeated unpredictable violence have often experienced sustained or frequent "crisis states" in which arousal is followed immediately and automatically by an action response. This tendency remains, so that even when the trauma or danger is past, arousal leads automatically to an action response without pause. As a result, an assessment of the value or desirability of the action is not possible.

The client can "slow down" the move from feeling to action or from feeling to thought through consideration of the three channels of emotional response: *Each of the component responses can be separated from the others.* The actual ability to do this can be developed and strengthened by using the various channel-specific strategies described above. Focused breathing can help reduce arousal. The impulse to act can be diminished by thinking, "I don't need to act," or "I have felt like this before with this person." These thoughts allow a client to step back from the emotion rather than being immersed or lost in it. Notably, these kinds of thoughts are different from thoughts such as "I really want to tell him off," which might work to heighten arousal and the tendency toward action. Lastly, if the tendency to act as the result of a negative emotion cannot be suspended, it can be transformed. So, for example, a move toward someone to hit him or her can be transformed into a handshake. If the tendency to speak cannot be suspended, saying something positive or neutral may slow down or diffuse a negative outcome.

INTRODUCE POSITIVE EMOTIONS AND PLAN PLEASURABLE ACTIVITIES

Review Rationale for Experiencing Positive Emotions

This session also introduces the goal of experiencing positive emotions through seeking out pleasurable activities. Emotional numbing is a frequent partner to hyperarousal, reflecting the "all-or-nothing" emotional responsivity of some trauma survivors. Some individuals describe being numb or "emotionally dead" most of the time, with occasional extreme reactions to mild stressors. The final task of this session is to highlight that emotional modulation means not only working toward reducing distress, but having opportunities to increase experiences of positive emotions. The therapist should review reasons to engage in pleasurable activities.

Positive Emotions Are a Reward for Distress Reduction Efforts

The therapist should convey to the client that emotional numbing may protect her from disabling arousal, but it also decreases or eliminates her opportunities for taking pleasure in ordinary events. People who have experienced chronic trauma often have only a limited capacity to respond to their environment, including the positive aspects of day-to-day life. Increasing skill at distress reduction will make time and energy available to the client to open up and engage in positive events. This may provide the client with a "reward" for her more taxing efforts in distress reduction activities.

Positive Emotions Are a Form of Distress Management

Developing skills in experiencing positive emotions is itself a form of distress reduction. Positive feelings can extinguish, cancel, inhibit, or attenuate negative feelings. Amusement can extinguish anxiety. A joke can cancel anger. Feelings of tenderness for someone can modulate disappointment.

Positive Emotions Direct Action

Just as distressing feelings of fear or anxiety do, positive emotions predispose a person to action. Positive feelings also support the development of discipline and perseverance, which are required for the completion of long-term goals. Enthusiasm for a particular goal or accomplishment keeps a person working on a variety of tasks, which are not of great interest in themselves but are necessary to reach the desired goal.

Positive Emotions Enhance Motivation and a Sense of Future Possibilities

As the preceding point indicates, positive emotions can be mptivation enhancers. Indeed, they can ultimately give people the mental and physical energy to tap into their creativity and to begin experiencing the possibility of developing and pursuing long-term life goals. This latter possibility may be overwhelming and intimidating to a person with chronic PTSD who is just trying to get through the day at hand; it may best be introduced at a later session.

Positive Emotions Produce Greater Self-Awareness and Connection to Others

Positive emotions inform us about our preferences and give us confidence in our decision making. Feelings of warmth toward certain other people inform us that we might want to spend more time with them. Feelings of enthusiasm for certain activities or places confirm for us what we would like to do or where we would like to go. Positive feelings provide us with a surer sense of who we are and greater certainty about personal decisions. Similarly, access to positive feelings increases attunement to others' needs and wants, and enhances our capacity to empathize with others more fully. The ability to read others' "social signals" helps us to negotiate the first steps in relationships and to maintain them successfully.

Identify Pleasurable or Positive Activities

A general strategy for modulating mood through enhancing positive emotions is to schedule pleasurable activities. The therapist can begin this process by simply asking clients what they enjoy doing or what things they do to make them feel happy. Although many clients can answer this question, this may not be as simple as it sounds for other clients. Some individuals may respond, "I don't know," or "I don't really enjoy anything." They may really need to take time in or out of session to think about this more. Is there something new they have always wanted to try? If such a client can't imagine enjoying anything, she should be asked to think back to a time in her life when she did get pleasure out of activities and start from there. The therapist may provide suggestions or resource guides as a way to get the client thinking about specific activities (see Handout 12.2).

REVIEW MISCONCEPTIONS
ABOUT EMOTION REGULATION WORK (AS NECESSARY)

Some clients resist learning emotion regulation. This resistance often stems from fears or misconceptions about its nature and consequences. Emotion regulation is not intended to be or produce any of the circumstances below. The therapist should review each point as necessary for a particular client.

Distress Reduction Requires Rejection or Denial of Feelings

Some clients think that modulating emotions means not having them at all, or if they have them, not showing them. The developmental perspective can help clients understand that emotions, both positive and negative, are typical parts of being human. What clients are trying to learn, therefore, is not to turn off their emotions, but to cope with them in healthier, more effective ways.

Distress Reduction Trivializes Feelings

Some clients feel as if their pain is so great that using some type of "coping skill" will merely trivialize it. If so, the therapist should take time to make clear that the aim of the strategies is to give a client control over her feelings, and some choice in how and when to tolerate distress. We are not suggesting that simply thinking positive thoughts will make everything fine, but it does offer a way out of unproductive ruminating or self-criticism and escalating emotional distress.

Distress Reduction Invalidates Abuse Trauma

Even if clients come to believe that these strategies could make them feel better and improve their lives, they may need to hold onto their suffering as a testament to what was done to them. They may think, "If I feel good, it means the abuse was not that bad." The therapist will need to assess this resistance and gently address it, emphasizing that obtaining relief from suffering does not trivialize or invalidate it. In treatment, we commonly use the example of a scraped knee. We ask such clients, "What would you do if you had a scraped knee?" Clients will easily answer that they would clean it, put a bandage on it if necessary, and take an over-the-counter medication for the pain if necessary. We then ask, "What if the reason you had the scraped knee was that someone pushed you? Would you treat your knee any differently? Would you go without relief?" Clients will of course answer that they would not. The therapist can then make the analogy that if a client were pushed and fell and scraped her knee, putting some cream on the wound would not take away the right to be angry at the person who pushed.

Positive Emotions Are Inconsistent with Life Experience

In response to being asked to engage in pleasurable activities, some clients respond, "I don't have enough time." For clients who view engaging in pleasurable activities as a luxury, the therapist will need to reframe it as an essential part of recovery from childhood abuse and discuss in more detail how the clients can carve out some time. Other clients may say, "I don't have enough money to do anything nice for myself." For that reason, it is important that at least some of the activities scheduled should not cost money. The therapist should work with each client to create a list of at least three pleasurable activities she can incorporate into her life. The client can expand on this list of ideas over the course of treatment and keep it handy. The therapist explains that since the client is doing hard work by facing distressing aspects of her life, she should also take the opportunity to reward herself by building in positive activities. At first this may feel forced, but if she makes the effort in the beginning it will become easier and more natural. This intervention provides a way for clients to expand their range of feelings, with the idea that by allowing for and tolerating negative feelings, the clients will also become more open to positive feelings that have been cut off as a result of avoidance.

Positive Emotions Are Inconsistent with Self-Image

It is important to keep in mind that a client may not feel she deserves to enjoy or nurture herself. If so, the therapist should explore this issue with the client and discuss how feeling like a "bad person" or having low self-worth is a common reaction to childhood abuse and/ or neglect. Not engaging in pleasurable or soothing activities further confirms the client's negative self-image and perpetuates the damaging idea that she is not entitled to positive experiences.

Doing Things to Create Positive Emotions Feels "Fake"

Finally, a client attempting to pursue pleasant activities may report, "It feels fake." If so, the therapist can suggest continuing to do so as an experiment during the treatment. The therapist should explain that low self-esteem and poor self-image are common reactions to abuse. Some clients find the analogy of friendship helpful. The therapist can ask such a client, "If a friend of yours is going through a hard time, and you want to encourage her and make her feel better, what would you do?" The client will answer that she would spend time with the friend doing things they both like to do, maybe buy her a small gift, or the like. The therapist can suggest that the client think of engaging in pleasurable activities for herself similarly: The client is learning to encourage and support herself while she is doing something difficult. Often over time, the client will find that engaging in pleasurable activities begins to feel more natural.

CASE EXAMPLE: MOVING TOWARD EMOTION REGULATION

Cathy was sexually and physically abused by her mother and stepfather. As an adult she experienced overwhelming feelings of sadness and anger, often flying into violent rages, which took a toll on her physically as well as on her relationships. She recalled that her mother and other family members regularly invalidated her feelings. On one occasion, Cathy came home crying after being teased at school. Rather than comforting her, Cathy's stepfather slapped her saying, "No daughter of mine will be a sissy! Next time you better fight back!" Cathy claimed that she never cried in front of anyone in her family again.

THERAPIST: In the last session, we talked about starting to identify feelings—that is, learning to know what you are feeling when you are feeling it. In this session, we are focusing on emotion modulation—that is, how you cope with negative or difficult feelings. So let's start with a general question: When you feel bad, what do you do to make yourself feel better?

CATHY: I don't know. I feel bad most of the time. Nothing I do really seems to work; that's why I am here. I feel hopeless.

THERAPIST: I can understand why you feel that way, given everything you have tried. Part of what we will be doing is helping you learn new ways of coping with difficult feelings that are more effective. But before we do that, we need to understand what you do now when you feel badly. Let's start with something you brought up earlier in the session—the negative evaluation you received at work. On the Self-Monitoring of Feelings Form, you said that after you met with your boss, you felt really depressed and hopeless.

CATHY: Yes, that's how I feel most of the time. But I felt even worse after I received that bad review.

THERAPIST: What was your boss critical about?

CATHY: She said that she and the other partners noticed I had been late for work a lot. She said my work had lots of errors in it, was often late, and wasn't the quality they were used to from me.

THERAPIST: Let's start by identifying what you were feeling when your boss said this. Do you remember last week when we talked about the three channels of emotion—physiological, cognitive, and behavioral? What did you feel in your body while your boss was speaking?

CATHY: I felt anxious as soon as she started, because I knew the review wasn't going to be good. My heart was racing, and I had butterflies in my stomach.

THERAPIST: What were you thinking?

CATHY: I thought, "I've screwed up again. I can't do anything right. I should just quit now before they fire me."

THERAPIST: And how were you behaving in the meeting?

CATHY: I just sat there and didn't say anything. My boss even asked if anything was going on with me personally that would explain my performance. She actually looked concerned. But I just shook my head no and left. I think it might have come across like I didn't care about the review at all.

THERAPIST: What did you do after you left the meeting?

CATHY: I went back to my office, slammed the door, and punched the wall. One of my colleagues heard me, because he came by to see what was going on. Then I yelled at him and stormed out. I did not show up for work yesterday or today.

THERAPIST: So you were angry.

CATHY: Yes.

THERAPIST: And you did a number of things in response to being upset about your review. You slammed the door, you punched the wall, you yelled at your colleague, and you have avoided going to work.

CATHY: Yes.

THERAPIST: And did these things make you feel better?

CATHY: Yeah, I felt like I was getting back at them. But now I am worried that I will get fired because of how I behaved and because I missed work. I can't lose this job! And I feel guilty, because I actually like and respect my boss a lot, and she was right about what she said. I haven't been performing well at work

THERAPIST: Okay. Well, it's understandable from your history why you responded the way you did. Remember when we talked about the time you were teased at school—the last time you cried in front of your family? What were you told to do?

CATHY: Fight back.

THERAPIST: So, actually, we should be thankful that you had enough self-control not to fight your boss in the meeting. If you had followed your stepfather's example, you would have punched her!

CATHY: I never thought about it that way.

THERAPIST: So let's replay the situation. You are angry because your boss has criticized you. What could you do to make yourself feel better?

SUMMARIZE THE GOALS OF THE SESSION

Not all clients will take to all coping strategies. The therapist should encourage a reluctant client to give things a try, but convey that she can focus on those strategies finds most helpful. Some clients are "doers"; they find it helpful to engage in activities such as making lists of things to do, washing their hair and getting dressed, or watching television. Others are "thinkers"; they cope by telling themselves that their distress will only last for a small while, or by trying to think of happier things. Still others seek social support by going out to dinner with friends or doing something nice for someone. In some cases, the therapist may omit certain skills and encourage others, based on his or her understanding of the client. For example, a very avoidant client may not be encouraged to use attention shifting. We have described these strategies in the form of a handout for the client (Handout 12.1).

ASSIGN BETWEEN-SESSION WORK

For homework, the therapist should have the client continue to fill out the Self-Monitoring of Feelings Form once a day including the section on "Response/coping strategy." The client should also perform focused breathing twice a day, and should identify three coping strategies for emotion modulation that she will practice during the week. We recommend that the client also engage in pleasant event scheduling at least once per week (see Handout 12.2). In assigning homework, it helps if the therapist is as specific as possible. That is, the therapist should help the client identify specific times the homework tasks will be performed and which coping strategies will be practiced. Ideally, the client will also have made verbal commitments in session about which pleasurable activities she will schedule and when.

Examples of Emotion Regulation Skills for the Three Channels of Emotional Responding

THREE CHANNELS OF EMOTION

For the purposes of problem solving, we can think of our emotional experiencing as directed into and expressed through three channels: "physiological," "cognitive," and "behavioral." The physiological channel is what you feel physically in your body. For example, when you are feeling anxious, you may notice that your breathing quickens, your heart rate increases, and you sweat or shake. The cognitive channel is what you say to yourself, your thoughts, and the attributions you make. For example, when you are feeling anxious, you may think to yourself, "I'm such a loser," or "I can't trust anyone." These thoughts contribute to and maintain your distress. Finally, the behavioral channel consists of what you actually do in response to the distress. For example, when you are feeling anxious, you may overeat, get into a fight with someone, or distract yourself with another activity.

COPING STRATEGIES FOR EACH CHANNEL

Because these channels are interconnected, intervention can be targeted at any one channel, with the expectation that they will have an impact on the other channels as well. People differ in terms of the channel in which it is easiest for them to intervene. Not all people are helped by all these coping strategies. By trying these strategies, you will find which skills work best for you.

In the physiological channel, focused breathing helps to reduce the bodily symptoms of distress. Other relaxation techniques can also be used to help in this way.

In the cognitive channel, attention shifting can be effective. Examples of attention-shifting activities include cleaning your home, calling a friend, planning a vacation, recalling pleasant past events, and counting backward by sevens. Positive imagery can also be used to intervene in the cognitive channel. This technique involves calling to mind a situation or setting (real or imagined) in which you feel calm and good. To get the maximum benefit from positive imagery, you should make the image as clear as possible by imagining what the place looks like, smells like, and so forth. Another cognitive intervention is making positive self-statements. When your thoughts are self-critical, it can be useful to counteract those negative self-statements by formulating positive responses. For example, in response to the thought "I'm a loser," you may tell yourself, "I'm doing my best."

In the behavioral channel, time out and alternative activities are helpful interventions. Time out involves leaving a stressful or difficult situation for a period of time in order to reduce distress before responding. For example, if you are having a fight with a friend, you can tell your friend that you will finish the discussion with him or her in an hour, and then go out for a walk to give yourself time to calm down. Engaging in alternative activities entails doing a pleasurable or neutral activity to distract yourself from distress.

Suggestions for Pleasurable Activities:
Regulation of Positive Feelings

Emotion regulation includes not only the capacity to reduce overwhelming distress, but also the capacity to enhance positive feelings. Below are some activities that may help you experience and enjoy positive feelings.

Aromatherapy

Bike riding

Browsing in a bookstore

Camping

Cooking

Creating a scrapbook

Dancing

Decorating your living space

Drawing

Exercising

Exploring on the Internet

Gardening

Getting a massage

Getting hair or nails done

Going for a drive

Going hiking

Going on a picnic

Going to a library

Going to a museum

Going to a play or concert

Having lunch/dinner with
   a friend

Jogging

Journal writing

Lifting weights

Lighting candles

Listening to music

Making a collage

Meditating

Painting

"People watching"

Photography

Playing music

Playing with pets or children

Reading

Relaxing in the park

Riding a bus

Singing

Sitting in a coffee shop

Taking a long hot bath

Taking a walk

Taking an interesting class

Talking on the phone with
   a friend

Viewing beautiful scenery

Visiting friends

CHAPTER 13

~

SESSION 4

Emotionally Engaged Living

To the degree that our emotions get in the way of or enhance our ability to think and plan, to pursue . . . a distant goal, to solve problems and the like, they define the limits of our capacity . . . and so determine how we do in life.

—DANIEL GOLEMAN (1995, p. 80)

OVERVIEW

For many abuse survivors, the only alternatives to living a painful and out-of-control life are emotional avoidance, social withdrawal, limited pleasure in daily activities, and severely limited actualization of their potential. In this session, a client is encouraged to identify positive goals for herself, to articulate her desires and wishes, and to consider ways in which she may realize them. Leaving the familiarity of an avoidant lifestyle requires support from the therapist and skills development centered around making sound choices of which goals to attempt, pacing the pursuit of goals, and weighing the costs and benefits of any new experience. The concept of "distress tolerance" and the skills associated with it are introduced as key interventions in this effort.

The concept of distress tolerance may seem counterintuitive to both therapists and clients. As one client said, "I have spent my whole life being distressed. I don't want to tolerate it any more. I want to learn to stop it!" What we have found, however, is that clients are often not tolerating distress when doing so would actually be helpful to them. Rather, they have developed ways of avoiding distress that feels overwhelming and out of control. The primary goal of Session 3 has been to help clients feel empowered by developing coping strategies for emotion regulation. Now that clients are beginning to learn to manage their

173

BOX 13.1
Theme and Curriculum for Session 4:
Emotionally Engaged Living

THEME

This session introduces the counterintuitive idea that tolerating and even accepting some emotional distress can be healthy and advance the client toward improved life functioning. A clear distinction is made between distress that is the result of abuse and distress that is accepted as part of reaching one's chosen goals. This session provides clients with practice in identifying goals, determining the value of this goal in relation to unaviodable distress, and making a decision to reject or accept the goal and attendant distress. Emotion regulation strategies are recruited to manage the distress. Lastly, the client is encouraged to value positive feelings as a guide to goal identification and to engage in "approach behaviors" toward positive life experiences.

PLANNING AND PREPARATION

Review concept of distress tolerance. Bring extra copies of the Self-Monitoring of Feelings Form (Handout 11.2). Prepare several examples of tolerating distress in pursuit of valued goals that may be relevant to your client in the treatment.

AGENDA

- Perform emotional check-in and review of between-session work.
- Present concept of distress tolerance.
- Assess the client's distress tolerance skills.
- Connect distress tolerance to client's goals.
- Present and practice method of assessing pros and cons.
- Match distress reduction strategies to goals.
- Introduce practice of distress tolerance during life's "random moments."
- Discuss role of positive feelings in pursuing goals.
- Prepare client for work on interpersonal problems.

(continued)

BOX 13.1. *(continued)*

- Assign between-session work:
  - Complete Self-Monitoring of Feelings Form once a day.
  - Practice focused breathing twice a day.
  - Identify three emotion regulation strategies relevant to client's needs, and practice one each day.
  - Schedule one pleasurable activity per week.

SESSION HANDOUTS

Handout 13.1. What Is Distress Tolerance and Why Should I Do It?
Additional copies of Handout 11.2. Self-Monitoring of Feelings Form

---

emotions, this session focuses on enabling clients to accept their feelings and tolerate distress for an important purpose: *the pursuit of valued goals.*

Clients will often balk at this idea, for the reasons mentioned above. It is therefore very important for the therapist to link the concept of distress tolerance to the pursuit of valued goals. Clients have often lived with distress that had no discernible purpose or personal value, but was simply the result of having the impulses and the will of others imposed upon them. Now clients are introduced to the idea that tolerating distress not only can at times be healthy itself, but is a process that clients will be asked to engage in to reach goals *they have set for themselves.* Rather than being victims of their distress, clients can choose distress tolerance in order to reach self-identified goals. In addition, and as an extension of the previous session's introduction to positive emotions, this session encourages clients to value positive feelings as a guide to goal identification and to engage in "approach behaviors" toward positive life experiences. Box 13.1 outlines the theme and curriculum for Session 4 of treatment.

PRESENT CONCEPT OF DISTRESS TOLERANCE

The therapist can introduce the idea of distress tolerance as follows:

"Distress tolerance is the ability to endure pain or hardship without resorting to actions or behaviors that are damaging to yourself or others. Distress tolerance is a necessary skill that most of us practice on a daily basis. For example, you practice distress tolerance when you effectively control your anger in confronting a friend who you feel has wronged you. In your work life, successful distress tolerance may involve managing your anxiety when you are receiving a performance review from your supervisor. By managing your anxiety, you can be open to what your supervisor is saying and can calmly assert yourself when you feel he or she is mistaken. Skillful distress tolerance is particularly important during periods when we want to make changes in our lives. Change, by its nature, often creates anxiety, fear, and other strong feelings in ourselves and in those around us. Managing these feelings in order to make the changes that are important to us requires distress tolerance."

Once the therapist has explained what distress tolerance is, the next step is to work with the client to help her understand why she should learn to recognize and tolerate distress. Below, we have outlined some of the reasons we talk about distress tolerance with clients.

1. *Distress is a catalyst.* Distress is a catalyst for change in recovering from childhood trauma. For example, it is often distress that prompts clients to come for treatment. These feelings of distress are signals of what is wrong and indicate areas of the clients' lives that they need to attend to or change. It is important to help clients understand that preparing to make significant changes in life is very likely to involve some anticipatory anxiety and discomfort. If clients do not allow themselves to be in touch with this distress, there will be no motivation to make important changes.

2. *Avoiding distress saps energy.* Clients who were abused as young children have often developed fairly elaborate ways of avoiding distress that involve a great deal of energy to maintain. For example, one client who became very distressed when she was alone at night always worked the night shift. Not only was this draining to her physically, but her schedule also impeded her from developing relationships. She spent her energy organizing her life around avoiding uncomfortable feelings, rather than spending it pursuing things that were important to her.

3. *Avoiding distress restricts positive feelings.* Learning to tolerate more negative, difficult feelings has the benefit of allowing a person to be more open to experiencing positive feelings as well. When clients avoid feelings, these usually include positive as well as negative ones. As a result, many survivors of childhood abuse have a very restricted range of emotions; they often report feeling "numb" and unable to enjoy things in their life.

4. *Avoiding distress interferes with achieving desired goals.* Enduring some degree of distress is necessary if people want to accomplish goals that are important to them. Clients coming to treatment will often have limited their lives and experiences in many ways, in order to avoid distress—and, in the backs of their minds, to reduce their chances of being hurt again as they were hurt as children. This is often most apparent in their interpersonal relationships, particularly their romantic relationships. Abuse survivors were often hurt by caretakers on whom they most depended and with whom they were most vulnerable. Being in an intimate relationship raises these feelings of vulnerability and fears that if they let themselves trust someone, they will be hurt again.

5. *Avoiding distress contributes to PTSD symptoms.* One important treatment goal many trauma clients have is to get rid of their PTSD symptoms. Given that the second half of the present treatment focuses on strategies for PTSD symptom resolution, a reminder of the value of distress tolerance in regard to this goal is relevant. Avoiding trauma memories contributes to the continued presence of PTSD symptoms. Distress about traumatic child-

hood abuse is inevitable, but ignoring or denying this distress or the trauma does not make the distress go away. Although attempts to avoid or escape this distress are understandable, they unfortunately typically result in prolonging and exacerbating pain and suffering. Not having the opportunity to develop coping skills certainly puts one in the position of having both more severe and chronic distress. Learning distress management strategies and confronting the emotional pain of the trauma will lead to an alleviation of this suffering. Indeed, the second part of this treatment program (NST) will require a client to tolerate the distress associated with confronting the traumatic memories, in order to move toward the goal of resolving her PTSD symptoms.

ASSESS CLIENT'S DISTRESS TOLERANCE SKILLS

Identify Successes

The therapist should work with clients to identify specific situations in their lives where they chose to tolerate distress and where doing so produced a positive outcome. All clients have tolerated distress successfully in some aspects of their lives at some time. Often clients can easily identify the areas of their lives where they need work, but have little awareness of areas where they are successful. For example, a client who has managed to complete education or training in a demanding area has had to tolerate and manage her anxiety related to performing on exams. Or a client who has a child has had to tolerate the distress of pregnancy and childbirth. In coming to therapy, a client has tolerated the distress of sharing her abuse history and some of her most intimate feelings with a stranger, in the hopes of feeling better and improving her life. Linking the concept of distress tolerance to the client's past successes will make the concept seem less frightening.

Identify Maladaptive Strategies

Once therapist and client have identified ways in which the client has successfully tolerated distress in the past, the therapist should work with the client to identify ways in which she avoids distress. Examples of this can be drawn from Session 3, in which the client's coping strategies for negative mood regulation have been reviewed. In our experience, clients tend to move between two extremes of tolerating distress: externalizing behaviors and avoidance.

Externalizing Behaviors

Common externalizing behaviors include using alcohol or drugs; self-injurious behaviors, such as cutting, burning, or hitting oneself; binge eating and purging; and unsafe, violent, or aggressive behaviors. Clients whose behaviors in these areas are extreme enough that they put their safety or that of others at risk—such as current alcohol dependence, anorexia, or bulimia—will need to have those issues addressed first. However, many clients with childhood abuse exhibit some of these behaviors and can benefit from this treat-ment as a means by which to resolve these problems.

For example, one patient in our study had the tendency to binge-eat when she became very anxious, including in anticipation of or following a date. Because her binge eating was clearly a reaction to a specific trigger and was not frequent enough to pose a risk to her health, the treatment was appropriate for her. Work on emotion regulation helped her replace binge eating with healthy behaviors, including moderate exercise and calling sup-portive friends. In addition, she accepted that the distress she experienced, if managed in a healthy way, was worth the opportunity to have a social life.

Avoidance

Clients with PTSD symptoms related to childhood abuse have often arranged their lives to avoid reminders (e.g., particular thoughts, feelings, or places) of the abuse. Avoidance of reminders also enables them to avoid confronting distressing feelings associated with the abuse. Clients may report prematurely breaking off relationships when conflict arises, because it makes them so distressed. Clients may also have limited their professional lives by not taking advantage of opportunities or by not advocating for themselves, because of the fear that if they assert themselves they will be harmed. Clients must learn to tolerate distress in order to make changes in their lives and reach goals that are important to them.

CONNECT DISTRESS TOLERANCE TO THE CLIENT'S GOALS

One of the main aims of this treatment is to teach skills for distress tolerance in relation-ship to identified goals. Instead of learning to tolerate distress for its own sake, the empha-sis is on determining whether the client's goals for improving or changing how she functions are important or beneficial enough that tolerating some discomfort and distress in the process of attaining the goals is manageable and worthwhile.

Identify Specific Goals

At this point, the therapist will have at least some idea of what brought the client to treat-ment and what her long- and short-term goals are. In this session, it is important to identify a couple of goals that can be accomplished or can begin being addressed in the treatment in a substantial way.

Some clients may have difficulty identifying specific goals. For example, it is not uncommon for a client to say, "I just want to feel better." While it is likely that the client will feel better by the end of the treatment, it is important for the goals to be specific, so that both the therapist and the client can evaluate whether or not the treatment is succeed-ing. If the client is being vague, the client might ask, "Why do you want to feel better?", "What would be different in your life if you felt better?", or "Describe what you would be doing/who you would be if you felt better." Most clients will have unspoken ideas about

---

BOX 13.2
Examples of Specific Treatment Goals

Asking for a raise

Performing music in front of an audience

Beginning a romantic relationship

Ending a romantic relationship

Finding a new job

Creating better boundaries with mother/
  father

Improving parenting skills

Losing weight

Confronting partner about spending habits

Sharing abuse history with a close friend

Performing poetry in public

Going back to school

Starting an exercise program

Asking someone out on a date

Recontacting an estranged son or daughter

Reestablishing an old friendship

Attending a high school reunion

Helping other trauma survivors

Meeting with a lawyer about custody issues

---

specific ways in which their life would be different if they "felt better." By verbalizing what they hope for, the client can begin to make a list of goals. The client's goals can be of any type in any area of her life. Box 13.2 contains some examples of goals our clients have worked on in treatment.

Clients often have many things they would like to change about themselves and their lives. This is one of the reasons they are in therapy. The greater difficulty will be choosing which goals to work on. The first two priorities in choosing a goal are (1) its importance to a client and (2) the positive consequences of pursuing the goal. In order to identify which goal is most important to the client, the therapist can have her identify what she would change first, which goal is most immediate, or which goal would have the greatest impact on other areas of her life.

PRESENT AND PRACTICE METHOD OF ASSESSING PROS AND CONS

Introduce Method

Assessing pros and cons is a strategy that can aid the client in determining whether it is worth tolerating distress to reach a goal. Assessing pros and cons involves selecting a significantly distressing or anxiety-producing situation related to reaching an important goal, and identifying a comprehensive list of pros and cons of tolerating the situation or the feelings associated with it. The point of this exercise is that the client should not think she is being asked to tolerate distress for no purpose; rather, she should realize that she is learning to tolerate distress because it is inevitable and worth the effort of working toward her goal. The concept of linking the presence of distress with identified goals is particularly important when goals require long-term work and the benefit or relief is not immediate.

Identify the Goal

Sometimes a goal that a client proposes will need to be reworked or broken down into more focused goals for which specific implementation strategies can be identified. For example, a client named Alice reported, "I become very scared when I am asked to show my artwork. When I get scared, I stop working, start avoiding appointments, act irresponsibly, become depressed, and ruin the show." Her goal: "I want to be a famous artist." Alice's desire to be a famous artist was problematic for the treatment, because it was not something within her direct control and was dependent on too many outside forces, including luck. Through discussion with her therapist, Alice was able to restate the goal more concretely: "I want to show my artwork publicly, and ultimately be able to support myself financially as a full-time artist." This goal could then be broken down into smaller steps that could be addressed in the treatment, including finding a studio space, joining a support group for local artists, contacting gallery owners who had shown interest in her work, and working regularly to prepare for a show.

Evaluate the Necessity for Distress

Before working through the pros and cons of a goal, the client may first consider whether there is indeed any distress necessarily involved in reaching this goal. The concept of "necessary suffering" can help clients evaluate whether they are tolerating distress that is necessary to reach a goal, or whether they are tolerating unwarranted distress. Clients can ask themselves, "Is it really necessary to tolerate distress to reach this goal?"

Clients who are unclear about the answer to this question might ask a friend for his or her thoughts on the situation. An alternative strategy is to use displacement. A client can imagine that someone she cares about is tolerating a distressing situation to reach a valued goal. Does she see an alternative way for her friend to reach the goal? Does she think her friend has to stay in the situation to reach the goal?

For example, one client wanted to become an architect. Part of the training involved an extensive apprenticeship with someone in the field. This particular client got a placement with a very prominent architect. She was elated and started working. Quickly, however, it became apparent that the architect she was working for was very abusive. The situation only became worse over time. Initially, the client thought she had to tolerate the distressing situation in order to reach her goal of becoming an architect. After discussing her situation in therapy, however, the client realized that she might be tolerating unnecessary suffering. She decided to look into getting another placement with someone who was known to be a good mentor.

Identify Pros and Cons

The therapist can write out the identified goal on the top of a clean sheet of paper and divide the sheet into two columns: "Pros" and "Cons." In her review of the pros and cons, the client first determines the level of distress she will experience, and the strategies she has for managing or reducing the distress. Then the client determines whether the remaining distress is worthwhile. In addition to providing a specific example of how to use skills, this exercise is a productive way to prepare and enlist the client in facing challenges inherent in the treatment.

If the client has difficulty with generating pros and cons for an identified goal, the therapist can review a particular goal of the treatment—for example, reducing PTSD symptoms. The client can be prompted to ask herself questions such as "Why am I putting myself through this?", "What is my ultimate goal here?", and "Will I get enough positive results out of this situation that tolerating the distressing feelings will be worth it?" The associated pros might be better daily functioning, improvement in relationships, and better sleep, while the cons might be reliving painful memories.

CASE EXAMPLE:
IDENTIFYING GOALS AND GENERATING PROS AND CONS

Beth was a 40-year-old woman with a history of sexual abuse and violation in the context of intimate relationships. In childhood her uncle, a central caregiver, had repeatedly molested her. She described a "special" relationship with him and noted that prior to the abuse, she had trusted and loved him very much. In college she was raped by a boyfriend—again, a person with whom she had previously felt closeness and trust. Beth felt that these experiences influenced her choice at age 26 to marry a man whom she did not find sexually attractive, and who did not express much interest or initiative in a sexual relationship with her. She divorced several years later and since that time had not been involved in any romantic relationships. Although she had felt unfulfilled in many ways over the past 10 years, she also described feeling safe and well protected by "the wall" that she had built to keep others (both men and women) from getting too close.

At the beginning of treatment, Beth shared that Doug, a friend she had known for a few years, had recently told her he was interested in her romantically. She expressed tremendous ambivalence and anxiety about this. Beth was aware that getting closer to Doug would create anxiety and upheaval in her life. She also stated that she liked and felt comfortable with Doug, and feared that if she didn't try to get closer to him, she would regret it and might not get another chance. As part of treatment, it was suggested that Beth use the strategy of assessing pros and cons in order to help her decide whether tolerating the distress and anxiety that would arise in this situation would be manageable and worthwhile for her.

Beth initially identified that ideally, her highest goal would be to develop a wonderful relationship with Doug and maybe get married. The therapist suggested that they shift the focus away from this overwhelming and uncontrollable goal to a more realistic and manageable set of smaller subgoals. These included developing a more intimate relationship with Doug, learning to be more open, and becoming close to another person in a healthy way. Breaking down the highest goal into more realistic and immediate subgoals was an intervention in itself, as it helped reduce Beth's anxiety. She was then able to generate a

Goals: Developing a more intimate relationship with Doug, learning to open up, becoming close to someone in a healthy way.

Cons	Pros
Making myself vulnerable	Companionship
Risking getting hurt	Developing an important connection
Feeling foolish and anxious	Having somebody to depend on
Having to deal with sexual problems	Learning to enjoy sex
Having to confront the abuse	Being with someone who is supportive
Risking a good friendship	Developing a deeper relationship

EXAMPLE 13.1. Beth's pros and cons list.

useful list of pros and cons of committing herself to these smaller goals. This list is presented in Example 13.1.

Beth's pros and cons list helped her to identify how her abuse history was getting in the way of her potentially having a rewarding relationship with Doug. She decided it was worth tolerating some distress for the possibility of developing a closer relationship with Doug. For the next week, she decided that as a step toward meeting this goal, she would ask him to go see a movie he had mentioned they should see together.

MATCH DISTRESS REDUCTION STRATEGIES TO GOALS

The next step is to identify the type of strategy that will be most effective in managing the particular type of distress the client is experiencing and that will support or facilitate her success in getting to the goal.

Some strategies are general, in that they will contribute to a client's overall ability to regulate her mood; others are more situation-specific. General strategies include what is commonly referred to as "self-care": getting adequate rest, eating a well-balanced diet, drinking alcohol moderately, exercising regularly, addressing medical issues, managing money responsibly, and so forth. All of these will contribute to the client's being less emotionally reactive and distressed overall.

In order to reach desired goals, clients need to learn to apply negative mood regulation strategies in specific situations. For example, if a client is anxious before a meeting with her boss, she might use focused breathing several times during the preceding days to maintain her calm. She might also keep her anxiety in check by engaging in activities consistent with her goals that she finds anxiety-reducing, such as taking a relaxing bath, preparing/writing out what she plans to say, and doing laundry or otherwise making sure she has clean and appropriate clothes for the meeting. Talking late into the night on the phone with friends might reduce her distress but might not be consistent with her goal, which includes being alert and attentive at her meeting.

INTRODUCE PRACTICE OF DISTRESS TOLERANCE DURING LIFE'S "RANDOM MOMENTS"

Describe Rationale for Acceptance of Negative Feelings

Up to this point, the emphasis of this session has been on tolerating distress that is associated with clients' active pursuit of specific, identifiable goals. However, the therapist can note that feelings of distress also frequently emerge during more or less "random moments" in people's lives. They may experience episodic anxiety, sadness, and frustration during everyday unexpected hassles, during difficult interactions with others, or simply as a result of dysregulated biological rhythms (e.g., disrupted sleep–wake cycles). Also, despite efforts at proactive management of PTSD symptoms, there will be inevitable occasions where symptoms occur unexpectedly and are not controllable. For example, a client's reliving and hyperarousal symptoms may be triggered automatically by environmental stimuli that unconsciously remind her of her traumatic experiences.

In these and other similar circumstances, the therapist can note that it isn't always possible to change and decrease negative emotions. Indeed, there are occasions where it may be preferable not to work toward changing the negative feelings. Rather, some negative emotional states can be accepted as common, typical, and necessary parts of human life. Indeed, exercising acceptance of negative emotions during difficult events paradoxically often culminates in clients' feeling less distress.

Provide Examples of Acceptance of Negative Feelings in Everyday Life

The therapist can identify situations where acceptance may work well for the client. For example, it is easy to feel anger or anxiety while having to wait in a long line of customers at a grocery store or bank. In this situation, through simply being mindful of feelings of anger and anxiety, the client can learn to tolerate increasing levels of this type of everyday life distress. The therapist can suggest that the client explore this option. The client can perceive or simply be aware that "this is what anger/anxiety feels like," but can do so without directly responding to, acting on, or identifying with her feelings. Acceptance is an experience of being aware of feelings without trying to change, reject, or suppress them. Clients may find that if they simply observe their emotional symptoms with a sense of detached awareness, their symptoms will often be more short-lived than if they try to avoid their feelings altogether or engage in self-destructive behaviors in an attempt to make their feelings go away. In fact, by observing but being accepting of a certain degree of negative affect, clients will typically find that negative emotions will abate on their own.

Provide Examples of Acceptance of Intense Feelings and Moods

The therapist can also note that clients often experience intense feelings and then engage in behaviors to minimize or rid themselves of the feeling—behaviors that result in perpetuating the negative feelings or putting the clients into worse circumstances. For example, a client might wake up in an intensely sad state and in response stay in bed all day, missing work and other responsibilities. This client might then feel guilty and berate herself for missing work. She might also be in trouble with her boss. As a result, she might start feeling depressed. The client's response to her feelings might thus make her feel worse instead of better.

An alternative approach is for the client to accept her state. If the client had tolerated her sadness and gone to work, she would not have experienced the cascade of guilt and depression that followed her decision to stay in bed. The therapist can remind the client that often intense feelings are changeable, and that no matter what mood she is in at one time, her mood will change. Emotions are sometimes described as waves that rise up to a peak and then eventually wane. This image may be helpful to the client, because what she is feeling at any one moment may seem unbearable—but the feeling will not last forever.

Identify Potential Long-Term Benefits of Distress Tolerance: Increased Well-Being

Lastly, the therapist can note that the more a client feels able to tolerate negative emotions during the random moments of her everyday life, the more confident she is likely to be in her ability to tolerate distress while actively engaging in the pursuit of newly set positive goals in her life. In keeping with this session's theme of the pursuit of goals, exercising distress tolerance during random moments can be regarded as being consistent with a major goal: that of increasing overall psychological health and well-being.

DISCUSS ROLE OF POSITIVE FEELINGS IN PURSUING GOALS

Although negative emotions have the capacity to disrupt the pursuit of important goals and daily functioning more generally, it is also important to review with the client the ways in which experiences of positive emotions can *enhance* functioning. This discussion is an extension of the work from Session 3, in which the client has been invited to engage in pleasurable activities and to explore, accept, and modulate (as necessary) positive feelings.

Improved functioning can be obtained by increasing exposure to novel and positive experiences. This aspect of improved functioning may be somewhat foreign to abuse survivors. The tendency to engage in "approach behaviors"—even toward things, situations, or people that appear interesting, elicit curiosity, or generate warmth—may have been undermined by repeated negative and hostile feedback in the past. However, positive feelings can guide a person toward discovering hidden talents and interests. By recognizing and following feelings of pleasure and positive excitement, clients can discover what they truly like to do, and even discover some latent talents and abilities that have lain dormant. In addition, the acknowledged pleasure or satisfaction to be had in reaching a goal can help sustain a person's commitment and discipline during more difficult periods of the effort toward the goal.

Positive Feelings as Guides to Selecting Goals

The therapist should ask the client whether there are any skills or activities that she is drawn to or that spontaneously engage her. Eliciting excitement and interest about an idea, problem, or circumstance can help confirm and consolidate a client's interest in a goal. Acknowledged positive feelings and enthusiasm for a goal can help motivate the client to persist in the face of setbacks. They have another function as well: They provide the client with feedback about herself. As the client becomes aware that she is a person who likes certain things and dislikes others, she becomes a more substantial and specific person in her own eyes.

Goals as Intrinsically Pleasurable and Engaging

Selecting a goal in which the client has a positive interest is also likely to lead to skills practice and mastery. Such goals can be any number of things: learning a dance, completing a sculpture, fixing a bike, learning to read music, or writing poetry. However, if the client is occupied by the goal and experiencing some success, an additional and more profound benefit emerges, which is the experience of feeling engaged in living.

PREPARE CLIENT FOR WORK ON INTERPERSONAL PROBLEMS

The next several sessions will focus on the client's interpersonal relationships. At first glance, it may seem like a challenge to help the client develop her emotion regulation and distress tolerance skills while at the same time working on her interpersonal relationships. However, as becomes obvious from examining Box 13.2, almost all clients' goals involve an interpersonal aspect, even if their goals are not specifically focused on a relationship. For example, a client's goal of asking her boss for a raise does not seem on the surface to be interpersonal. However, actually talking to her boss about a raise requires that the client manage her feelings toward her boss, tolerate her anxiety about asking for the raise, and practice her interpersonal skills so that she can ask her boss for a raise in an appropriate way.

ASSIGN BETWEEN-SESSION EXERCISES

Before assigning home exercises, the therapist should ask the client about her thoughts and feelings in response to the idea of tolerating distress in pursuit of valued goals. Does the idea make sense? Does it sound doable? Is the pros and cons technique useful? The therapist should determine whether any concepts or examples need clarification, and ask the client if she thinks she will be able to assess the pros and cons of tolerating distress every day. If the client seems hesitant, the therapist can help her come up with examples of possible situations to use. Some of the situations can be mundane (e.g., asking a friend to drive the client to the airport), as the important thing is to practice the skill. The therapist should spend some time planning the pros and cons exercises with the client, encouraging her to be specific about when she will do the designated "steps" to reaching a goal, and helping her decide which coping strategies will be practiced. In addition, the therapist can suggest to the client that she allow herself to simply be aware and accepting of feelings as she plans her goals. To the extent that the client experiences anxiety at "random moments" or moments she has no power to change right now, she can simply be interested in the feeling and note when it happens and why. Finally, the therapist should remind the client that part of the rationale for distress tolerance is that such skills will be important in the second part of the treatment when the client will be working on confronting her trauma history. Handout 13.1 provides a useful summary for the client of all the points that have been covered in this session.

What Is Distress Tolerance and Why Should I Do It?

RATIONALE FOR DISTRESS TOLERANCE

Distress is a catalyst for change in recovering from childhood trauma. Preparing to make any major change in yourself or your life will involve some anticipatory anxiety and discomfort. If you do not allow yourself to be in touch with this distress, you will not become motivated to make important changes. Allowing feelings of distress to come to the surface can be frightening and upsetting, but it can also be very enlightening. Distress can serve the function of telling you that something is wrong. Distress can also tell you about areas in your life you may need to attend to or change. It can also provide relief, as you may be expending tremendous emotional energy trying to avoid distress and find that you are still suffering anyway. Lastly, learning to tolerate more negative, difficult feelings has the benefit of allowing you to be more open to experiencing positive feelings as well. When you avoid feelings, the result is that most or many feelings are cut off, not just negative ones. As a result, you—like many other victims of childhood abuse—may have a very restricted range of emotions, and may report feeling "numb" and unable to enjoy many things in life.

TOLERATING DISTRESS IN THE CONTEXT OF IDENTIFIED GOALS

One of the main aims of this treatment is to teach skills for distress tolerance in relationship to identified goals. One of the tasks for you and your therapist is to identify your goals, and then realistically assess whether distress is necessary and then whether the cost in distress is worth the benefits of reaching the goals. Trauma survivors become used to and even expect hardship and distress in reaching goals. So the first step is determining whether the identified distress is actually necessary, or whether there are alternative and easier routes to reaching the goal. If some distress is intrinsic to the goal, you and your therapist then review the expected and inevitable challenges and obstacles that will arise when you are working toward these goals, and identify ways for you to effectively manage and even master the associated distress. This concept is particularly important in situations that require long-term work toward a goal where the benefit or relief is not immediate. The emphasis is on determining whether the goal is important or beneficial enough that tolerating some discomfort and distress in the process of attaining this goal is manageable and worthwhile.

ASSESSING PROS AND CONS

Assessing pros and cons is a strategy that can aid you in determining whether a distressing situation is worth tolerating. Assessing pros and cons involves selecting a significantly distressing or anxiety-producing situation and identifying a comprehensive list of pros and cons of tolerating the situation or feelings

(continued)

associated with it. After the pros and cons are enumerated, the next step is for you to assess and weigh each side, asking questions such as "Why am I putting myself through this?", "What is my ultimate goal here?", and "Will I get enough positive results out of this situation that tolerating distressing feelings will be worth it?"

MATCHING DISTRESS REDUCTION TO DESIRED GOALS

Another skill you will be working on is that of identifying the type of strategy that will be most effective in managing the particular type of distress you are experiencing. The strategy you choose should be the one that will best facilitate your success in achieving your goal. Some strategies are general in that they will contribute to your overall ability to regulate your mood; others are more situation specific.

General strategies include what is commonly referred to as "self-care": getting adequate rest, eating a well-balanced diet, drinking alcohol moderately, exercising regularly, addressing medical issues, managing money responsibly, and so forth. All of these will contribute to your being less emotionally reactive and distressed overall.

In order to reach desired goals, you will also need to learn to apply negative mood-regulation strategies in specific situations. For example, if you are anxious before an early morning meeting with your boss you might use focused breathing several times during the preceding days to maintain your calm. You might also keep your anxiety in check by engaging in activities that you find relaxing, such as taking a hot bath, preparing/writing out what you plan to say, and doing laundry or otherwise making sure you have appropriate clothes for the meeting. Talking late into the night on the phone with friends might seduce your distress but might not be consistent with your goal of being attentive and alert at your meeting.

ACCEPTING DISTRESS THAT OCCURS DURING "RANDOM MOMENTS"

It isn't always possible or even preferable to intentionally try to change and decrease negative feelings. Indeed, some negative emotional states are common, typical, and necessary parts of human life. These include minor irritations such as anxiety while waiting in a line, or even unexpected PTSD hyperarousal symptoms resulting from an unanticipated trigger. Simply being mindful of feelings of anger and anxiety can paradoxically lead to these feelings' resolving more quickly than if you make an active effort to reduce, avoid or suppress them. Practice this strategy in random moments such as waiting in a line, waiting for a train or bus, or reacting to a negative remark someone makes toward you.

CHAPTER 14

⌢

SESSION 5

The Resource of Connection
Understanding Relationship Patterns

> Through our relationship with the [caretaking person] . . ., we develop a working
> model of ourselves and our parents . . . that gives a model for how we treat each other
> and ourselves. This model determines what information is attended to, which
> memories are evoked, what behaviors are employable. It is the basis for our sense of
> self and other.
> —SANDRA L. BLOOM AND MICHAEL REICHERT (1998, p. 135)

OVERVIEW

Interactions with other people shape how we see ourselves in the world and what we come to expect from our environments. From infancy through adulthood, our relationships and our beliefs about these relationships are constantly exerting influence on our thoughts, feelings, and behaviors, even when we are not aware of their impact. Based on our early experiences, we develop models of relationships and test these out over time, continually elaborating and adapting them to fit our current realities. Among abuse survivors, the process of using past experience to guide current expectations can often lead to negative outcomes. The primary goal of Session 5 is to focus on helping a client understand how "interpersonal schemas," or models of relationships she developed in her early life, continue to influence her feelings and interactions with others as an adult.

The first component of this session involves introducing the idea of an interpersonal schema in ways that are understandable and relevant to the client. The second component of this session entails introducing and working with a specific tool (the Interpersonal Schemas Worksheet I) to help the client draw out or abstract from her life experiences the core interpersonal schemas that effectively describe her beliefs in interpersonal situations. Given that many trauma survivors have difficulty remembering or keeping hold of insights from one week to the next, this tool creates a record of distilled insights that can be referred to in later sessions. Box 14.1 outlines the theme and curriculum for Session 5 of treatment.

BOX 14.1
Theme and Curriculum for Session 5: The Resource of Connection—Understanding Relationship Patterns

THEME

Interpersonal schemas are structures formed early in life in the context of relationships with caregivers. These schemas reflect ideas about the self and others, and about how the relationships between the self and others work. The task of developing these schemas for relationships is disrupted and distorted by childhood abuse experiences. Because these schemas guide behaviors and expectations in relationships, and because they are automatically activated, patterns set down in childhood can lead an adult toward repeating relationship dynamics that may not be adaptive in the present.

PLANNING AND PREPARATION

Bring copies of the Interpersonal Schemas Worksheet I (Handout 14.1).

AGENDA

- Complete emotional check-in and review of between-session work.
- Provide psychoeducation: What are interpersonal schemas?
- Introduce Interpersonal Schemas Worksheet I as a tool to identify core schemas.
- Practice using Interpersonal Schemas Worksheet I.
- Assign between-session work:
  - Complete the Interpersonal Schemas Worksheet I once a day; include emotion regulation skills as relevant to the situation.
  - Practice focused breathing twice a day.

SESSION HANDOUTS

Several copies of Handout 14.1. Interpersonal Schemas Worksheet I

BOX 14.2
What Are Interpersonal Schemas?

1. Children are biologically driven to attach themselves to their caregivers for purposes of survival, so they will quickly learn specific behavioral contingencies that are associated with establishing and maintaining connections to their caregivers.

2. "Interpersonal schemas" are organizing models formed early in life in the context of relationships with caregivers.

3. Interpersonal schemas reflect ideas about the self and others, and about how the relationships between the self and others work.

4. These schemas guide behaviors and expectations in relationships and are automatically activated in interpersonal situations.

5. The task of developing these schemas for relationships is disrupted and distorted by childhood abuse experiences, because when interpersonal schemas are constructed in an abusive environment, survival becomes linked with abuse.

6. People bring their interpersonal schemas into adulthood. Though interpersonal schemas are initially formed in the context of relationships with parental figures, they are also later applied to more general interpersonal situations.

7. Interpersonal schemas that were adaptive in childhood may be maladaptive in adulthood and can inadvertently lead an adult toward repeating negative relationship patterns.

8. Interpersonal schemas continue to play a central role in shaping thoughts, feelings, and behaviors throughout life, since people's expectations about relationships (interpersonal schemas) lead them to behave in ways to prepare for the imagined outcomes.

9. Interpersonal schemas are often redundant and can be difficult to disconfirm.

10. However, interpersonal schemas are modifiable. Once patterns are identified and assumptions about relationships are more critically evaluated, there is room for trying out alternative ways of interacting, which could significantly improve current relationships.

Interpersonal Schema Theory

The therapist should be familiar with the basic principles of interpersonal schema theory, which are elucidated in Chapter 2. It may be useful for the therapist to review this chapter for a refresher prior to this session. We also provide a summary of key points in Box 14.2, which is intended for the therapist's use as a guide when discussing interpersonal schemas with the client in this session.

Repetition of Relationship Patterns

Clients will often present for treatment with tremendous distress and confusion about such repeated negative relationship patterns with friends, coworkers, and partners. Though they may be well aware of the cyclical nature of their relationships they often describe being bewildered about why similar situations recur with different people and feeling helpless about how they can break this cycle, which has come to feel inevitable.

Peoples' expectations about relationships, and about the responses they are likely to receive from others, lead them to behave in ways to prepare for the imagined outcomes. Consequently, interpersonal schemas are often self-fulfilling, even when the relationship result is one that a person does not want. For example, a young woman from an abusive family who has developed the understanding that interpersonal relatedness is contingent on sexual behavior may be likely to engage in or initiate sexual activity as a way of emotionally connecting to others, whether she is interested in sex or not and whether or not her partner is actually expecting sex.

Individuals often erroneously use relationship outcomes as confirmatory evidence that their original expectations were founded and accurate. In this way, interpersonal schemas are perpetuated with little awareness of how the expectations themselves, which may or may not have been based in current reality, have influenced an interpersonal sequence. One useful and common example the therapist might share with the client involves expectations of rejection, which often lead to perceived and even actual rejection. If a client typically expects to be rejected in relationships, she is less willing to engage with others and generally behaves in a self-protective manner by maintaining distance and avoiding intimacy. Others interacting with her will be unaware of this basic assumption and are likely to interpret her behavior as lack of interest or openness to interpersonal contact. As a result, most people will not initiate or pursue involvement with her. She in turn will see this as confirming evidence of rejection in relationships, and will remain unaware of her own role in perpetuating this negative cycle.

Limited and Rigid Interpersonal Repertoires

Not only do individuals with childhood abuse histories tend to have negative expectations in relationships, but they also often have a limited and rigid repertoire of interpersonal schemas from which to select. They may say something like this: "I can't move out of this pattern, because I don't know where to go next." When individuals are not exposed to varying interactions, there is a higher degree of redundancy in their interpersonal relationships, and maladaptive interpersonal schemas are difficult to disconfirm (Carson, 1969). Thus having a constricted range of schemas and engaging in these regardless of the actual situation further perpetuate the self-confirming cycle and limit possible responses from others.

One common maladaptive schema is the victim–abuser relationship, which can be reflected in domestic violence situations and even in the therapy relationship. Sometimes the survivor takes on the victim role, experiencing abuse at the hands of a partner, boss, friend, or therapist. At other times, the survivor can take on the role of the aggressor with significant others. Many women fear falling into the trap of taking on either role, but the problem is that they have very few alternative ways of thinking about themselves and others.

In sum, interpersonal schema theory and research indicate that the tendency to generalize the application of predominant schemas to new experiences should be viewed as a general principle of interpersonal functioning, rather than as a pathological process associated with abuse survivors.

PROVIDE PSYCHOEDUCATION:
WHAT ARE INTERPERSONAL SCHEMAS?

In introducing the client to the concept of interpersonal schemas, the therapist should emphasize and flesh out the points in Box 14.2. The therapist should periodically ask the client whether or not these concepts make sense and seem relevant; ideally, doing so will facilitate some meaningful dialogue and get the client thinking about how these concepts relate to her life, including any recent situations.

The therapist should also highlight for the client the role of feelings in her present-day interpersonal problems, and describe how intense emotions related to interpersonal schemas that were developed in the context of early relationships can derail current interpersonal goals. In a current interaction, strong feeling states from the past may be triggered and then drive a client's behavior, regardless of important ways in which the present situation may be different or may call for a different response. Women with abuse histories often experience such derailments in situations that elicit power and control schemas—particularly when there is a power differential or imbalance, as these are central dynamics of abuse.

If possible, the therapist should use an example from the client's life to illustrate this point. If none are forthcoming, however, the following example may be useful: A client may feel overworked at her job and taken advantage of by her boss, who has not given the client the raise she deserves. This scenario may remind her of her childhood exploitation and may quickly give rise to intense feelings of anger and grief. This is a situation in which the client is vulnerable to acting on strong feelings that belong to the past, instead of responding to demands and aims of the current interpersonal situation. Clearly, the feeling of anger at her boss is legitimate and understandable, but the client's level of feeling and the way in which she handles these feelings are what will dictate the outcome. If the client's behavior is driven by her feelings and schemas related to the past, it is unlikely that she will be able to meet her interpersonal goals in the current situation. In response to the boss's perceived exploitation and abuse, the client may withdraw and become passive, or she may alternatively counterattack by expressing anger inappropriately to her boss in an effort to defend herself. Neither of these approaches is likely to result in meeting her goal of getting a raise and improving her status at work.

The therapist should communicate to the client that a primary goal of this treatment is to help her identify the interpersonal schemas that are coming into play in her current relationships and causing problems in her interpersonal functioning. The client will first learn how to recognize when she is being influenced by expectations and strong feelings from the past, and then how to catch and manage these feelings before they interfere with her present relationships. Becoming aware of these issues will ultimately give the client more control and choice in terms of how she responds, and will make it more likely that her interpersonal goals will be met.

When addressing distinctions between strong feelings from the past and current interpersonal goals, the therapist must be sure to emphasize that choosing not to act on these strong emotions does *not* invalidate them or imply that they are inappropriate. Many individuals with abuse histories are quick to feel ashamed, discounted, or invalidated. The goal is not to increase a client's sense of distrust in her own perceptions, but rather to help her become aware of ways in which feelings that belong to the past are being activated and are not working in her favor now. Although the client will still be vulnerable to having these feelings triggered in various interpersonal situations, ideally she will feel more aware and in control of them, and can make choices about the extent to which these reactions should dictate current behavior.

INTRODUCE INTERPERSONAL SCHEMAS WORKSHEET I

The Interpersonal Schemas Worksheet I is designed to help clients identify and understand their interpersonal schemas (which represent assumptions about the self–other dyad) and the ways these schemas come to bear on current interactions. This analysis is framed within a cognitive model, which includes two parts: beliefs about the self, and beliefs about others' perceptions of the self. With this intervention, the concepts described earlier can be concretized and personalized for each client. The initial goal is to help the client get in touch with experiencing herself as a "self" with expectations, beliefs, and feelings. Next, the client needs to become aware that she brings a set of expectations, beliefs, and feelings about others into relationships.

Given that this is likely to be the first time many clients have tried to articulate these complex concepts, it is critical to describe this worksheet and its rationale thoroughly. By this point in the treatment, the client should be comfortable completing the Self-Monitoring of Feelings Form (Handout 11.2). The therapist should present the Interpersonal Schemas Worksheet I (Handout 14.1) in a similar way, highlighting its value and importance for discovering important information that includes the dimension of interpersonal relationships. The purpose of this handout is to help the client articulate her key interpersonal schemas and to identify ways these schemas are negatively affecting her current relationships. In Session 6, an expanded version of this handout (the Identification of Interpersonal Schemas Worksheet II; Handout 15.1) is presented. It may be helpful to inform the client now that the goal of the next session will be to begin creating and testing alternative schemas—that is, alternative ways of thinking, feeling, and behaving in relationships. However, it is not necessary, or even of much value, to move directly into the generation of alternative schemas. Initially, it is enough for the client to identify interpersonal schemas that are represented in specific interactions. As time goes by, the articulation of a schema will become more refined and will become linked to a list of other schemas.

PRACTICE USING INTERPERSONAL SCHEMAS WORKSHEET I

The therapist should then take time in the session to fill out a copy of Handout 14.1 with the client, and to answer any questions about how the client should proceed in using the form on her own. At the end of the session, the therapist should give the client the completed copy as a reference point.

The therapist should begin by eliciting an example from the client of a recent problematic interpersonal situation. Preferably this situation will have taken place over the past week, so that the details and emotional relevance will be fresher in the client's mind. If the client cannot think of a recent example, the therapist can provide one, based on information discussed in previous sessions. The therapist should prompt the client to respond to queries raised in each column of the form, and record her answers:

> "What happened in this situation? Who was involved? What did you feel and believe about yourself in this situation? What did you feel and believe the other person thought of you in this situation? How did you expect the other person would respond to you? What action did you take, and what was the result?"

CASE EXAMPLE: IDENTIFYING AN INTERPERSONAL SCHEMA

Below, we provide a dialogue that took place between a client and therapist as they worked through completing Handout 14.1 (see Example 14.1 for the client's completed copy). The client, Renee, was in her late 20s, with a history of childhood sexual abuse by her uncle and neglect by her parents. In her family there were many "secrets," and the clear message was that these should be kept quiet. Family members rarely discussed their feelings or problems openly, as this was seen as a sign of weakness or self-indulgent complaining. Renee's parents frequently responded to her with statements such as "Snap out of it," "Pull yourself together," or "A lot of people have it worse than you; there's nothing to complain about."

In treatment, Renee shared that she was beginning a new relationship. Her past romantic relationships had been short-lived and disappointing. Previous boyfriends had told Renee that she was "hard to get close to." Despite Renee's wish to become more open and emotionally close, she found herself repeating the old pattern in this new relationship and came into the session upset about a specific situation. The therapist used this situation to demonstrate use of the Interpersonal Schemas Worksheet I.

Interpersonal situation	Feelings/beliefs about self	Expectations about other	Resulting action
• What happened? • Who was involved?	• What did I feel/believe about myself?	• How did I expect the other person to act/respond to me?	• What did I do? • What was the result?
I was upset and stressed out because of fight with my sister. Rob (boyfriend) asked me what was wrong.	I should handle this better without feeling so upset. I am too emotional.	If he really cared, he could ask me again. If I tell him what is wrong, he will think I am a pain and not want to deal with it. He will think I am being overly emotional.	Didn't tell him about it, kept it to myself, shut him out. Felt even more stressed out, because things were awkward between us.

EXAMPLE 14.1. Renee's filled in Interpersonal Schemas Worksheet I.

THERAPIST: In this session, we have been talking about interpersonal schemas—how they develop and are maintained in your current relationships. The situation you mentioned earlier with your boyfriend seems like a familiar one for you, and it caused you some distress. Let's use it as an example to break down the pattern, so we can understand more clearly what happens and how your interpersonal schemas may come into play. This is also a good way for us to practice using the Interpersonal Schemas Worksheet I, so I am going to record the information on a copy of this worksheet. Can you tell me a little more about what happened in this recent situation?

RENEE: Well, I was very upset about the fight I had just had with my sister. I was still really stressed out about it and in a bad mood by the time Rob came to pick me up, but I was trying not to show it. I guess he could tell something was bothering me, even though I was trying to act like it wasn't. He asked me what was wrong.

THERAPIST: How did you respond?

RENEE: I said that nothing was the matter, that I was just tired, and so he left me alone. But then that made me feel even worse, like he didn't really care but just asked to be polite.

THERAPIST: OK, so I'm going to write down in the "Interpersonal situation" column that you were upset and stressed out about your fight with your sister, and Rob asked you what was going on. Is that right?

RENEE: Yeah, that's what happened, even though part of me wanted to tell him I didn't.

THERAPIST: OK, so let's work it through with the form. Identify the specific sequence. Now that we know what happened, let's think about the next column: What feelings and beliefs did you have about yourself in this situation?

RENEE: I felt like I was too emotional—that I shouldn't be so upset about the thing with my sister and should not let it ruin my time with Rob.

THERAPIST: What did you think Rob thought or felt about you in this situation?

RENEE: I don't know. He probably thought I was being moody and ignoring him.

THERAPIST: How did you expect him to respond?

RENEE: Well, if he really wanted to know, he could have asked me more about it.

THERAPIST: What did you expect he would have done if you had told him what was the matter?

RENEE: I figured he would probably be nice about it, but he would not really feel like dealing with it and would think that I was overreacting—that I am overly emotional.

THERAPIST: OK, so you had an expectation that he would feel burdened if you had actually told him.

RENEE: Yeah—that he would have found it a pain to have to deal with a girlfriend who was so emotional.

THERAPIST: OK, so what did you do in the situation? How did you act?

RENEE: Like I said, I didn't tell him what was wrong, so we drove in silence the whole way to his house.

THERAPIST: And what was the result? How did you end up feeling, and what happened between the two of you?

RENEE: I ending up feeling even worse that there was awkwardness between us.

THERAPIST: Good job filling in the details. How did it feel going through this exercise?

RENEE: It was fine, but I don't always remember things in such detail.

THERAPIST: That's OK. Just do your best, and also the sooner you fill out the form after you have a situation like this or some other relationship situation, the easier it will be to remember details. Did you learn anything from what we just did?

RENEE: Basically, just that I tried to act in a way that I thought would be better for the relationship, and it ended up that I still felt bad and then he felt bad.

THERAPIST: Right. Well, I think it is a good example that gives us useful information. We can start to really see how your feelings about yourself—that you are too emotional, and your belief that others will also see you this way and find you a burden—really dictate how you choose to act. Even in a situation where someone cares about you and wants to know what is going on, you keep them at a distance and maybe miss an opportunity to feel better and also closer.

After completing an example such as this with the client, the therapist should ask her how doing this exercise felt and whether she learned anything. The therapist should share his or her own observations about how the identified feelings, expectations, and beliefs of self and other may have contributed to the situation's outcome.

ASSIGN BETWEEN-SESSION WORK

The therapist should ask the client if she thinks she can try applying the Interpersonal Schemas Worksheet I to specific interpersonal situations that may arise over the week. Ideally, she should try to complete it once daily. The therapist can remind her again of the rationale—for example:

"In addition to helping you with PTSD symptoms, another central way this treatment can be useful is by helping you improve the quality of your relationships. In order to do so, we need to begin with specifics as to what is actually happening in your day-to-day interactions with others."

The therapist should also discuss any potential problems or concerns that the client might encounter in trying to do this work between sessions. For example, the therapist will want to make sure that the client doesn't feel pressure to complete the form "correctly." Instead, the client should be encouraged to view it as an experiment—to see how it feels to use it on her own.

Interpersonal Schemas Worksheet I

Interpersonal situation	Feelings/beliefs about self	Expectations about other	Resulting action
• What happened? • Who was involved?	• What did I feel/believe about myself?	• How did I expect the other person to act/respond to me?	• What did I do? • What was the result?

From *Treating Survivors of Childhood Abuse: Psychotherapy for the Interrupted Life* by Marylene Cloitre, Lisa R. Cohen, and Karestan C. Koenen. Copyright 2006 by The Guilford Press.

CHAPTER 15

~

SESSION 6
Changing Relationship Patterns

> In emotional life as in much of history, we are only doomed
> to repeat what has not been remembered, reflected upon
> and worked through.
>
> —ROBERT KAREN (1998, p. 408)

OVERVIEW

The focus of Session 5 has been on educating the client about interpersonal schemas and working to identify them. The next step, which is the focus of Session 6, involves helping the client to develop alternative and more flexible interpersonal schemas that will allow for positive expectations of others in relationships and the possibility of effectively and adaptively negotiating interpersonal difficulties. This work is done during the session in two ways. First, the therapist and client begin by role-playing difficult interpersonal situations. The client will have the opportunity to try out different ways of relating, with feedback from the therapist. Second, the therapist and client will work through possible alternative scenarios, in order to distill what seems to work best for the client. These alternatives will be registered on the Interpersonal Schemas Worksheet II, which the client can use as a tool to expand her range of possible responses in interpersonal situations. The therapist will want to predict for the client that making these changes can be quite challenging, because of the pervasiveness and powerfulness of interpersonal schemas and associated feelings. Box 15.1 outlines the theme and curriculum for Session 6 of treatment.

PROVIDE RATIONALE FOR ROLE-PLAYING EXERCISE

The therapist shares with the client that one of the ways they will continue to work on building relationship skills in this session is to use role-playing exercises. These exercises will involve her taking on the role of herself and other people in situations she anticipates

BOX 15.1
Theme and Curriculum for Session 6:
Changing Relationship Patterns

THEME

Once the client's key interpersonal schemas have been identified, the next step is to begin generating alternative and more flexible interpersonal schemas. Though this is not an easy process, there are ways to build new schemas and experiment with new ways of relating in interactions with others. Role playing and covert modeling are useful ways to develop and practice new interpersonal skills.

PLANNING AND PREPARATION

Bring copies of the Interpersonal Schemas Worksheet II (Handout 15.1).

AGENDA

- Complete emotional check-in and review of between-session exercises.
- Provide rationale for role-playing exercises.
- Conduct role plays.
- Give feedback on interpersonal style.
- Describe covert modeling.
- Introduce Interpersonal Schemas Worksheet II.
- Assign between-session exercises:
  - Initiate at least one interpersonal situation and practice an alternative approach.
  - Complete the Interpersonal Schemas Worksheet II once a day; include emotion regulation skills as relevant to the situation.
  - Practice focused breathing twice a day.

SESSION HANDOUTS

Several copies of Handout 15.1. Interpersonal Schemas Worksheet II experiencing or has already experienced and would like to analyze in more detail. The therapist should communicate the rationale and potential benefits of role-playing exercises as described here. We have found role playing to be a very useful way for clients to begin experimenting with different ways of interacting in relationships. In this way, the therapy can serve as an "interpersonal laboratory" in which the client can practice difficult interactions live with the therapist and receive immediate feedback on the process in a safe environment. Role playing also gives the therapist and client a shared sense of what a particular situation is actually like. Then the therapist and client can talk more effectively about aspects of the client's approach that may hinder or derail her from reaching her interpersonal goals. The therapist can also highlight aspects that are particularly effective for getting a specific message across.

CONDUCT ROLE PLAYS

The therapist asks the client to identify one or two difficult/challenging interpersonal situations. Ideally, the client will have come to the session with some specific examples from the past week that she has recorded on her Interpersonal Schemas Worksheet I. One or more of these examples should be used in the role plays, as they are most likely to be fresh in the client's mind. If the client did not complete any copies of this form, then the therapist will need to reiterate the rationale for between-session work and ask the client to think about some recent interpersonal situations to use in this exercise. Situations with moderate distress levels should be chosen to start with, so that they are emotionally salient to the client without being overwhelming.

In order for the therapist to respond in a realistic and helpful way during the role plays, basic background information (e.g., the context for each specific interaction, the nature of the client's relationship with the other person in the interaction, the client's main goal in this interaction) should be elicited from the client prior to beginning. Once the clinician has a sense of each identified interpersonal situation and has provided the client with a rationale for the exercise, the role playing can begin.

First, the client should act as herself and the therapist as the other person in the interaction. This initial role play will give the therapist an opportunity to see how the client has addressed (or plans to address) this situation, rather than relying solely on the client's description. After this role play has been completed, the therapist can ask questions, share observations, provide feedback, and make suggestions for improving the communication.

Most clients can benefit from general tips about communication, and especially about how to express feelings without putting the other on the defensive or getting caught up in side issues. For example, the therapist can explain that it is usually more effective to use "I" statements and focus on one's own feelings than to focus on the other's behavior or potential motives. Emphasizing how a person's feelings cannot be "wrong" or "invalid" is also important, as is observing ways in which the client may undermine her communication. For instance, many clients will be overly apologetic or use disclaimers before even beginning, such as "I know this may seem like I'm making a big deal of this, but . . . " or "I don't mean to be picky, but . . . " Describing to such a client how this is a "set-up" for her to be minimized can help her to make important shifts. Alternatively, some clients will communicate with a more aggressive style. The clinician will want to make such a client aware that this type of approach could be off-putting and could obscure her message. These issues are discussed in more detail in the next chapter.

The therapist's feedback can then be modeled in the next role play of the same situation, with the therapist now playing the role of the client and the client taking the role of the other person. After this run-through, it is important to ask the client how it sounded to her and whether she could realistically picture herself using this approach. The goal is to help the client come up with a style of communication that fits for her, rather than having the client rotely adopt the therapist's particular way of wording a response. In this role play, the therapist's approach should be presented as just one alternative rather than as "the right way." In this spirit, the client should be encouraged to discuss what may or may not work about the way the therapist managed the situation in the role play. It is also helpful for the therapist to validate how challenging it can be to respond in certain situations, especially when emotions are strong and there is conflict. The therapist will be in a good position to comment on this after having had the experience of playing the role of the client (e.g., "I can really see how having your mother say those things would feel pretty intimidating").

Finally, the therapist and client reverse roles again, giving the client the opportunity to play herself a second time. In this role play, the client is encouraged to try out the therapist's feedback and to experiment with an alternative approach. Afterward, the therapist should ask the client to describe how the role play felt this time, as compared to the first time she did it in the initial role play of the situation. Ideally, the client will notice some differences when incorporating the feedback. The situation can be practiced both within and outside the session until the client feels a sense of mastery. Box 15.2 outlines the basic steps of the role-playing exercise for the therapist.

GIVE FEEDBACK ON INTERPERSONAL STYLE

Giving feedback to any client on her interpersonal style can be a challenging task. Many abuse survivors in particular have an enhanced sensitivity to perceived disapproval. If a client feels she is being criticized, she may become defensive and/or feel ashamed—neither of which is conducive to practicing new interpersonal skills. In order to minimize the risk of a client's feeling judged or misunderstood, it is important for the clinician to keep the following guidelines in mind when providing feedback:

- Reiterate that interpersonal skills are learned—we are not born with them—and that learning any new skills takes practice. It is likely that the client did not have role models for effective communication or opportunities to practice these skills in

---

BOX 15.2
Basic Steps of the Role-Playing Exercise

1. Provide rationale for role playing.
   - It is a method for "trying on" and fine-tuning different ways of interacting in interpersonal situations.
   - It provides an opportunity to get immediate feedback from the clinician.

2. Identify a relevant interpersonal situation.
   - If possible, use an example client has recorded on the Interpersonal Schemas Worksheet I between sessions.
   - Otherwise, ask client to describe a recent relevant interpersonal situation.
   - Choose a situation that had a moderate distress level.

3. First role-play sequence: Have client play herself, and you (clinician) play the other person.
   - After initial sequence, get any needed clarification on client's goals in interaction, share observations about role play, provide feedback, and make suggestions for improving the communication.

4. Second role-play sequence: Have client role play other person, and you (clinician) play client.
   - Afterward, ask client for feedback on your approach. Does she have any suggestions or observations? Can she see herself using this alternative approach?
   - Share experience of playing role of client in this situation.

5. Third role-play sequence: Again, have client play herself and you (clinician) play other person.
   - Afterward, ask client to describe how the role play felt this time, as compared to when she did it in the initial role play of the situation.
   - Discuss how client can continue to practice.

---

her childhood environment. These factors probably make managing current interpersonal situations more challenging for her.
- Put the emphasis on generating alternatives, as opposed to rejecting the client's current approach. Communicate explicitly that there is no "right or wrong" way to express oneself, but rather a range of options the client can choose from, depending on the interpersonal message she would like to convey in a given interaction.
- Provide information about both strengths and weaknesses in discussing the client's style of communication, and be as specific as possible.
- When addressing problems or sticking points, provide the potential experience of the other person in the interaction rather than directly using your own perceptions,

as the latter might be overwhelming or confusing to the client. You might say, for instance, *"A person in this situation might feel rejected by your comment that you don't really care what she thinks."*

- Ask the client how it felt for her to receive feedback, and whether there were things with which she agreed or disagreed.

CASE EXAMPLE: ROLE PLAY

During the course of treatment, Kayla found herself experiencing an increase in feelings of irritability, sadness, and anxiety. She felt concerned that friends would not understand or be tolerant of her "moodiness," nor did she know how to explain it to them. She began to withdraw from and avoid social interactions even more than before. Kayla then received a message from her closest friend, Amy, who sounded angry and frustrated about not hearing from her. Kayla experienced guilt and anxiety. She described feeling "paralyzed" and unable to respond, but also fearful that she was destroying an important friendship.

Kayla shared this situation with her therapist. They discussed possible options for how Kayla might manage the situation. One option was for Kayla to continue to avoid Amy and run the risk of damaging the friendship. Kayla became upset and told the therapist that she did not want to lose the friendship. Alternatively, the therapist suggested that Kayla could share with her friend some of what was going on and how she was feeling. Initially Kayla responded, "I couldn't do that. What would I say?" Kayla felt that she could not possibly explain "the whole story" to Amy because it was too overwhelming. She feared her friend would think she had "serious problems" and ultimately reject her. The therapist suggested a role play as an experiment, to give Kayla a chance to think through safe and comfortable ways she could share with her friend without alienating her.

> THERAPIST: I think this is a good situation to use for the role-play exercise. Again, the goal here is to try out possible ways to express yourself before you are actually in the situation. If we do it like we are actually in the conversation, I will be in a position to see how it feels on the other end. That way, I can give you some feedback on what I'm hearing and how I think your message is coming across. Why don't we start with you being yourself and me playing the role of Amy?
>
> KAYLA: OK, so I should start as if I am talking to Amy—but I'm not sure what to say.
>
> THERAPIST: That's OK. You don't need to have it all worked out. In fact, the whole point of this exercise is to help you work through some options and come up with something that feels right and gets your point across in a way you want to be heard. Remember, there is no risk here because you are not actually speaking with her. So just start with what you think you would want to say, and then we can fine-tune it.

KAYLA: (*Beginning the role play*) You sounded kind of mad on your message.

THERAPIST: Well, I think it's rude that you have not been calling me back and have just sort of disappeared.

KAYLA: I know I haven't been good with calling back. It is really not personal, and I don't want you to take it that way.

THERAPIST: It is personal when I leave you a lot of messages and tell you to call me back, and then I don't hear from you.

KAYLA: Really, I have been avoiding everyone, not just you.

THERAPIST: That doesn't make me feel better. I don't care about everyone; I'm talking about me. How would you feel if I started avoiding your calls?

KAYLA: I don't know. I'm so sorry that I have been such a horrible, horrible friend. Please do not be mad.

THERAPIST: I really don't understand what is going on with you and why you are acting this way. It is frustrating, and it's making me feel like you don't care about our friendship any more.

KAYLA: No, it's not that at all. I do really care about our friendship and would never want you to think otherwise. A lot is going on, and I have a lot of problems I haven't told you about. My family is very crazy, and things happened that have really screwed me up. I'm really a big mess right now, and I didn't want anyone to know that I have finally lost it.

In providing feedback, the clinician first focused on Kayla's strengths.

"I think it was good how you started by acknowledging Amy's anger rather than trying to avoid it or make small talk. I also felt that you expressed clearly that you value the friendship and feel bad if your actions made it seem otherwise. Additionally, even when I got upset you listened and did not get angry or defensive, which can often escalate."

The clinician then shared some points she felt Kayla could work on:

"Telling your friend not to take it personally could lead her to feel brushed off or disregarded rather than reassured. This response doesn't leave a whole lot of room for dialogue. It might be more effective to start by saying you can understand how she might feel this way, and then reassure her that it is not your intention. What do you think of this suggestion?"

The clinician also noted that Kayla's profuse apologizing and presentation of herself as a "mess" might put more distance between herself and her friend. Her friend might feel taken off guard and not know how to respond, which in turn could lead Kayla to feel self-conscious and rejected—her worst fear. The clinician wondered whether Kayla might feel more comfortable if she initially did not disclose so much but waited to see how her friend responded.

Next, the therapist played the role of Kayla, and Kayla played the role of her friend Amy. The therapist modeled an example of how Kayla might communicate without pathologizing herself or offering more information than she felt comfortable, while at the same time not sounding vague or impersonal:

> "I'm aware that I have not been available lately, and I'm sorry for not returning your calls sooner—I did not mean to upset you. I really appreciate your concern and want to let you know what's been going on with me. I have recently begun therapy in order to address some long-standing family issues, and as a result have been dealing with some painful and difficult feelings. I guess I felt unsure how to let you know, so I kept it to myself."

The therapist asked Kayla how this sounded to her. Kayla replied, "It sounds good. I didn't know you could put it that way. I'm not sure I can remember to say all that, though" The therapist then switched roles again with Kayla, to allow her to incorporate the feedback in a way that felt natural and comfortable for her.

DESCRIBE COVERT MODELING

Next, the therapist introduces the concept of "covert modeling" to the client. This technique is the same as role playing, except that the client is asked to imagine the situation and then describe and discuss it in detail with the therapist, rather than acting it out. The therapist can prompt the client by asking questions (e.g., "What could you say to this person?", "How do you think you can best communicate your feelings to meet your goal in this situation?", "How do you think you would handle it if he got angry?") and suggesting that the client try on various approaches "for size."

This method is particularly useful for clients who are too self-conscious to engage in role playing, or for use with situations that don't lend themselves to effective role plays (e.g., sexual intimacy). If a therapist observes that a particular client is struggling with the role play or that it does not appear helpful for the client, covert modeling may be the preferred method of generating alternative scenarios, and the therapist can bypass role playing and start here.

Another strength of covert modeling is that clients can use this method to work through future distressing or difficult situations without the therapist's presence. Between sessions, clients can practice talking themselves through situations by asking themselves, "What could I say in this situation?" or "How would it sound if I said it this way?" This exercise can be particularly effective if a client has the capacity to use it in combination with positive visualization—actually imagining herself in the situation and picturing herself managing it successfully.

INTRODUCE INTERPERSONAL SCHEMAS WORKSHEET II

After role-playing and/or covert-modeling exercises, the therapist introduces the Interpersonal Schemas Worksheet II (see Handout 15.1). The client will already be familiar with the top half of this form, because it is identical to the Interpersonal Schemas Worksheet I (Handout 14.1, covered in Session 5). The therapist should describe the purpose of the new form, especially its bottom half:

> "Last time we worked on identifying interpersonal schemas and breaking down how they might come into play in certain relationship situations. Now we want to expand on this by adding a new set of columns, which will facilitate generating alternative ways of seeing the situation and alternative ways of responding."

After orienting the client to Handout 15.1 and describing how to complete the bottom half, the clinician should use one of the examples from the session to complete the form with the client in the session. This step will serve as a way to solidify work done in this session on the process of generating alternatives, and to illustrate how the client should use the form over the week. In particular, the therapist should prompt the client to respond to queries raised in each new column of the form, discuss the meaning of the question if necessary, and record her answers:

> "What are your interpersonal goals in this situation? What else could you feel and believe about yourself in this situation? How else could you expect the other person to act or respond? What other actions could you take in this situation?"

See Example 15.1 for a filled-in example of Handout 15.1, based on the clinical illustration presented above (the case of Kayla).

ASSIGN BETWEEN-SESSION WORK

After completing a copy of Handout 15.1 with the client, the therapist should ask her how doing this exercise felt and whether she learned anything. The therapist should then ask the client if she thinks she can try this exercise out over the week, as a way to build on the work she did outside of session last week and in session this week. Ideally, she should complete the Interpersonal Schemas Worksheet II once a day, in order to detail interpersonal situations that have arisen. If necessary, the therapist should remind the client again of the rationale for between-session work, and discuss any possible things that could interfere with her being able to utilize the form.

Interpersonal situation	Feelings/beliefs about self	Expectations about other	Resulting action
• What happened? • Who was involved? My friend Amy left a message. She sounded upset and annoyed that I had not called her back in several days.	• What did I feel/ believe about myself? I can't deal with this. I can't let her know I'm weak. I can't tell her how many problems I have.	• How did I expect the other person to act/ respond to me? If I tell her what is going on, I will scare her off; she won't want to be friends any more.	• What did I do? • What was the result? Nothing. Felt paralyzed and anxious about losing my friend, but still didn't call her back.

Interpersonal goals	Alternative feelings about self	Alternative expectations	Alternative action
• What are my goals in this situation? To keep this friendship—it's important to me. To be honest and find out if she really is a good friend.	• What else could I feel/believe about myself? I'm going through a hard time right now, but I'm getting help and trying to make positive changes.	• How else could I expect the other person to act/ respond to me? If she knew what I was going through, she would probably be understanding and supportive.	• What else could I do? Call her back; tell her a little about what has been going on and why I have been isolating myself lately.

EXAMPLE 15.1. Kayla's filled-in Interpersonal Schemas Worksheet II.

Interpersonal Schemas Worksheet II

Interpersonal situation	Feelings/beliefs about self	Expectations about other	Resulting action
• What happened? • Who was involved?	• What did I feel/believe about myself?	• How did I expect the other person to act/respond to me?	• What did I do? • What was the result?

Interpersonal goals	Alternative feelings about self	Alternative expectations	Alternative action
• What are my goals in this situation?	• What else could I feel/believe about myself?	• How else could I expect the other person to act/respond to me?	• What else could I do?

CHAPTER 16

⌒

SESSION 7
Agency in Relationships

A person comes to feel that "I am the doer who does, I am the author of my acts," by being with another person who recognizes her acts, her feelings, her intentions, her existence. . . . As life evolves, assertion and recognition become the vital moves in the dialogue between self and other.
— JESSICA BENJAMIN (1988, pp. 21–22)

OVERVIEW

In Session 6 the client has been encouraged to experiment with different ways of approaching and interacting with others. Through role plays and between-session practice, it often becomes apparent how difficulties with assertiveness can hinder a client's efforts to communicate more directly and successfully. Thus Session 7 focuses on this specific interpersonal area. We define "being assertive" as advocating for one's own rights and needs without trampling on the needs and rights of others. Though this may sound basic, behaving assertively can be quite difficult for many people—and especially daunting for individuals with abuse histories, whose needs and rights were blatantly disregarded. Many if not most abuse survivors did not have the option of behaving assertively. As a result of these early experiences, problems in being both underassertive (passive) and overassertive (aggressive) are quite common among survivors in adulthood. In order to reach an effective and comfortable middle ground between submissive and controlling approaches, a survivor needs to understand her assumptions about assertiveness, to learn about potential benefits of behaving assertively, and to have opportunities to learn and practice specific assertiveness skills. Box 16.1 outlines the theme and curriculum for Session 7 of treatment.

BOX 16.1
Theme and Curriculum for Session 7: Agency in Relationships

THEME

In many abusive families, family members often model denying or hiding their feelings and needs, or forcing them aggressively on others. Assertiveness entails standing up for one's rights and presenting one's needs or wants in a way that is respectful of both oneself and others. In assertive behavior, the person expresses her legitimate rights and needs, but without violating the rights of others. Assertive behavior may lead the person to feel confident, self-respecting, and good about herself.

PLANNING AND PREPARATION

Bring several copies of Interpersonal Schemas Worksheet II (Handout 15.1), as well as one copy each of Handouts 16.1, 16.2, 16.3, and 16.4 (see below).

AGENDA

- Complete emotional check-in and review of between session exercises.
- Provide psychoeducation: What is assertive behavior?
- Identify specific problems with assertiveness and control.
- Review basic assertiveness techniques.
- Identify interpersonal schemas related to assertiveness.
- Conduct role plays with focus on use of assertiveness skills.
- Assign between-session exercises:
  - Review Basic Personal Rights handout (Handout 16.2).
  - Identify upcoming assertiveness situation, or select/initiate situation from Assertiveness Practice Situations handout (Handout 16.4).
  - Complete Interpersonal Schemas Worksheet II (Handout 15.1). Once a day with focus on assertiveness skills, and include emotion regulation skills as relevant to the situation.
  - Practice focused breathing twice a day.

SESSION HANDOUTS

Handout 16.1. What is Assertiveness?
Handout 16.2. Basic Personal Rights
Handout 16.3. Assertiveness Skills
Handout 16.4. Assertiveness Practice Situations
Additional copies of Handout 15.1. Interpersonal Schemas Worksheet II

PROVIDE PSYCHOEDUCATION:
WHAT IS ASSERTIVE BEHAVIOR?

The therapist should not assume that the client has the same ideas about the meaning of assertiveness. Instead, the therapist should begin by asking the client what she thinks being assertive means. This will provide a jumping-off point for the session and will give the clinician information about the client's assertiveness beliefs, as well as any of her assumptions about assertiveness that may need to be challenged. There are numerous misconceptions (e.g., "Being assertive means being impolite, demanding, or selfish," "In order to be assertive, you must be prepared for fights or confrontations," "If you assert yourself, you will be disliked or punished"), and many people, especially women, have been taught that assertiveness is a negative quality. This is especially true of individuals with abuse histories, who have been actively discouraged from asserting their rights and needs, whose personal boundaries have been violated, and who may have been penalized for trying to stand up for themselves.

The therapist should give the client the handout defining assertiveness (Handout 16.1), so she can follow along during the review of the information below. The clinician can begin this review by emphasizing that assertiveness entails standing up for one's rights and presenting one's needs or wants in a way that is respectful of both oneself and others. Assertive behavior must be distinguished from nonassertive and aggressive behavior, and brief general examples of each should be provided. It may be helpful to ask the client to provide some brief examples of her own or of others' nonassertive, aggressive, and assertive behavior, to make these concepts more personally meaningful.

In "nonassertive behavior," a person disregards or does not directly express her own rights, needs, and desires. She often acts passively or submissively and permits others to violate her rights. Nonassertive behavior may lead the person to feel hurt, resentful, angry, frustrated, anxious, ignored, and/or disappointed in herself.

In "aggressive behavior," a person acts upon her rights at the expense of others through intimidation and bullying. She may behave in ways that are manipulative, openly hostile, and/or demanding; at the extreme end, these can lead to threatening and/or inappropriate outbursts. Aggressive behavior may lead the person to feel angry, out of control, frightened, and/or guilty.

It is important to note that the same person may at different times display both nonassertive and aggressive behavior, and that these often occur cyclically. For example, a person who typically has difficulty being direct and setting limits with others is likely to become more and more resentful and frustrated over time. This type of emotional buildup that comes with being consistently overcompliant makes the person more vulnerable to losing control at some point and reacting angrily or aggressively in a situation that does not necessarily merit such a strong response. This type of reaction in turn may elicit defensiveness and anger from others—the very thing that the nonassertive individual was so desperately trying to avoid.

In "assertive behavior," on the other hand, the person consistently stands up for her rights in a way that does not infringe upon the rights of others. Assertive behavior may lead the person to feel more confident and powerful, is likely to open the door to more choices, and can also result in increased intimacy and honesty in relationships. These potential benefits provide the rationale for the focus of the exercises in this session: identifying specific assertiveness problems and related interpersonal schemas, and developing assertiveness skills.

IDENTIFY SPECIFIC PROBLEMS WITH ASSERTIVENESS AND CONTROL

After defining assertiveness and differentiating it from other behaviors, the next step is to identify more specifically the individual client's typical beliefs and interpersonal schemas with regard to assertiveness.

Review Basic Personal Rights

In order for an individual client to initiate assertive behavior in which she advocates for her own welfare, she must have a sense that she is entitled to basic personal rights. Unfortunately, abuse survivors are often taught the opposite—that they do not have personal rights. Thus it is important for the clinician to introduce this concept by giving the client a list of Basic Personal Rights (see Handout 16.2). The therapist should review these rights briefly with the client, and ask what she thinks of them and where she may have difficulties. It is important for the clinician to keep in mind that though these personal rights may seem straightforward and self-explanatory, to many trauma clients these rights represent a departure, and reviewing them can be an extremely meaningful experience. The client is asked to review Handout 16.2 more carefully at home between sessions.

Clarify the Historical Basis for the Client's Assumptions about Assertiveness

The therapist now encourages the client to give examples of how needs and wants were communicated and responded to in her family of origin. The goal of this discussion is for the therapist and client to have a concrete understanding and clear examples of the client's typical thoughts, feelings, and behaviors centering around assertiveness and control. These examples also provide elaboration of the more subtle aspects of how the client's interpersonal schemas work; as such, they can help clarify to the client her own personal history and provide detail for use in the role plays later in the session. Linking her assertiveness difficulties to these experiences will help reduce any sense of blame or irrationality that the client may be feeling about her maladaptive ways of acting and thinking.

The following questions can be helpful in generating specific links between the client's current difficulties with assertiveness and experiences she had with her family of origin:

- "How did people in your family model assertive, nonassertive, and aggressive behaviors?"
- "How did you generally communicate your needs and wants, and how did family members respond to these requests?"
- "How did family members respond to your attempts to be assertive?"

Frequently, abuse survivors come from families in which assertive behaviors were not a viable option for communicating needs and wants. In these families, needs are often met through violent and aggressive means (e.g., by an abusive father) or are denied and downplayed (e.g., by a passive mother). For example, an abused child may be the target of a parent's aggressive style of getting his or her "needs" met, and many abused children also witness the abusive parent behaving aggressively toward other family members as well. In an abusive environment, a child may see the mother responding passively to the abusive father, or the mother may tell the child, "Don't bother your father with that, or he'll get angry." In addition, abuse survivors have often experienced negative consequences of attempts at assertiveness. For example, a child's protest against the abuse often leads to additional maltreatment. Often only models of aggressive and nonassertive behavior are available in these families. There is typically neither any model of assertiveness nor any opportunity to learn that negotiation of needs is possible. Instead, children who grow up in this kind of family environment come to believe that getting needs met is an all-or-nothing process: One person gets what he or she wants at another's expense.

REVIEW BASIC ASSERTIVENESS TECHNIQUES

Now that the importance of being assertive and the specific difficulties in this area have been reviewed, the clinician can provide the client with information on how to develop more effective assertiveness skills. First, the client should be given Handout 16.3 as an outline of the main points reviewed below.

"I" Messages

As briefly described in Session 6, effective "I" messages are important assertiveness tools because they promote communication with another person about the effects of the other's behavior. For the client, the purpose of "I" messages is to focus on the negative impact of the other person's troubling behavior on the client, instead of blaming the other person him- or herself. As a result, the other is less likely to feel attacked. An "I" message has three parts: "behavior," "feeling," and "consequence." The following formula can be helpful:

Behavior: "When you [state the behavior] . . . "
Feeling: "I feel [state the feeling] . . . "
Consequence: "because [state the consequence for the client] . . . "

An example of an "I" message is "I felt frustrated when you didn't pick me up, because I missed my appointment." Or "When you yell at me, I feel hurt and upset, and it makes me not want to talk to you." The therapist should model for the client how she might use an "I" message in a recent interpersonal interaction, and then have her practice using the skill.

Making Requests

Asking for something that a client needs or wants is one of the most important assertiveness skills for the client to master. Asking for something assertively does not guarantee that the client will get it, but it is highly unlikely that she will get what she wants without asking. To make a request assertively, the therapist should instruct the client to do the following:

- Make the request specific, and state it clearly and simply (e.g., "I would like you to come to the doctor's appointment with me").
- Couch the request in "I" language ("I would like . . . " vs. "You need to . . . ").
- State the positive consequences of the other's compliance with the request (e.g., "If you take care of that errand for me, I will have more time to spend with you this evening") and/or the negative consequences of the other's noncompliance (e.g., "If you don't do that errand for me, I won't make it on time for our dinner date tonight").
- Avoid making excuses, downplaying or apologizing for the request, or blaming the other person (e.g., "I would like you to help me with my move" vs. "It's a shame that I'm going to have to move all alone," "I know you probably don't have time, but if you have nothing better to do, would you maybe be able to help me move?", or "You are so inconsiderate. You never do anything for me").

Another important assertiveness tool is to leave or temporarily put off the situation if the other person responds aggressively (e.g., "I can see that you're angry right now. Let's talk about this after lunch").

Saying No

For many women raised in abusive environments, it can be difficult to say no assertively. In cases when a client is dealing with a person with whom she does not want to foster or maintain a relationship, it is often sufficient to say, "No, thank you," in a firm and respectful tone. If the other person persists, the client should repeat herself while maintaining eye contact and slightly raising the tone of her voice.

A useful technique for dealing with someone who will not take no for an answer is the "broken record." In this technique, the client simply repeats a concise sentence over and over without backing down or getting sidetracked by other issues. For example, if a salesperson keeps badgering the client to buy something she does not want, she can keep repeating, "I understand what you are saying, but I'm not interested."

In situations involving a person with whom the client does want to maintain a relationship, it can be useful to begin by acknowledging the request by reflecting it back to the other person. Without apologizing, the client should give a brief explanation of the reason for turning him or her down and then say no. If possible, the client can end by suggesting an alternative plan in which both her and the other person's needs will be met. For example, in response to a friend's request to help him move, the client could say, "I understand that you need help with your move. Unfortunately, I have other plans for that day, so I won't be able to help you. If it would be helpful to you, I'd be happy to help you pack boxes the day before." If saying no is an especially difficult problem for a client, it can be useful to build in time before responding to a request. This can help counter the tendency to automatically agree to others' requests before the client has considered whether they are in her own best interests (e.g., "I need to check my availability and so will let you know tomorrow").

It is important for the therapist to point out that behaving assertively does not guarantee that people will respond positively to the request or statement. Sometimes people will respond negatively, no matter how assertive or respectful the client is. The therapist should explain to the client that she may still receive some negative or unhelpful responses to her assertive behaviors, but that she will be more generally successful in her interactions.

IDENTIFY INTERPERSONAL SCHEMAS
RELATED TO ASSERTIVENESS

At this point, the clinician probably has a good sense of the types of problems the client has in being either overassertive (i.e., aggressive), underassertive (i.e., passive), or both. The top half of the Interpersonal Schemas Worksheet II (Handout 15.1) can be used to identify one or two specific problematic situations. In order to work with the client around real-life examples, ask her to think about recent times when she had trouble being assertive. As discussed above, typical examples of problem behaviors include avoiding or denying problems that really bother the client, which leads to feelings of anger and resentment; acting assertively, but feeling too aggressive; or aggressively attacking the other person in an effort to be assertive.

Having identified specific situations in which the client has difficulty behaving assertively, the therapist should work with the client to identify the maladaptive interpersonal schema or schemas that these situations reflect. As discussed above, often the current maladaptive schema that emerges will involve a stark "either–or" picture in which assertiveness is equated with being either the victim/exploited or the bully/abuser. The client should list the beliefs about self, expectations of others, and consequences as prompted on Handout 15.1.

The next step is to help the client start generating healthier and more flexible interpersonal schemas for assertive situations. In such alternative schemas, the self and other are viewed as two individuals negotiating about something. Both people have strengths, weaknesses, and rights. Such a schema indicates that the goal of the interaction for the client is to present her request or needs in a way that is both direct and respectful of herself and the other. Her belief about herself is that she has the right to ask for what she needs and wants. Her expectations of others are that they may or may not be able or willing to grant her request, but that they will not punish or reject her for asking assertively.

Using the second half of the Interpersonal Schemas Worksheet II as a guide, the therapist should help the client begin to question her maladaptive interpersonal schemas and to articulate alternative possibilities. Applying an alternative schema to one of the specific problem situations identified earlier, the therapist works with the client to see how this schema would change her feelings about herself, her expectations about the other, and her actions in that situation. The client should be helped to identify the potential benefits and challenges of actually trying to use the new schema in this and other assertiveness situations.

CASE EXAMPLE: WORKING WITH ASSERTIVENESS-RELATED SCHEMAS

When asked to give a recent example in which she had difficulty with assertiveness, Caroline shared her experience with Paul, a new man she had met during the course of the treatment. Caroline described being interested in Paul but not ready to begin serious sexual involvement. Caroline felt that she had communicated this to Paul on their first two dates through her avoidance of situations in which they would be alone in private. On the third date, Caroline agreed to let Paul drive her home. When he asked to come in, she consented, even though she did not think it was a good idea. She became very uncomfortable when he told her that he was attracted to her, and felt confused when he began to kiss her. She let it go on for several minutes and then told Paul that she did not feel well; she apologized and said she thought she should get some rest. After Caroline had shared the specifics of the situation, the therapist talked through how to apply the Interpersonal Schemas Worksheet II in order to help identify assertiveness schemas and potential alternatives (see Example 16.1).

THERAPIST: How did you feel about yourself in this situation?

CAROLINE: I felt silly—like why should this be such a big deal? I am a grown woman and should be able to handle a man kissing me, but the reality is that I was nervous and confused and just wanted him to go so I could get my thoughts together.

THERAPIST: How did you expect him to respond to you asking him to leave?

CAROLINE: I didn't know how he would react—maybe get angry that I led him on by having him come up and then making him leave, or maybe just think I was nuts and never call me again.

THERAPIST: Neither of which were appealing outcomes. So what did you do?

CAROLINE: I was searching my mind for what to say without offending him or having to get into a whole thing about it. I waited until I couldn't handle it any more and then made up an excuse for why he needed to go.

THERAPIST: OK. What was the result of that action?

Interpersonal situation	Feelings/beliefs about self	Expectations about other	Resulting action
• What happened? • Who was involved? Allowed Paul to come in but then wanted him to leave when he started kissing me.	• What did I feel/ believe about myself? I should be able to handle this.	• How did I expect the other person to act/ respond to me? I thought he might get angry, feeling I led him on. He might think I'm nuts and never call again.	• What did I do? • What was the result? I waited until I couldn't handle it any more and made up an excuse for why he should go. I felt relieved, but also bad and guilty.

Interpersonal goals	Alternative feelings about self	Alternative expectations	Alternative action
• What are my goals in this situation? I wanted him to like me, to ask me out again. I did not want to get in a situation where sex was a possibility.	• What else could I feel/believe about myself? That I wasn't crazy. That it was okay that I wanted to continue the relationship without being sexual.	• How else could I expect the other person to act/ respond to me? That he might be nice and understanding about it.	• What else could I do? I could tell him the truth about how I felt instead of making up an excuse.

EXAMPLE 16.1. Caroline's filled-in Interpersonal Schemas Worksheet II.

CAROLINE: Well, he did leave, so I felt relieved, but I also felt bad and guilty.

THERAPIST: What did you feel badly about?

CAROLINE: Everything—I didn't handle it right and blew a chance with someone I liked.

Caroline and the therapist spent time talking about how in this particular situation, Caroline's beliefs about herself and about Paul, what she expected, and the result were all related to some of her core beliefs about assertiveness identified earlier in the session. Caroline was aware of her long-standing difficulties in being able to assert her needs, especially in the face of others' competing needs. In thinking about how assertiveness was typically managed in her family, Caroline noted that she and her siblings were "not allowed" to say if there was something they didn't like: "If my mother even thought she saw a sour look, she would threaten to smack it off our faces."

Caroline seemed to have coped with this environment by learning to distance herself from her feelings and needs. As she put it, "we just learned not to have opinions," which made going along with her parents' demands easier. What she also learned was that her needs were really not important and that it was best for her not to show them. Thus she did not have much experience with tuning in to her needs, let alone trying to effectively express them to other people. The sense that it was better to go along than to fight for what she wanted was further confirmed by the times she did try to assert herself: "People either don't listen—act like they didn't even hear me—or I have been told that I am making things complicated."

The therapist then shifted to working with Caroline on the potential for other scenarios, despite the fact that it was hard for her to imagine any.

THERAPIST: Let's just experiment with the possibility of other options, starting with identifying what your goals were in this situation with Paul. What did you want in terms of the relationship in this interaction?

CAROLINE: I wanted him to like me, and I wanted him to ask me out again.

THERAPIST: All right, we've identified that you wanted to continue the relationship. That's important, because (as we said earlier) if you did not want continued contact, that would change your approach. What else, including what you did *not* want in this particular situation?

CAROLINE: What I did not want is exactly what happened. I didn't want to get in a situation where sex was a possibility. I wouldn't have minded a quick kiss, but I knew I wasn't ready for anything more.

THERAPIST: OK, so you wanted to maintain the connection but didn't want it to get sexual.

CAROLINE: Yes—but I'm not sure if that's even possible with a man, if he would put up with that.

THERAPIST: Right. Well, it seems like that assumption is part of what made it hard to be direct. What else could you have felt or believed about yourself in this situation?

CAROLINE: That I wasn't crazy or ridiculous?

THERAPIST: Yes—that your wish to continue the relationship without getting sexual at this point was valid instead of shameful. What about your expectations of Paul? You feared he would get angry or reject you if you said something. What else could you have expected from him?

CAROLINE: I guess to not get mad or reject me, but that seems unlikely.

THERAPIST: Again at this point you don't have to believe the alternative. Just try to stretch your mind to let yourself think of other possibilities.

CAROLINE: OK, I could expect him to be nice and understand—that's what I would have wanted.

THERAPIST: Now if you had these alternative beliefs and expectations that your feelings were valid and that Paul might understand them, what other action could you take besides what you did?

CAROLINE: If I really believed he would not have a bad reaction, I guess I could tell him what was actually going on with me, instead of giving an excuse.

THERAPIST: Right. At least if you believed that there was a possibility of him being understanding, you could take the risk and be more direct about what was really going on. Also, you may have been able to tell him right off the bat that you didn't want him to come up to your apartment without being apologetic or guilty.

CAROLINE: Maybe, but even then I don't know if I could say it in the right way.

THERAPIST: Right. Well, that might take some practice since these are new skills you are learning. That's why we are going to do a role play.

This case example illustrates the process by which trauma survivors can begin developing new ways of expressing themselves and interacting with others. As the case study portrays, abuse survivors may initially err by being too passive in expressing their needs. Caroline's difficulty in looking out for her own interests came up repeatedly during subsequent sessions, as Caroline continued to work on developing ways of feeling more confident and powerful. Typically, role plays and covert modeling will have to be practiced many times and with a variety of situations until the client feels natural, comfortable, and effective in enacting appropriate assertive behavior in a real-life situation.

CONDUCT ROLE PLAYS WITH FOCUS ON USE OF ASSERTIVENESS SKILLS

The therapist and the client should now complete a role play of one of the problematic interpersonal situations identified. Initially, the client should act as herself and the therapist as the other person. This first role play will give the therapist the opportunity to see how the client has assimilated the assertiveness skills presented. After the role play has been completed, the therapist can then share observations and provide suggestions for improving assertiveness. As noted in Session 6, it is important for the therapist to acknowledge the client's strengths and weaknesses. When addressing problems or sticking points, the therapist should provide the potential experience of the other person in the interaction rather than directly using his or her own perceptions, to avoid overwhelming or confusing the client. For instance, the therapist might say, "A person in this situation may feel attacked by your comment."

The therapist's feedback is modeled in the next role play of the same situation, with the therapist now playing the role of the client and the client taking the role of the other person. After this role play, it is important to ask the client how the therapist's approach sounded to her and whether she could realistically picture herself using it.

Finally, the therapist and client reverse roles again, to give the client the opportunity to play herself again and fine-tune her skills in this role play. The client is encouraged to try out the therapist's feedback and experiment with assertiveness skills. Afterward, the therapist should ask the client to describe how the role play felt this time as compared to the first time. The therapist again provides feedback to the client regarding her assertiveness, and makes suggestions for ways to address any lingering trouble spots in this situation.

Challenges in Conducting Assertiveness Role Plays

Communicating anger assertively is often an especially difficult, even threatening task for abuse survivors. Abuse survivors have witnessed firsthand the dangerous consequences of anger through the aggressive acts of their abusers, and they are often unaware that anger can be communicated in a way that is safe and useful. As a result, survivors often deny or minimize their anger, leading to feelings of powerlessness, frustration, and rage. Alternatively, survivors can also express their anger aggressively, leading to feelings of intense guilt, anxiety, and fear. Role playing and covert modeling can be useful in helping the client to develop new ways for communicating her anger appropriately and assertively.

Having the therapist take on the role of a person with whom the client fears interacting (e.g., a critical boss) can be unnerving and distressing to the client, especially if the therapist is effective in role-playing the critical attitude. The client can become convinced that the therapist harbors negative feelings toward her, which may shake her sense of trust in the therapeutic relationship. If this is a major concern, the therapist can decide to use covert modeling instead of role playing to explore alternative assertive behaviors. Covert modeling will give such a client a greater sense of safety and distance from the situation, while allowing her to practice alternative behaviors.

ASSIGN BETWEEN-SESSION WORK

The most important task for the week is to practice effective assertive behaviors. The therapist should ask the client to identify a likely activity, meeting, or interaction that will require assertive behavior. If the client is unable to identify an upcoming situation, she should select exercises from the list of Assertiveness Practice Situations (Handout 16.4) and commit to engaging in one or two of them. Prior to approaching a specific situation, the client should review Handouts 16.1, 16.2, and 16.3 in more detail.

The Interpersonal Schemas Worksheet II (Handout 15.1) should be filled out once a day, with a focus on situations that require assertiveness and practice of assertiveness skills. The client should use Handout 15.1 to record any other significant interpersonal situations as well.

What Is Assertiveness?

"Assertive behavior" means standing up for your legitimate rights and presenting your needs/wants in a way that is respectful of both yourself and others. Assertive behavior may lead you to feel confident, self-respecting, and good about yourself.

In many abusive families, family members often deny or hide their feelings and needs or force them aggressively on others. As a result, there are no models for appropriate assertive behaviors.

"Nonassertive behavior" means ignoring or not expressing your own rights, needs, and desires. Nonassertive behavior may lead you to feel hurt, resentful, anxious, disappointed, and/or angry.

"Aggressive behavior" means expressing your own rights at the expense of others through inappropriate outbursts or hostility. Aggressive behavior may lead you to feel angry, indignant, out of control, and/or guilty.

Basic Personal Rights

1. I have the right to ask for what I want.

2. I have the right to say no.

3. I have the right to feel and express my feelings, both positive and negative.

4. I have the right to make mistakes.

5. I have the right to have my own opinions, convictions, and values.

6. I have the right to be treated with dignity and respect.

7. I have the right to change my mind or decide on a different course of action.

8. I have the right to protest unfair treatment or criticism.

9. I have the right to expect honesty from others.

10. I have the right to be angry at someone I love.

11. I have the right to say, "I don't know."

12. I have the right to negotiate for change.

13. I have the right to be in a nonabusive environment.

14. I have the right to ask for help or emotional support.

15. I have the right to my own needs for personal space and time, even if others would prefer my company.

16. I have the right not to have to justify myself to others.

17. I have the right not to take responsibility for someone else's behavior, feelings, or problems.

18. I have the right not to have to anticipate others' needs and wishes.

19. I have the right not to have to worry all the time about the goodwill of others.

20. I have the right to choose not to respond to a situation.

Assertiveness Skills

"I" messages. These have three parts:

Behavior: "When you [state the behavior] . . . "
Feeling "I feel [state the feeling] . . . "
Consequence: "because [state the consequence for you]."

Making requests. Be specific about what you want, and state it clearly and simply.

Couch your request in "I" language.
State positive consequences of the other's compliance with your request, and/or the negative consequences of the other's noncompliance.
Avoid making excuses, downplaying your request, or blaming the other person.
Delay the situation if the other person responds angrily or aggressively.

Saying no. The strategies you choose will depend on your interest in maintaining the relationship.

If you do not want to maintain the relationship:
Say, "No, thank you," in a respectful, firm tone.
If the other person persists, repeat yourself while maintaining eye contact and slightly raising the tone of your voice.
Or use the "broken record" technique: Repeat a concise sentence over and over without getting sidetracked by other issues.

If you do want to maintain the relationship:
Acknowledge the other person's request by repeating it.
Without apologizing, give a brief explanation of your reason for declining.
If appropriate, suggest an alternative plan in which both your and the other person's needs will be met.
If saying no is especially difficult, give yourself some time before responding to a request.

Remember: Behaving assertively does not guarantee that people will respond positively. Though you may sometimes receive negative or unhelpful responses to your assertive behaviors, you will be more generally successful in your interactions with other people.

Assertiveness Practice Situations

1. Go to a library and ask the librarian for assistance in finding a book. Alternatively, ask a salesperson to help you find something.

2. In a drugstore or convenience store, ask for change for a $1 bill without buying anything.

3. Call and make an appointment to have your hair cut. Call back later and cancel the appointment. Alternatively, make and cancel dinner reservations or airline reservations.

4. Ask the pharmacist for information on an over-the-counter drug.

5. Ask for a substitution on the menu when ordering a meal.

6. Ask coworkers or classmates to do a favor for you (e.g., get you a cup of coffee while they get their own, give you an opinion on some aspect of your work).

7. Disagree with someone's opinion.

8. Ask a friend for help in fixing something.

9. Ask a person who is making too much noise to be quieter.

10. Ask your landlord to fix a problem in your apartment.

11. Ask a person to stop doing something that bothers you.

CHAPTER 17

~

SESSION 8
Flexibility in Relationships

Restrictions in human living might be tolerable were it not
for the fact that they lead to further complications.
—HANS H. STRUPP AND JEFFREY L. BINDER (1984, p. 32)

OVERVIEW

In Session 8, the work of identifying maladaptive interpersonal schemas and developing
alternative ways of approaching and processing relationships continues. The focus, however, is narrowed so as to address the specific difficulties childhood abuse survivors can
have in being flexible in their relationships. As previously discussed, abuse survivors
may often rely on a restricted range of schemas and apply them across the board to most
interpersonal situations. Yet successful social functioning requires people to have multiple potential schemas at their disposal, since different situations and types of relationships are imbued with different degrees of intimacy, emotional expectations, and power
balances. Reaching a particular interpersonal goal or conveying a particular message
cannot be separated from the emotions and emotional tone conveyed in the exchange.
Difficulties in appropriate personal and emotional engagement are often most apparent
in interpersonal situations involving issues of power. The main aim of this session is to
help clients engage with others in a flexible and emotionally authentic and respectful
way, within a variety of interpersonal contexts. This involves having clients move away
from the tendency to apply an "all-or-nothing" view of power in their relationships.
Instead, an approach that emphasizes the importance of different balances of power and
intimacy in relationships is presented. Box 17.1 outlines the theme and curriculum for
Session 8 of treatment.

BOX 17.1
Theme and Curriculum for Session 8:
Flexibility in Relationships

THEME

Child abuse survivors often have a limited and rigid repertoire of interpersonal schemas that are typically based on negative expectations in relationships. Different types of relationships require different types of communication, however. A person's approach to and expectations of interpersonal situations should consider the power balance in the relationship and the goals for the interaction. Dealing with power dynamics and differentiating various goals in an interpersonal interaction are two specific areas that require flexibility, and thus are often particularly difficult for abuse survivors in their relationships.

PLANNING AND PREPARATION

Bring extra copies of Interpersonal Schemas Worksheet II (Handout 15.1).

AGENDA

- Complete emotional check-in and review of between-session work.
- Provide psychoeducation: Why is flexibility so important?
- Describe types of power balances in relationships.
- Discuss common stumbling blocks in each type of relationship.
- Review skills for getting better balance.
- Identify interpersonal schemas in different types of power relationships.

- Conduct role plays with focus on negotiating power balances.
- Prepare for transition to second phase of treatment.
- Assign between-session work:
  - Complete Interpersonal Schemas Worksheet II (Handout 15.1) once a day on ways of relating differently to people, including emotion regulation skills relevant to the situation.
  - Make list of questions and concerns about next phase of treatment.
  - Practice focused breathing twice a day.

SESSION HANDOUTS

Additional copies of Handout 15.1. Interpersonal Schemas Worksheet II

PROVIDE PSYCHOEDUCATION:
WHY IS FLEXIBILITY SO IMPORTANT?

The therapist will want to open the session by discussing with the client the advantages of being flexible in relationships. This discussion will set the stage for the work of building skills in assessing various goals and power balances in different types of relationships. In considering the importance of interpersonal flexibility, the therapist can begin by briefly reiterating some of the information presented in Session 5 about the tendency of childhood abuse survivors to have limited and rigid relationship schemas, and the potential negative consequences of maintaining these schemas in their current lives. It is also helpful to engage the client by asking her how she thinks difficulties with flexibility have influenced her relationships specifically. Using the client's perspective as a jumping-off point highlights ways that inflexibility can interfere with effective social functioning. For example, the therapist can say, "Since different interpersonal situations require different types of communication, rather than a 'one size fits all' model, we need to consider the nature of and goals for each relationship and vary our approaches accordingly."

The therapist can share with the client that for many abuse survivors, differentiating various goals in an interpersonal situation is quite challenging. They may focus solely on maintaining a relationship with the other person, which leads to sacrificing immediate needs completely. Alternatively, they may focus exclusively on getting immediate needs and wants met through the other person, without considering the impact this will have on the relationship.

The therapist can also describe how inflexibility can contribute to difficulties in managing power dynamics in relationships. Abuse survivors' experiences often lead them to equate power with abuse and disregard for the needs and rights of others. As a result, it is common for them to feel that there are only two options in a relationship: to be a powerful abuser or the powerless victim. Clearly, both of these roles can create serious problems in a client's relationships.

DESCRIBE TYPES OF POWER BALANCES IN RELATIONSHIPS

Describe to the client the three central kinds of power balances in relationships, presented in Box 17.2.

• *Type I.* In the first type, the self has the same amount of power as the other person in the interaction. Typical examples of people in this power balance are colleagues, friends, and siblings. How we interact with individuals in an equal power balance depends upon our goals for the interaction. With friends and siblings, our ultimate goal may be to maintain or strengthen the relationship, which may lead us to be more willing to compromise on our immediate wants or needs. In contrast, we may be less concerned about promoting a close relationship with colleagues, because our ultimate goal in the relationship is to secure their cooperation in getting work done. These different goals

---

BOX 17.2
Three Types of Power Balances in Relationships

- *Type I*. Self and other have equal power: friend, sibling, coworker, partner.
- *Type II*. Self has more power: parent, teacher, employer, supervisor.
- *Type III*. Self has less power: child, student, employee.

---

determine how willing we are to be confrontational and/or compromising in an interaction.

- *Type II*. In the second kind of power balance, the self has more power than the other person, as is the case when the self is an employer or a parent. In such a relationship, the self typically takes a more active role in setting the agenda and has the expectation that the other will respond to requests because of the power differential. The types of demands made vary according to the goals for the interaction. With a child, the goals for the interaction may center on protecting and nurturing the child and promoting the relationship with the child. With an employee, on the other hand, promotion of the relationship is often less of a focus than ensuring that work goals are being met.

- *Type III*. In the last kind of power balance, the self has less power than the other person, as is typically the case when the self is an employee or a child. In these relationships, the self tends to be more submissive and often takes the role of responding to the requests of the other. How we communicate in this role and how we respond to the other person's demands again vary according to our goals. In our relationships with employers, the typical goal for an interaction may be to keep our job and to increase our chances of advancement through recognition of our work. While these goals often require that we have a positive relationship with our employers based on mutual respect, promoting the relationship itself is usually not the primary goal in these interactions. In our relationships with parents, our goals for interactions often focus on maintaining and promoting a relationship with them, while ensuring that our own needs are met. For people who were abused by their parents, the goal may instead be to minimize a connection with the parents in order to protect themselves.

To demonstrate the differences among the three types of power balances, therapists may find it useful to use the following illustration. While this example is somewhat silly, it illustrates the different ways we can respond to the same request coming from different people, based on the power balance between us and the other person.

> "If your child says he or she wants chocolate cake for lunch, you would be likely to say no firmly, without entertaining the possibility. If your partner says he or she wants chocolate cake for lunch, you may choose to say, 'How about a sandwich instead? Chocolate cake isn't such a healthy choice.' Finally, if your boss says he or she wants chocolate cake for lunch, you may choose to say, 'Excellent choice!' "

DISCUSS COMMON STUMBLING BLOCKS
IN POWER RELATIONSHIPS

The therapist should now discuss with the client common stumbling blocks in each of the three power relationships described below and provide examples.

• *Type I*. Although the power balance is equal in these relationships, abuse survivors may be prone to see themselves as having more or less power than the other person, due to their childhood experiences. For example, they may relate to work colleagues as abusive parents and have difficulty seeing that their colleagues do not hold that kind of power over them. On the other hand, survivors may act as if they hold more power in the relationship for fear of being "victimized" or taken advantage of by the other person. The case examples below illustrate both of these types of problems in Type I relationships.

At the beginning of treatment, Angie, a 20-year-old student, described tremendous anxiety in interactions with most of her friends. She constantly feared letting her friends down or making them angry with her. When there was any issue or conflict, she would become uncomfortable and distressed, which would lead her to call and smooth things over regardless of the situation. Despite the reality that Angie was (or should have been) on an equal footing with her friends, she certainly did not feel or act this way, which continued to fuel her anxiety and obsequious behavior.

In contrast, Joanne came into treatment because she feared losing her boyfriend of several years. He had threatened to break up with her because of her "bossiness," saying that he could no longer stand her efforts to control him. When Joanne and her therapist examined these relationship interactions, it became apparent that Joanne often treated her boyfriend as though he was a child. She would often tell him what to eat, pick out his clothing, and even make plans for him. Rather than being a girlfriend, Joanne had taken on the role of an intrusive mother. Although initially her boyfriend had felt taken care of, over time he began to feel resentful.

• *Type II*. Because of experiences in past relationships, abuse survivors may not understand that they have more power in these types of relationships, or they may deny that they do for fear of what it means to be powerful (e.g., power may be equated with aggression). In contrast, some abuse survivors find themselves taking on the role of abuser in this power situation, becoming literally or figuratively abusive. Behaving abusively in these interactions can lead a survivor to feel frightened, anxious, guilty, and disgusted with herself. The case examples below illustrate both of these types of problems in Type II relationships.

Jen, a high school teacher, was distressed by the fact that her students did not seem to respect her. She felt ineffective and embarrassed by her reputation as a pushover. When her therapist asked her more about what was going on in her classroom, Jen described an atmosphere in which she gave her students tremendous freedom and imposed minimal limits. She was surprised and hurt when students disregarded assignments, but she had difficulty giving consequences. Though Jen appeared to be a skilled teacher, her discomfort in taking on the role of an authority figure was having a negative impact on her professional life and self-esteem.

At the opposite end of the spectrum, Becca, the eldest of three children, was named executor of her mother's will; this included overseeing the sale of her mother's properties and ensuring that each of the three children received an equal percentage of the profits. Rather than implementing her mother's plan and involving her siblings in the process, Becca became very secretive and manipulative. She delayed putting the properties on the market; she also made important decisions without talking to her sisters and refused to provide them with updates, saying that since she was the one chosen to handle things, she should not have to run things by her sisters for their approval. Becca acknowledged that she felt entitled to more than her two sisters because she was taking on more responsibility, noting that this had always been the case. In this way Becca was using this opportunity to fulfill her own agenda by unilaterally assuming power, instead of taking the lead while also acting collaboratively with her siblings, as her mother had intended.

• *Type III.* Type III relationships can be especially difficult for abuse survivors, because people in positions of power are often equated with abusive caretakers (or actually are abusive themselves). This association can leave survivors feeling angry, helpless, scared, and anxious in interactions with these people. The primary challenge of relationships in which we have less power is to try to achieve a balance between meeting the other person's demands or requests, while getting our own needs met in the relationship. The following case examples illustrate such problems in Type III relationships.

Beth had recently seen a doctor who had diagnosed her with a thyroid condition and had prescribed medication without giving much explanation or information. Shortly after she began taking the medication, she reported to her therapist that she felt fatigued and dizzy. Her therapist recommended she call the doctor to ask about possible side effects rather than waiting for her next appointment, which was scheduled for next month. Despite her discomfort, Beth felt hesitant to call the doctor, since it was not an emergency situation. She did not want to annoy or question the doctor, as she felt this might affect the quality of care he was willing to provide. Beth's therapist used this example to discuss ways Beth interacted with those she viewed as being in authority. She did not feel entitled to ask questions even when her own needs were being compromised. The therapist tried to provide a reality check and discussed with Beth that part of her doctor's job was to provide follow-up care and information.

Dawn worked as an assistant to a prestigious editor. Though she knew her job would include long hours and little pay, she had taken it because she knew the experience could further her career. However, when Dawn's boss asked if she could come in on a weekend in order to meet a pressing deadline, Dawn felt that she was being taken advantage of and needed to stand up for herself. She told her boss in no uncertain terms that she would not be treated like a slave and walked out of the office. In treatment Dawn identified that one of her major interpersonal schemas involved the assumption that those in positions of power would inevitably exploit her. In response to this expectation, she was always on the lookout for this possibility and likely to interpret others' behavior as fitting with this model, which at times caused her to take actions she later regretted. The therapist acknowledged the importance of Dawn's self-protective instincts, but also noted the need to develop other potential schemas in which abuse was not a given. The therapist also worked with Dawn on building skills (e.g., identifying relationship goals and considering pros and cons of continuing the relationship) that could help her assess current situations with authority figures more objectively, prior to taking actions.

REVIEW SKILLS FOR GETTING BETTER BALANCE

As we have emphasized throughout this chapter, in order to achieve better balance in relationships, clients need to become more adept at considering relationship goals and identifying power dynamics before reacting. Contextual information and awareness will also help clients determine the appropriate level of intimacy and assertiveness (e.g., avoiding traps of not being sufficiently assertive and being overly assertive) in interactions. One way to do this is to help clients draw on the skills learned in the previous sessions and apply them to the various types of power relationships. For example, a therapist can tell a client:

- "Remember to listen carefully."
- "Slow down, and clarify what is being expected of you."
- "Practice distress tolerance. Sit with your feelings, and realize that there will be opportunities to come back to the issue."
- "Identify your goals and examine your pros and cons. What are you trying to accomplish? Is it worth it?"
- "Get multiple perspectives before reacting."
- "When you are confused, get more data. Ask for feedback about power dynamics. Make sure that this is the kind of person you can safely talk to."
- "Remind yourself, 'This is part of my history.' Using this type of self-talk may help you contain your emotions and understand why you are reacting strongly in the moment."

IDENTIFY INTERPERSONAL SCHEMAS IN DIFFERENT TYPES OF POWER RELATIONSHIPS

In order to work on building flexibility skills in the session, the therapist should ask the client to think of examples of people in her life who are in the three types of power relationships with her. For one person in each type of relationship category, the client should briefly recall a recent interaction. Using the top half of the Interpersonal Schemas Worksheet II (Handout 15.1) as a guide, the client should identify the interpersonal schemas that she has for these different people. The therapist and client can then discuss her beliefs about herself and each other person, determine how these beliefs affect the relationship, and try to identify elements of her schema that are linked to maladaptive past relationships. Finally, using the bottom half of Handout 15.1, the therapist can work with the client to develop more adaptive and appropriate schemas, based on a thoughtful and realistic sense of the power balance and goals for these relationships.

CASE EXAMPLE: WORKING WITH POWER RELATIONSHIP

Julie identified two relationships with key people in her daily life that represented different power balances—her relationship with her boyfriend and her boss. The therapist asked Julie to describe recent experiences with both relationships, and used the top half of the Interpersonal Schemas Worksheet II as a guide to identify current interpersonal schemas and outcomes (see the top portions of Examples 17.1 and 17.2).

THERAPIST: Although these relationships are very different, there are some real similarities in these two examples. What do you notice?

JULIE: Well, in both cases I ended up feeling bad and feeling that everything I do is wrong.

THERAPIST: Yes, that does seem to be a theme. Also, in both cases you expected the worst from the other person. You anticipated that neither your boss nor your boyfriend would listen to you. Do you think these expectations affected your behavior in any way?

JULIE: Well, yeah. That's why I didn't try to talk to them about it.

THERAPIST: Which makes sense—if you expect no one will listen, then you are not likely to put yourself out there. Where do you think these expectations that you will not be heard come from?

JULIE: They come from people not listening to me.

THERAPIST: You have shared with me that this certainly was the case with your parents—that they would accuse you of something and not give you the chance to defend yourself.

JULIE: If I tried to explain, they would get mad and say I was being disrespectful. Usually I would get punished or even hit.

THERAPIST: In this context with your parents, it sounds like avoiding further discussion and leaving the situation before it escalated was an adaptive response and allowed you to avoid some negative consequences. However, in your current life, always expecting that you will be shut down and punished for trying to speak up has some potential negative consequences. Can you think of any?

Interpersonal situation	Feelings/beliefs about self	Expectations about other	Resulting action
• What happened? • Who was involved? In my latest meeting with my boss, she was not happy with my work. According to her, a recent report I wrote was done incorrectly.	• What did I feel/believe about myself? Embarrassed and useless—how could I have thought the report was done right? Also mad, because I don't think she explained the task well—I felt unfairly blamed.	• How did I expect the other person to act/respond to me? I thought she was going to blame me without giving me a chance to explain. I was worried that she would think less of me.	• What did I do? • What was the result? I didn't say much in the meeting. I listened to what she said and agreed. Then I went to the bathroom and cried. Felt like I wanted to quit.

Interpersonal goals	Alternative feelings about self	Alternative expectations	Alternative action
• What are my goals in this situation? Keep my job. Have my boss feel I am competent. Have her understand why I approached the assignment as I did.	• What else could I feel/believe about myself? That I am not stupid—that it was a misunderstanding I could explain.	• How else could I expect the other person to act/respond to me? That she would listen to my perspective. That she would give me a chance to correct it. That she would take into consideration my other work.	• What else could I do? Set up another meeting to talk to her about it, after I have had a chance to think about what I want to say.

EXAMPLE 17.1. Julie's filled-in Interpersonal Schemas Worksheet II
for her relationships with her boss.

JULIE: Well, yeah. I let people go on thinking whatever they want to think about me, even if it is wrong—but I would rather do that than try to convince them of something else.

THERAPIST: Yes, you are not inclined to try to clarify a misunderstanding or further discuss a situation, which leaves you unable to further discuss your intentions or understand the other person's perception of your behavior. Again, when you are dealing with someone who is toxic, this may be for the best—you avoid getting into a nonproductive interaction. But what about situations in which you are wrong in assuming the other person will respond negatively?

JULIE: Well, how do I know if this is going to be the case?

THERAPIST: True, you don't always know, so it involves some risk—but in certain cases it may be worth it. For example, there are likely to be situations in which others will not belittle or ignore your efforts to explain yourself. In these cases you don't let the person know what's on your mind, and you miss out on the opportunity to have an important conversation that may improve things in the relationship. This is the main limitation of applying expectations across the board in your relationships. Although it is more nuanced and complicated, ultimately it is more adaptive to take each relationship on a case-by-case basis, taking into account the goals you have for the relationship and the balance of power in that specific relationship. This will help you to consider what approach you might want to take. In your examples, you felt unheard by both your boss and boyfriend—but since they are different types of relationships, if you do decide to respond, you will want to approach them in different ways.

Using Julie's two examples, the therapist worked with her to identify and differentiate interpersonal goals and alternative schemas in each type of power relationship (see the bottom portions of Examples 17.1 and 17.2). Whereas with her boss the identified goal was to keep her job and be seen as competent, with her boyfriend the goal was to have him

Interpersonal situation	Feelings/beliefs about self	Expectations about other	Resulting action
• What happened? • Who was involved? My boyfriend snapped at me because I lost the car keys. He called me irresponsible.	• What did I feel/believe about myself? Stupid. Why am I always losing things? I can never get things together.	• How did I expect the other person to act/respond to me? He would not understand why I felt the way I did.	• What did I do? • What was the result? Went into the other room until he left for work. Was upset most of the day.

Interpersonal goals	Alternative feelings about self	Alternative expectations	Alternative action
• What are my goals in this situation? To apologize, but also to improve communication in the future. To tell him I don't like being snapped at.	• What else could I feel/believe about myself? I sometimes lose things, but I'm not the only one.	• How else could I expect the other person to act/respond to me? That he would hear my apology without being rude. That he might apologize for snapping at me over it if he knew this hurt my feelings.	• What else could I do? Talk to him about it. If he is a jerk, end the conversation.

EXAMPLE 17.2. Julie's filled-in Interpersonal Schemas Worksheet II
for her relationships with her boyfriend.

understand her feelings and to improve the relationship. The therapist and Julie also discussed specifically how the different power balances in these two relationships were relevant. For example, whereas Julie might want to get more into sharing her emotions with her boyfriend and discuss ways she did not feel heard, with her boss this level of communication would not be appropriate or likely to be useful. In the latter case, since Julie had less power in the relationship, she would probably be more effective if she followed her boss's lead and specifically addressed the concerns expressed about her work. In the former case, Julie might want to work on being more assertive: Although she shared power in the relationship with her boyfriend, she often behaved submissively, as though he was more of a parent figure.

After identifying goals and power balances, the therapist asked Julie to think about alternative ways of approaching each situation, alternative beliefs about herself and expectations of the other, and how these might lead her to take alternative actions. For example, if Julie believed that her boss might listen to her response without being punishing, Julie would feel less anxious about explaining her perspective (keeping in mind the goal and power differential). Also, if Julie believed that her boyfriend might not become more adversarial and would care about how she was feeling about their interaction, she might feel more confident about herself and be willing to share her feelings and ways she would like the relationship to improve.

CONDUCT ROLE PLAYS WITH FOCUS ON NEGOTIATING POWER BALANCES

The therapist and client now conduct two role plays using relationship examples provided by the client, each focusing on a person in a particular power balance. The selected examples should involve two different types of power relationships (e.g., the client's relationships with her employer vs. her child). As in Sessions 6 and 7, the first role play should have the client playing herself and the clinician playing the role of the other person. After the role play has been completed, the therapist can then share observations and provide suggestions for improving the client's communication in this power structure and clarifying her goals for the interaction. As noted in the description of role playing for Session 6 (see Chapter 15), it is important for the therapist to acknowledge both the client's strengths and weaknesses. When addressing problems or sticking points, the therapist should provide the potential experience of the other person in the interaction rather than directly using his or her own perceptions, to avoid overwhelming or confusing the client.

The therapist's feedback is modeled in the next role play of the same situation, with the therapist now playing the role of the client and the client taking the role of the other person. After this role play, it is important to ask the client how the therapist's approach sounded to her, whether she could realistically picture herself using it, and whether she has any feedback or suggestions.

Finally, the therapist and client reverse roles again, to give the client the opportunity to play herself again and fine-tune her skills in this role play. The client is encouraged to try out the therapist's feedback and to experiment with alternative interpersonal skills.

Afterward, the therapist should ask the client to describe how the role play felt this time as compared to the first time. The therapist again provides feedback to the client regarding her communication style, and makes suggestions for ways to address any lingering trouble spots in this situation.

The role-play procedure should then be repeated for the client's second example, in which the client is in a different power situation. Feedback, suggestions, and discussion here should focus on both building and refining communication skills, differentiating interpersonal goals, and identifying and understanding differences in communication in the two role plays. The therapist continues to emphasize the necessity for different types of communication in different situations.

PREPARE FOR TRANSITION TO NEXT PHASE OF TREATMENT

Acknowledge That This Session Marks the End of Phase I, and Review Progress

The clinician needs to allow time in Session 8 to acknowledge that this session marks the end of the first phase of treatment by doing the following:

- Briefly reviewing with the client the work that she has done in building emotional regulation and interpersonal skills.
- Asking the client to share her own thoughts about her progress and ways the treatment has been both helpful and unhelpful thus far.
- Congratulating the client on her hard work and progress during this first phase of the treatment, and emphasizing her strengths.
- Discussing together the areas in which she is continuing to grow and improve, and letting her know that work will continue on these areas during the next phase of treatment.

Review Format and Session Changes for NST Phase

The therapist should remind the client that in the NST phase of treatment (Phase II), their work together will shift toward helping her to process and integrate her traumatic memories. This goal will be accomplished by going through her traumatic memories repeatedly and coming to an understanding of their meaning for her now. The client should be told that during NST sessions, the first part of each session will be spent doing the exposure work, leaving the end to continue working on emotion management and relationship skills.

Elicit Client's Questions and Concerns about Transition to NST

The therapist should now ask the client whether she has any questions or concerns about the transition to NST. Is the format of this phase of treatment clear to her? Does she understand the rationale and procedure for NST? What are her concerns and fears about starting to do NST? The therapist should encourage the client to be frank about her concerns, and should also indicate that there will be more time to discuss her questions, concerns, and NST in general next session.

ASSIGN BETWEEN-SESSION WORK

The client's most important task for the week is to practice being flexible in situations with different people. Accordingly, the client should identify two people in different types of power relationships with whom she will interact during the week. She should then fill out the Interpersonal Schemas Worksheet II (Handout 15.1) for these interactions to chart the different schemas needed for these different situations. The client should also use Handout 15.1 to record relevant emotion regulation strategies responsive to the situation (e.g., positive activities, thought stopping, and positive statements) as determined by therapist and client.

Prior to the next session, the client should also make a list of any questions or concerns she has about the next phase of treatment. The beginning of the next session will be spent addressing these issues.

PHASE II

〜

Narrative Story Telling (NST)
Facing the Past and Imagining a Future

> What makes humans so extraordinary is that we have imagination; that we can think about creating worlds different from the ones we are in. If we are lucky, we use the misery that we go through to create better things. And we are fundamentally profoundly creative and transforming people.
>   —BESSEL A. VAN DER KOLK (2003)

It has often been said that PTSD is a disorder of memory, because the client cannot leave the past behind. It follows her wherever she goes, living side by side with her. But PTSD is also a disorder that steals the future. The client cannot leave the past behind, but she also cannot go forward into an imagined future. This is a result of many factors: of having had few or limited life experiences other than those defined by chronic abuse, of the consuming effort of getting through each day, and of the paralyzing expectation that the future will be much too like the past.

It takes courage to leap into the unknown—where, against all experience, a person imagines living a life that has never been, and allows herself the possibility of joining in a world in which she has never participated. It is our hope that by creating a sense of continuity between the past and present, and initiating a process of discovery about new and possible ways of seeing herself and others, the client will, after looking back, face forward and orient herself to an imagined future.

CHAPTER 18

~

Moving from Skills Training to Narrative Processing of Trauma
How Do You Know Your Client Is Ready?

My silences have not protected me. Your silence will not protect you.
—AUDRE LORDE (1984, p. 40)

The transition to focused attention on the trauma memories is often associated with increased anxiety and discomfort for a client, and sometimes for a therapist as well. Therapists often fear that their clients will get worse, suffer symptom exacerbation, or flee from the therapy when confronting painful memories. If not fearful of the task itself, therapists often uneasily inquire, "How will I know that my client is ready for narrative work?"

Both a therapist and a client need to keep in mind that some amount of increased anxiety in the anticipation of the task and in the initial efforts of confronting the memories is inevitable. It is frightening to face what one fears. However, it is our experience that narrative work is more difficult to think about than do. The anticipatory anxiety resulting from imagining the next steps often requires more emotion management than the actual effort involved when therapist and client structure, agree upon, and begin the task. The skills sessions have prepared the client and therapist for this work: The two of them have an established working relationship; the client has developed sufficient skills and confidence in herself to face difficult emotions; and she has some amount of trust in the therapist to guide her safely and effectively through the process. The initial skills training phase enhances two therapeutic features that are important to successful narrative work:

1. *Therapist's knowledge of the client.* First, the therapist is by now thoroughly familiar with the client's trauma history, symptoms, and coping skills. The therapist is aware of the severity of the client's fear and emotional reactivity; has a working knowledge of the client's general coping style and distress tolerance; and has been able to evaluate, facilitate, and observe the client's skills strengths and areas of vulnerability. All of this information helps the therapist proceed effectively in the therapeutic task during the narrative work, which is to modulate the emotional experience of the client. This includes both encouraging the client to provide more specific and extended articulation of feelings and beliefs than she otherwise would have, and helping the client ease up or move away from material that is overwhelming.

2. *A shared understanding and commitment.* The initial sessions also provide the template for the working relationship between therapist and client. The therapist's knowledge of the client described above is the result of a process in which the therapist identifies and characterizes the client's problems and skills, so that the client can confirm, correct, adjust, or extend the developing picture. This process engenders in the client a sense of being recognized and understood. The client develops confidence in the therapist's growing knowledge of her strengths and weaknesses. In addition, they develop a specific language for referring to and describing internal emotional states and the traumatic memories. Lastly, the treatment goals and the means to reach these goals are repeatedly reviewed and take concrete shape through the emergence of the client's specific vulnerabilities, emotional reactivity, and strengths. Ideally, the therapist and client will be in agreement toward the end of the skills training work that the next task is the narrative work, and will have a good sense of how this task will go. Agreement on goals and the means to reach these goals, based on solid knowledge of the client's symptoms, needs, and strengths, secures the therapeutic foundation and provides confidence in both therapist and client for successful narrative work.

GUIDELINES FOR REVIEWING READINESS
FOR NARRATIVE WORK

There are no hard and fast rules about "when" to begin narrative work. Some clients may be ready in the second session, while others may not be prepared to do so for many months. The more important question is whether an individual client is ready. The client and the treatment relationship should meet the criteria described above. This is a clinical judgment that therapists should make on a case-by-basis. The following basic questions may be helpful in assessing whether moving to the exposure phase is indicated and appropriate for a certain client at a particular time in treatment. The assessment of readiness is helped if both therapist and client keep in mind the core features of narrative processing of the trauma (see Box 18.1).

BOX 18.1
What Is the Purpose and Nature of Narrative Work?

The goal of trauma narration is for the client to experience trauma-related feelings with depth and with control. Understood in this way, trauma narration is not a direct reexperiencing of the past. Rather, trauma narration allows the client to visit the past with the tools of the present, in the safety of the present, and with the companionship of an ally from the present.

Through the use of emotion management techniques and awareness of the safety features of her current environment, the client reexperiences fear but without being overwhelmed by it. The client can come into contact with the feeling that there is no escape from traumatic events and memories, but that she has survived her past. The client can feel the anger and sadness of being betrayed or abandoned by important people in her life, but with the therapist's presence, she need not feel obliterated by this knowledge. This client can reveal the shame she feels about her abuse and feel comforted by the compassion of an empathetic therapist.

Is the Client Committed to the Treatment?

Before embarking on narrative work, the therapist must have a sense of the client's motivation, ability, and willingness. Psychotherapy in general, and trauma treatment in particular, are challenging processes that require considerable investment and effort on the part of the client (as well as the therapist) to be fruitful. Even with a high level of motivation facing often distressing and painful issues required to make changes is difficult for a client; without it, a therapist is fighting an uphill battle. This is not to say that the client cannot express hesitation, ambivalence, or even resentment that she has these problems as a consequence of abuse experiences. The client does not necessarily have to feel positive about or enjoy being in treatment. In addition, a client may go through periods during the treatment when it feels particularly difficult to sustain involvement (for any number of reasons). These and other potential obstacles are manageable if they can be raised and addressed in the context of the therapy, and if they do not interfere with a basic level of client compliance in treatment.

If there is doubt about a client's level of commitment or ability to participate fully in the narrative work, then the treatment direction and goals need to be reevaluated in a nonjudgmental and realistic way. The following considerations about past experience in working with a given client may be helpful in this regard: Up to this point, has the client demonstrated interest and motivation in the treatment? If not, has she been able to tolerate and participate in examining obstacles? Has the client made her treatment a priority, or does therapy tend to take a back seat? Has she behaved in ways indicating a belief that the treatment is valuable (e.g., keeping most appointments, being generally on time, not putting other activities before treatment, doing between-session work, being actively engaged during sessions)?

Is the Client Relatively Stable at the Present Time?

The client's mental status and symptom severity should be continually evaluated throughout the therapy, as they will affect the treatment's direction and focus session by session. However, at this juncture when the therapist is considering whether to begin the narrative phase, particular attention to assessing the client's current level of stability and her current strengths and weaknesses is indicated.

"Stability" is a relative and hard-to-define term, especially given that so many childhood abuse survivors deal with a host of ongoing psychological, physical, and social problems on a daily basis. Many of our clients have chaotic and overwhelming lives; indeed, this has become the norm rather than the exception. Also, feeling consistently overwhelmed, "edgy," and easily emotionally triggered are hallmarks of the PTSD diagnosis for which many clients qualify. These factors can make an accurate appraisal of a particular client's current level of stress, capabilities, and limitations challenging. It is important to keep in mind that for most of these clients there is no "optimal" time to begin narrative work, as there is typically some kind of disruption or crisis happening in their lives. Waiting until things are "calm" is unrealistic, as much of the chaos is perpetuated by the ongoing PTSD symptoms. If a therapist continues to move from crisis to crisis with such a client, it is the equivalent of continually putting out small fires rather than locating the main source of the fire, which will continue to rage. In fact, many of our clients have already had this type of experience in previous therapies, which did not systematically address the trauma memories and associated feelings at the root of their troubling symptoms.

However, if a clinician feels that a client is in a particularly vulnerable or precarious psychological state in which any additional stress may be intolerable or lead to decompensation, then engaging in narrative work (even in a modified format) is not indicated, as the potential risks outweigh the benefits. This type of situation most often arises when there are sudden major stressors or transitions in a client's life (e.g., unexpected death or loss of family/friend, recent diagnosis of serious medical condition, loss of job or housing, divorce/breakup), or when for some reason the client has a particularly pressing situation that requires immediate attention and a high level of functioning (e.g., work situation that may jeopardize employment status, acute family emergency). In these cases narrative work should probably be delayed, as it requires substantial effort and energy that may be in especially short supply. This is particularly relevant for patients who have a history of addictive or self-injurious behaviors.

Has the Client Demonstrated Some Capacity for an Alliance with the Therapist?

Addressing the client's capacity for a therapeutic alliance involves taking stock of how the client has worked with and related to the therapist up until this point. Specific key issues relevant to childhood abuse survivors must be considered. Specifically, most of our clients are struggling in building and maintaining healthy interpersonal relationships, and often this particular problem is what has brought them into treatment. A history of repeated violations by caretakers understandably has a negative impact on a person's ability to develop closeness and trust with others, particularly with those (such as therapists) who may be perceived as authority or parental figures. Thus if a client demonstrates guardedness, suspiciousness, anxiety, hostility, or fear at times with the therapist, it is not surprising and should not be taken in and of itself as an indication that she can't develop an effective working relationship. In fact, these difficult feelings in the therapy relationship can be used in a beneficial manner if the client can directly express them or tolerate discussion of them.

However, if the client has not developed some level of trust with the therapist, has not been able to take in feedback constructively, or cannot communicate her reservations, there is cause for concern about moving into narrative work. The client needs to have some belief, even if it is tenuous, that the therapist is competent and motivated to help rather than to violate her. If not, it is unlikely that the client will be willing to engage in exposure techniques, during which the therapist will be encouraging her to take risks by stepping outside her comfort zone. Or the client may agree to proceed with exposure but may feel that she is being coerced and victimized by the therapist rather than actively participating by her own choice. It is not uncommon in work with a trauma survivor for the therapist and client to find themselves in respective "abuser–victim" roles in the treatment. This dynamic does not have to be destructive if it can be processed in such a way that allows the client to recognize how this old interpersonal schema related to past abuse is being generalized to the current situation. However, if the client continues to feel predominantly controlled, manipulated, or coerced by the therapist, narrative work is likely to be untherapeutic at best and retraumatizing at worst. One option is to continue trying to process these issues, with the hope of developing a more collaborative relationship before reconsidering narrative work. Alternatively, if this type of dialogue is not possible and the relationship continues in a similar vein over time, the therapist should discuss the option of maintaining the treatment with a sole focus on developing STAIR skills or of referring the client to a different therapist or treatment.

Has the Client Been Able to Learn and Use Skills Presented in Phase I?

The STAIR/NST program is designed so that prior to beginning intensive and emotionally demanding narrative work, the client has had the opportunity to learn skills to manage affective and interpersonal difficulties. We have typically found in our research that a 2-month (eight-session) phase of skill-based interventions is an adequate period of time for most clients to develop a basic repertoire of techniques that they can experiment with in stressful situations. Of course, there are important individual differences—depending on how much time clients have devoted to practicing the skills both within and outside sessions, as well as their level of coping skills prior to beginning treatment.

It is not necessary or realistic to wait until clients demonstrate complete mastery over the skills they have been introduced to before making the transition to narrative work, especially given that continued work on skill building is integral to the narrative treatment phase. Rather, it is important that the clients have been able to learn basics and have begun to use them outside sessions to cope with difficult feelings or situations. If a client is not exhibiting some degree of competence and confidence in using skills, then the STAIR phase of treatment may need to be prolonged before narrative work begins. Questions to consider include the following: Has the client been interested in or found some value in learning the skills? Has she practiced skill exercises regularly between sessions? Has she made any modifications to skills that indicate an effort to integrate them into her own life? Has she used skills independently both within and outside sessions with some success? Since narrative work will require the client to draw on some of the skills she has learned in managing overwhelming emotions, it is important to review with her which particular techniques feel most beneficial and which skills need continued practice.

CHAPTER 19

≈

SESSION 9

Introduction to NST

I know this story well, because I have been stuck inside it. I have lived with its causes and effects, its details and indelible lessons my entire life. . . . And if I ever hope to leave this place, I must tell what I know.
So let me begin.

—MIKAL GILMORE (1994, pp. x–xi)

OVERVIEW

The goal of Session 9 is to orient the client to the narrative work that will begin in Session 10. The therapist provides a clear description and rationale for the use of the NST. The therapist and client also review coping skills learned in previous sessions and identify ways that they will support the goal of completing narrative work. Lastly, the therapist and client identify specific abuse memories that will be narrated, organizing them by the level of distress each of these memories causes, so that the narrative work can be planned with sensitivity to distress management.

Interwoven into these preparatory activities are the repeated reflections that, while painful, the task of revisiting and making sense of the traumatic past will allow the client to be freed of it. In telling about it, the client confronts, understands, and eventually masters the trauma. By critically examining its causes and harmful consequences, the survivor can summon the reasons and the will to change her beliefs and behaviors.

Lastly, because NST is explicitly a *narrative* process, it conveys the message that a life story is composed of a past, present, and future. The client's retelling of the abuse both establishes and reinforces its "pastness." Moreover, narration assumes a chronological structure that not only allows the trauma to be located placed firmly in the past, but

BOX 19.1
Theme and Curriculum for Session 9: Introduction to NST

THEME

The NST phase of treatment involves repeated telling of specific traumatic memories, organizing these memories into coherent life events, critically evaluating their meaning, and deliberating about their place in a life history. Confronting the memories leads to the realization that the traumatic images and thoughts are simply memories that have no real power over the client. In addition, telling about the trauma allows the client to organize the traumatic events in a way that helps her understand what happened and explore its meaning. The client identifies beliefs about herself and others (interpersonal schemas) that emerged from the narratives, with the goal of understanding that these beliefs belong to a particular life context—namely, a traumatic childhood. The circumstances of her life have changed, and with these, the necessity of living according to trauma-generated beliefs. The client is free to choose alternative strategies for living.

PLANNING AND PREPARATION

Bring a copy of the Overview of Narrative Story Telling handout (Handout 19.1), and several copies of the Interpersonal Schemas Worksheet II (Handout 15.1).

AGENDA

- Begin with emotional check-in and review of between-session exercises.
- Prepare client for move to NST.
- Review rationale for NST as a method to do the following:
  - Resolve fear and PTSD symptoms.
  - Organize traumatic memories.
  - Develop an integrated life story.
- Review application of emotion regulation skills during narrative phase.
- Initiate collaborative review of NST rationale and goals.
- Establish commitment to narrative work: number of sessions and timeline.
- Develop memory hierarchy.
- Wind down the session.
- Assign between-session exercises:
  - Read Overview of Narrative Story Telling handout (Handout 19.1).
  - Complete distress tolerance exercise (pros and cons) for engaging in narrative work.
  - Complete Interpersonal Schemas Worksheet II (Handout 15.1) at least twice during the week.
  - Practice focused breathing twice a day, and other emotion regulation skills as relevant.

SESSION HANDOUTS

Handout 19.1. Overview of Narrative Story Telling
Additional copies of Handout 15.1. Interpersonal Schemas Worksheet II

prompts the client to consider the present and imagine a future. Through narration, the client creates important links between her past and present, as well as potential relationships between the past, present, and an imagined future. Through NST, the client expresses herself and becomes owner of her life story. Box 19.1 outlines the theme and curriculum for Session 9 of treatment.

PREPARE CLIENT FOR MOVE TO NST

After checking in with the client about her feelings of anticipation about this next step, the therapist should begin by communicating that the purpose of this session is to introduce and orient her to the narrative work, so that she will know what to expect *before* beginning the process. Providing this structure is critical in giving the client the message that this work will be approached gradually, at a pace that will allow her to raise questions and concerns. This is particularly important for trauma survivors, as they commonly feel taken off guard and not in control of what is happening to them. It is also important that the therapist convey a sense of reassurance and empathy, because the client is likely to feel unprepared for narrative work. This is often the case no matter how much work clients have done on developing coping skills, or how clearly they have articulated alternative schemas for living in the here and now. The past is essentially uncharted territory. A critical part of the narrative process is that the client comes to feel strongly anchored in the present, and with the attitude that the resources she has within the context of the treatment are more powerful than the past. This feeling can be set in motion through a review of her coping skills, reassurance that the therapist is aware of her strengths and vulnerabilities, and promises that the therapist will be there to support and guide her in the process.

PROVIDE OVERVIEW OF NST

The therapist lets the client know that they will begin the narrative work in the next session. Although the client has been given the rationale for the narrative process at the beginning of treatment (Session 1), the therapist now reviews it in detail and describes the specific procedures involved in NST. The therapist should deliver the information as though he or she is providing it for the first time, because many clients may not have retained important parts of the information they were initially given. The therapist should also tell the client that she will be given a written version of this information at the end of the session, in the form of a "take-home sheet" on NST for her review (see Handout 19.1). A description of the purpose and implementation of each aspect of NST is provided below. NST has three goals: (1) to reduce the client's fear and PTSD symptoms, (2) to enable the client to organize the trauma memories in a coherent and meaningful way, and (3) to help the client deliberate about the place of these experiences in her life history.

NST WORKS TO REDUCE FEAR AND PTSD SYMPTOMS

Narrative work begins with repeated telling of trauma memories until they are no longer frightening. The therapist should review the rationale for this repeated telling of the trauma as a strategy to reduce fear and for the process by which it is accomplished, based in the logic of prolonged exposure (see Foa & Rothbaum, 1998; Rothbaum & Foa, 1999). It should be noted that talking about the memories is not identical to reliving them, as the client is in reality safe. This knowledge allows the task to be conducted with greater ease. The therapist can start by succinctly describing what the first step in narrative work will entail:

> "What we will be doing in the narrative sessions is revisiting your abuse experiences—the ones that continue to cause distress and disruption in your life. I use the word 'revisiting' rather than 'reliving,' because during this process the aim is not to submerge yourself completely in the past, but rather to have one foot in the past and the other grounded in the present. The ultimate goal is to help you make sense of these disturbing memories, so that you will no longer feel so controlled and overwhelmed by them. During the narrative sessions, you will be describing narratives of your traumatic experiences and repeating them as many times as needed, in order to diminish the level of anxiety and fear associated with them. I will be there to provide support and to remind you that no matter how intense it may feel, you are no longer in the abusive situation but are instead in a safe environment.
>
> "You will see that with repeated telling, your fear reactions to the event will diminish. This process is called 'habituation.' The more often you tell the story, the less frightened you will become, and the better this treatment will work. You will eventually experience that the memories of the past are *only* memories and cannot harm you."

Review Rationale for Audiotaping Narratives

The narrative will be tape-recorded during the session. The client will take the tape home, with the goal of listening to it at least once a day. This will contribute to her habituation to the fear-eliciting aspects of the narrative. It will also provide an opportunity for the client to reflect on her reactions to the story and its meaning to her, both when it happened and now. The taping of the narrative has been described in the first session, but a reminder of the rationale for taping will help the client orient herself to the work and elicit any specific concerns she might have:

> "When you narrate your abuse memories, we will audiotape them. Your between-session work will be to listen to the tape every day and make sure you make time to do this. You will learn that a memory is just that—a memory—and that you have nothing to fear from recalling these past events, although doing so is painful."

Respond to Client's Concerns

The client is likely to have a range of reactions to hearing the descriptions above (e.g., anxiety, disbelief, confusion, and curiosity). It is important to address these feelings and concerns. When presenting the rationale for repeated narration of the trauma, the therapist explains the basis for recommending the procedure to this particular client at this particular time. This involves reviewing how methods the client has used, such as avoidance, have not worked in the past and indeed may have exacerbated her symptoms. In addition, the past trauma has invaded her present, so that the trauma continues to shape her current behaviors in negative ways.

The therapist should be mindful that the client may have some strong reactions to hearing that her ways of dealing with trauma may in fact have resulted in an *increase* of symptoms and problems. The therapist will want to "normalize" this way of managing painful experiences and provide a sense that the client has been coping as best she could. Doing so will minimize the possibility that the client will feel criticized or judged for using avoidance or other unsuccessful strategies. Instead, the therapist should emphasize to the client that her efforts have been attempts to cope with very stressful life circumstances, but that there are other, more effective ways of coping, including the narrative process she is about to use.

In the service of building the client's willingness to trust the therapist in this new phase, it is useful for the therapist to acknowledge that processing the memories connected with the abuse may be frightening at first. It is equally important for the therapist to provide assurance and belief in the narrative process by communicating that it will get easier, and that the client is likely to see both a decrease in the fear and distress related to the abuse memories and positive changes in her attitudes toward herself and her relationships.

Narrative Work Helps Organize Trauma Memories

The therapist can also describe the narration of the trauma as a technique for making sense of abuse memories. This activity has two functions: It contributes to the reduction in PTSD symptoms, and it represents the first "story" that will contribute to the identification of the trauma-generated beliefs and life themes.

Organizing Memories Contributes to PTSD Symptom Reduction

The clinician can reintroduce and expand on the information presented in Session 1. The therapist can also highlight the contribution of developmental stage to the impact of trauma in childhood. That is, the therapist can remind the client about the particularly disorganizing force of trauma occurring during childhood, when cognitive and emotional resources to respond to trauma are limited. In addition, it is unlikely that the survivor had social resources in terms of parental or other social support in understanding or making sense of the trauma. The therapist can say something like this:

> "Childhood abuse, like all traumas, is an event that overwhelms a person's senses. In times of extreme stress or danger, the typical mechanisms we have in place to interpret and process experiences can become overwhelmed. We are particularly vulnerable to this type of disruption if we are faced with traumatic events during childhood, when these capacities for handling incoming information have not yet

been fully developed. As a result, the memory of the abuse is often a disorganized, fragmented mess—parts of a puzzle in a heap. Many symptoms of PTSD, such as nightmares and intrusive images, reflect the disorganized nature of a trauma in the person's memory. The process of putting the pieces of the puzzle together includes organizing the images into a coherent memory. We will be doing this by organizing the events chronologically and putting words to the experience."

Individuals who experience trauma in childhood may have difficulty in putting the pieces of their memories together, as the experiences may have been mislabeled or the attributed contexts in which the abuse happened may have been described in misleading ways by the perpetrators. Furthermore, children rely heavily on parents as interpreters of experience and as the central sources of names for things. In cases where children's parents are their abusers, the parents rarely have the motivation or ability to label their experiences correctly or to discuss them coherently. Lastly, reliance on other adults may have been of little value. Childhood abuse is frequently stigmatized; it is an event that is not typically part of mainstream conversation in many educational and social environments. As a result, the event does not get named or understood. Abused children often cannot even describe what has happened, let alone make sense of what has happened and why. The experience remains a mystery as to its reason, purpose, and impact. It is a life event that is essentially "unreal" and incoherent—often disregarded by the child, but influential all the same. The therapist can describe the situation as follows:

> "Meaning is often made by putting words to our experiences. This capacity is disturbed during traumatic events, leading some to describe trauma as a 'wordless horror.' The process of organizing memories with words may be particularly difficult for childhood abuse survivors. Children learn and understand life experiences through communication and discussion with their parents. If their parents were the abusers, the children are at a particular disadvantage in making sense of their experience, as their parents may mislabel or deny the experience. In addition, opportunities to make sense of the event (such as disclosing or fully describing the experience to others) are often not options, since abuse is often a stigmatized experience that adults may feel uncomfortable discussing. As a result, the impact of these experiences on the children's beliefs and feelings remain unexamined and disconnected from the rest of life. Still, they continue to influence thoughts, feelings, and behaviors, in ways that are often outside of awareness or control."

Organizing Memories Sets the Stage
for Identifying Abuse-Related Interpersonal Schemas

As the discussion above suggests, if a child's memory of abuse is not organized or appropriately labeled, it remains disconnected from the rest of the child's life experience and meaning system. Narrative work helps integrate the abuse experience into the context of the individual's life experience, particularly the impact that it has had on beliefs and life themes. The therapist can initially characterize this notion by reference to the often-used "file cabinet" analogy for memory organization. The analogy can be described as follows:

> "The mind can be viewed as a kind of 'file cabinet' in which experiences are organized and stored. When something has its place in the file cabinet, the information in the file and the feelings that go along with it are more manageable, and new experiences can be integrated in the future.
>
> "For example, we have files for things like 'school,' where we store information about how to act in school, what other people have told us about school, and our memories of school-related experiences. Over the years, a child accumulates knowledge of what school is like, how one is supposed to behave, what is expected at school, and so on. Parents, siblings, peers, and others help the child label and process these experiences by communicating about school.
>
> "In contrast, there are no clear or accurate labels or organizing systems in which abuse experiences can be meaningfully filed. There may be no label on the file, or perhaps one that is vague ('Special Times with Dad') or inaccurate ('Things That Everyone Does with a Drama Coach'). The files are placed in some separate drawer, or, if they are mislabeled, exist as part of another set of experiences in which they truly do not fit. As a result, these experiences do not become integrated with all other information about one's childhood. Rather, they remain apart from it, or they create an inaccurate and distorted sense of some of life's themes."

Narrative Work Helps Organize a Life Story

The narrative process also involves identifying ways in which the trauma has shaped the client's beliefs about self and others (interpersonal schemas) and the ways in which these beliefs influence her current behavior.

Identification of Abuse-Related Interpersonal Schemas

The general content of the schemas has often already been articulated during the STAIR phase of treatment. However, the identification of the source of the schemas as the client's traumatic experiences helps resolve the mystery of her current behavior. Her past is connected to her present through the use of trauma-generated schemas in daily living. Her current behavior no longer appears frighteningly irrational and nonsensical. The client now understands the motivation for her behavior.

The circumstances of the trauma articulated in the narrative allow the client to understand the logic of her schemas and their source in powerful if not overwhelming experience. This often elicits sympathy for her past self and understanding of the power of the schemas to intrude into her current life. The therapist can provide an explanation like this one:

> "The belief system you now live with is one of the ways your trauma continues to influence you. Often you will recognize the schemas from the work we have done in STAIR. Others will be new but will make sense, given the particulars of your

trauma as you talk about what happened. One of the most valuable aspects of the schema identification work is that it will help you make sense of your current behaviors. Often abuse survivors feel themselves to be crazy because they do not understand why they behave the way they do, particularly when the behaviors seem at odds with their desired goals. These behaviors are often driven by schemas formulated in the context of your abuse and are accurate reflections of your trauma circumstances The identification of schemas often solves the mystery of what appears to be nonsensical or irrational behaviors. You have a reason for acting the way you do."

Changing Schemas: Recognizing Differences between Current and Past Life Circumstances

The therapist should also note that the schemas from the traumatic past will be critically examined and directly contrasted with the schemas that have been generated and tested in the STAIR phase of the treatment. This direct comparison will help the client distinguish beliefs based in the past from beliefs adaptive for the present. This comparison will help the client separate the traumatic past from the present. It is intended to give the client a sense of freedom from her past and a sense of choice about how she may live in the present.

Contrasting the internal and external resources of the traumatic past with those of the present will provide good examples of the fit between an environment and an appropriate schema. For example, trauma narratives will often include themes of powerlessness, vulnerability, incompetence, and dependence, and these themes will be reflected in the client's interpersonal schemas. However, the current life circumstances of clients in this treatment are often far improved, and each client should be reminded of essential differences as they pertain to her particular situation. Examples may include such differences as these: A client no longer lives in close proximity to her past abuser; she does not rely on the abuser for food or shelter, but has some (even if limited) resources of her own; she is much stronger both physically and mentally than she was during the abuse; she is able to fend for herself in work and can sleep through the night without expectation of intrusion or abuse; she can come and go out of her dwelling as she pleases.

Recognizing differences between the context of her present and her past will provide the client with additional motivation and confidence in adopting new schemas and expectations. Awareness of the distinction between the past and the present will reduce automatic repetition of trauma-based behaviors and functioning. When the client recognizes that many of her current maladaptive feelings and beliefs have their origins in the trauma, it will be much easier for her to develop awareness of their anachronistic and generally counterproductive nature and to be motivated to develop present-focused feelings, beliefs, and behaviors.

Validating the Past by Understanding Rather than Living It

Many abuse survivors have difficulty giving up certain trauma-generated behaviors, because they are among the few (or the only) forms of validation that the traumatic past actually happened. Because abuse survivors were often in circumstances where telling about what happened was punished or threatening, these behaviors, though maladaptive and painful, are recognized by abuse survivors as evidence of their own experiences. For some abuse survivors, to give up these behaviors would mean to "betray" their own past and their former selves.

The development and articulation of abuse-related interpersonal schemas constitute a healthy and powerful alternative means by which to acknowledge and respect the past trauma. Awareness of changes in her circumstances can allow a client, with the help of her therapist, to develop and test new schemas. The identification of schemas generated by her abuse, and the development of alternative schemas for her life in the present, can be placed side by side and examined for how they mark the evolution of change in her sense of self and opportunities for engagement with life. The therapist may explain narrative analysis to the client in the following way:

> "Narrative telling is the experience of going back to the past, with the final goal of creating an alternative assessment and understanding of that experience for living in the present. During the narrative, you will experience the many emotions and perceptions from the past as you felt them as a child, but will simultaneously be viewing the experience from your position as an adult. An adult is a person with additional life experiences and an experientially based understanding of the differences between the needs and abilities of children and those of adults. Given this additional perspective, the meaning of the traumatic event as it was formed during the trauma is available to you for reassessment.
>
> "This process is not intended to distort or minimize the trauma, or to diminish its importance. The goal is for you to have respect for your past, but an emerging awareness that you are not the same person as you were in childhood and need not have the same feelings or beliefs about your trauma as you did then."

REVIEW APPLICATION OF EMOTION REGULATION DURING NARRATIVE PHASE

The therapist should refer back to techniques the patient has learned over the course of treatment to cope with anxiety, as a way to remind the client that she is actually more equipped to do the narrative work than she may feel. The therapist will want to encourage the continued use and practice of these coping skills, especially focused breathing, which will be called on during the narrative process. For example, this is an opportune time to revisit the concepts presented in Session 4 about distress tolerance (see Chapter 13). During this session, the idea of making the *choice* to tolerate distress in the service of trying to reach an identified higher-level goal has been introduced. Having the client apply these techniques to the narrative (identifying the goal as well as the pros and cons of tolerating associated distress) before beginning is another powerful way to provide inspiration for the work ahead. The therapist may suggest that the client do this on paper before the next session, so that it can be referred to when sustained motivation is needed throughout the process. Also, by anticipating potential obstacles and distress, both client and therapist can begin to think of ways the client might approach these challenges before they arise.

The therapist can mention again that the client will set the pace of the narrative work, and that the therapist will follow, support, and encourage her. The therapist may also enumerate the client's strengths and convey a sense of her vulnerabilities, so that the client feels that the therapist truly understands her. The therapist should inquire whether there are any other aspects of the client's strengths or vulnerabilities that either she or the therapist may have overlooked.

Finally, it is important for the client to keep in mind that narrative sessions include continued commitment to maintaining good functioning in the here and now. The therapist should remind the client that throughout all the narrative sessions, the work on further developing and refining interpersonal skills will continue. This work will be particularly highlighted as the interpersonal themes picked up in the narrative work are further characterized and refined. Experientially based alternative schemas will be explored and contrasted with these old beliefs associated with traumatic events. The therapist should reassure the client that all interpersonal tasks will be based on the resources available to the client for success.

INITIATE COLLABORATIVE REVIEW OF NST RATIONALE AND GOALS

After presenting all of the information described above, the therapist should check in with the client to see if she has understood the main points and encourage her to share her reactions and questions. It is expected that the client will still have some anxiety and uncertainty about beginning the narrative; however, at this point she should be clear about its purpose and goals. The narrative work should not proceed until the rationale is generally understood and accepted by the client, because otherwise ongoing and active collaboration between the clinician and client is not possible. Both the rationale and the therapeutic alliance need to be established before this work begins, as these are essential tools in sustaining the client's motivation and participation in this challenging yet potentially powerful process.

ESTABLISH COMMITMENT TO NARRATIVE WORK: NUMBER OF SESSIONS AND TIMELINE

Once the client expresses an adequate understanding and acceptance of the process and goals of the narrative technique, it is recommended that the therapist discuss "making a commitment" before turning to the specifics of abuse memories. This entails a verbal contract in which the patient and therapist agree to use the narrative for a set number of sessions (at least three or four). The duration and intensity of the narrative during these sessions should remain flexible and will depend on the individual client's needs and reactions, but the minimum number of the narrative sessions should be clearly established before beginning. The impetus for this intervention is to put a structure in place that will encourage both the therapist and client to give the narrative work an adequate trial. The initial narrative sessions in particular tend to be the most challenging. It is not uncommon for client and/or therapist to want to retreat after an emotionally intense and difficult narrative session. This could, however, lead the client and therapist to abandon the treatment too early, based on the erroneous conclusion that the client is not actually ready to proceed.

In our experience, it is not only ineffective but can in fact be detrimental to start the narrative and then end it prematurely within a session or within the treatment. The process of starting and then abruptly stopping the narrative may significantly raise the client's anxiety level, because not enough time has elapsed to allow for habituation to occur. This type of experience could inadvertently confirm the client's belief that approaching the traumatic memories is dangerous and that she is incapable of managing the emotions associated with them. This could in turn result in an increase of symptoms, particularly phobic avoidance of trauma-related cues, and fear of engaging in future treatment.

DEVELOP THE MEMORY HIERARCHY

During the pretreatment assessment, the client has probably reported the general nature of her abuse experiences, but has not provided a series of specific memories. At this point, the therapist will need to assist the client in identifying several memories for use in the narrative work. The client does not need to go into extensive detail at this time, as the present goal is to identify the most critical memories for later work, not to conduct a narration of the event. The development of a hierarchy of distress is a common cognitive-behavioral technique; its application to trauma memories has been developed and nicely described by Foa and colleagues (see Foa & Rothbaum, 1998; Rothbaum & Foa, 1999). The procedure has three steps. First, the therapist elicits several traumatic memories from the client (the number of these typically ranges from 4 to 10), taking brief notes so that each memory can be referred to later. Once this list is complete, the client assigns a number that reflects the level of distress provoked by each memory, using a scale from 0 (no distress) to 100 (highest possible distress). The units on this scale are typically referred to as "subjective units of distress" (SUDs). The memory hierarchy is completed when the memories are rank-ordered, with revision as necessary following the SUDs ratings provided by the client. This process usually takes about 20–30 minutes. An organized and clean copy of the memory hierarchy sheet can be completed by the therapist after the session. Before starting to develop the hierarchy, the therapist can explain to the client:

"Before beginning the narrative work, we need to decide which memories it makes the most sense for us to focus on. In order to do so, I am going to ask you to identify your most important abuse memories and how they continue to affect you emotionally. In addition, you may want to identify additional memories of traumatic experiences other than those of childhood abuse that occurred later in life. The goal here is not to go into extensive detail about your memories at this point, but rather to identify and generally describe what you believe are the most significant trauma memories, so we can have a road map for future narrative sessions. So I would like you to think and tell me about the particular memories that are most disturbing and disruptive to you in your current life."

The clinician must encourage the client to discuss trauma memories in enough detail that they can be briefly recorded and referred to individually (e.g., "the time my father locked me in the closet"), but not in so much detail that the client feels overwhelmed. Achieving this balance requires the clinician to be active in containing the client during the session, so that she does not open up without having time to process traumatic memories within the session.

The clinician is encouraged to keep probing to a minimum in the process of developing the memory hierarchy. If a client is having trouble, the clinician may want to ask some simple and specific questions about the perpetrator, the client's age when the abuse occurred, and/or her emotional reaction, in order to help the client articulate basics that she does remember. Through the narrative process, the client may or may not be able to remember more details. The communication to the client should be that whatever she does remember is a good starting point, and that specific details about content are not likely to be as important as her emotional experience of the event(s).

Challenges

The Problem of Lengthy or Overly Elaborated Reporting of Memories

If the client is having trouble containing her description of an important memory, the clinician should sensitively redirect the client to talking more briefly and generally about what happened and moving on to another memory, by saying something like this:

> "The information you are sharing with me is very important, and I appreciate your willingness to do so. We will have the opportunity to process it in our narrative sessions. However, right now we need to focus on identifying and briefly describing relevant memories, so that we have a sense of the big picture before getting into the specific details."

The Problem of Few and Fragmented Memories

Some clients may have the opposite problem with this task: They have difficulty spontaneously providing specific information about their memories, and can only relay brief and vague snippets. This may be because the details of the event were never encoded due to dissociation at the time of the trauma, or because they have strenuously avoided thinking about the distressing memories for so long. Whatever the reason, it is important to assure the client that having incomplete or fragmented memories of traumatic experiences is common and will not prevent the client from doing and benefiting from narrative work.

The Problem of Abundant and Diverse Trauma Memories

Many clients will have long and complicated trauma histories, which makes developing a hierarchy of memories particularly challenging. It is important for the clinician to be aware that this could be overwhelming; in such a case, the therapist should explain to the client that she is not being asked to specify every memory, but rather to identify the ones that feel the most significant in the present. This will decrease the likelihood of the client's becoming flooded with anxiety or becoming detached in the face of intense emotion. However, the clinician still may need to check in repeatedly about how the client is feeling during this process.

Clients who have been repeatedly abused over a long period of time may describe a composite or confluence of many different episodes. This is to be expected. Again, such a client should be encouraged to report what she does remember, rather than worrying about teasing apart the specificity or sequence of the memories at this point. If it is clear, however, that in the process of relaying one specific traumatic memory the client moves into talking about another specific memory, the clinician should sensitively ask the client to stay focused on the first memory; after completing that description, she can return to talking about the second memory. It is reassuring for clients who have numerous traumas to be aware that often work on one memory will carry over to other memories—ones that involve similar types of abuse and/or similar emotional responses to the abuse.

Introducing the SUDs Rating Scale

Completing the Memory Hierarchy

The therapist should tell the client that the SUDs ratings will be used in making decisions about which memories to focus on during narrative sessions and in what sequence. Before using the SUDs scores to rate memories, the clinician should operationalize the meaning of these scores with each client, to ensure that it can be used meaningfully and consistently. This is done by generating anchor points with the client, using her own words and descriptions as a guide. For example, 0 might be "no distress whatsoever" or "a totally neutral state in recalling this memory"; 50 might be "moderate distress" or "very aware of feeling but definitely manageable"; and 100 might be "severe distress and discomfort" or "I can't manage." Using the analogy of a thermometer can be helpful. The therapist can explain: "The SUDs scale is used to get a quick read on your current level of distress and anxiety, in much the way that a thermometer is used to gauge temperature."

It is important to emphasize that the client should be using the SUDs scores to rate the level of anxiety/distress she is currently feeling while describing the memory, rather than to rate the level she may have experienced at the time of the traumatic event. After creating the list of traumatic memories and obtaining their associated SUDs ratings, the clinician will want to check in with the client to be sure that the memories rated with the highest scores are in fact the most distressing. In cases where more than one memory is given the highest rating, the clinician and client will want to think further about which of these memories is the most disruptive in her current life.

Use of SUDs Ratings in Narrative Work

The therapist should discuss with the client that the SUDs rating will also be used during the narrative work itself, as a way for the client to indicate how she is feeling immediately before she begins, during the telling of the story, and immediately after the narrative is complete. During each session that the SUDs scores are used, the client should be reminded that the scores are based on how she is feeling in the present, rather than how she felt in the past.

WIND DOWN THE SESSION

The process of memory elucidation, although not part of the formal narrative, can be quite overwhelming in its own right, particularly if the client has many abuse memories to describe. Though it can cause distress, creating a list of significant trauma memories and having to view them as a whole can also be quite powerful, especially for those clients who lack compassion for themselves and/or minimize the extent of their abuse. It is critical to allow some time at the end of the session to check in with the client about how it felt to review the memories in this way. If the client is still aroused or anxious, the therapist should use this as an opportunity to practice coping skills (e.g., focused breathing or distraction techniques) before ending the session. It is also important to give the client feedback and encouragement about the fact that she was able to complete an important first step in the narrative work. The therapist should remind the client that it would not be surprising if between now and the next session she finds herself thinking more about her abuse experiences than usual.

ASSIGN BETWEEN-SESSION WORK

Ask the client to read the Overview of Narrative Story Telling take-home sheet (Handout 19.1). This material will be useful in future sessions. The therapist should also assign the distress tolerance exercise (i.e., evaluating pros vs. cons)in relation to beginning the narrative treatment. Finally, the client should continue completing the Interpersonal Schemas Worksheet II, practicing focused breathing, and engaging in relevant emotion regulation strategies (e.g., positive activities, thought stopping, and positive statements) as determined by therapist and client.

Overview of Narrative Story Telling

Beginning in the next session, you will carry out narrative exercises in sessions and every day at home for the duration of the treatment program. This is very likely to be one of the most difficult parts of your treatment program. However, it will help to bring about long-term relief from your distress and to facilitate positive changes in the way you think about yourself and relate to others. It is important, therefore, that you do your best to do the narrative work and resist urges to avoid doing it. To assist you, this handout reviews the rationale and instructions for the Narrative Story Telling (NST) phase of treatment.

RATIONALE

The purpose of the narration of the trauma is to have you revisit and reorganize your childhood abuse memories. It is not easy to understand and make sense of traumatic experiences. When you are reminded of the abuse, you may experience extreme anxiety or other negative feelings. So you may tend to push away or avoid these painful memories. You may tell yourself, "Don't think about it," or "I just have to forget about it."

But as you have discussed in therapy, no matter how hard you try to push away thoughts about the abuse, the experiences come back to haunt you through nightmares, flashbacks, phobias, and negative beliefs about yourself and others. These symptoms serve as signals that the abuse is still "unfinished business." This is because avoidance prevents you from processing the thoughts and feelings that go along with the memories. After a traumatic event, your mind begins the work of organizing the experience. When various aspects of the experience are organized into a story, this process is completed. Additionally, your feelings are organized within the context of the story and as a result become more manageable. The meaning of the event—particularly beliefs about yourself and the world—is evaluated and placed in the larger context of other life experiences. If, however, the process is interrupted, the story never gets organized, and the emotions remain intense and unmanageable. Powerful and emotionally charged fragments of a story never settle into a sensible or coherent account of what happened or how it affects you. The unanchored memories dominate your internal experience, leaving you feeling fragmented, disorganized, hostile, out of control, and fearful. Relationships are equally fragmented and undermined by strong and unexpected emotions. These reactions are often intrusions of unsettled feelings from the past. They may have little to do with the present.

The goal of this phase of treatment is to help you process the memories connected with the abuse and to create a life story that helps you understand the impact that the trauma has had on your feelings and relationships and also allows you to put the past in its place. As you confront the memories and experience the intense emotions that go with them, the emotions will become less distressing. This process is called "deconditioning" or "habituation." It is important that you repeat the habituation process many times in the session and at home, because this repetition is essential for you to reduce the distress you now experience.

(continued)

In addition, the process of narrating the trauma will help you distinguish the feelings and beliefs that are results of the abuse from your current desires, wishes, and plans for yourself in the present. By identifying the interpersonal schemas in your narrative after you finish it or finish listening to a tape, you can explore how those beliefs influence your functioning in the present, whether they are helpful to you, and how relevant they are to your current goals. While these schemas were consistent with and highly adaptive to your abusive environment, they are not likely to help you now that you are out of the abusive environment and have goals other than avoiding, escaping, or confronting threat. Awareness of these schemas and their lack of relevance to your current life will help you recognize when you are using them and help you disengage from them. Practice and success with the alternative schemas that you have developed in the STAIR phase of treatment will gradually replace behaviors generated from the trauma-related schemas.

PROCEDURE FOR BETWEEN-SESSION NARRATIVE REVIEW AND ANALYSIS

To help you carry out the narrative work you will do between sessions, your therapist will provide you with audiotapes of the narratives you have completed in your treatment sessions. Listen to the tapes of the narrative conducted with your therapist in the session, and use the material from the session to guide you through the narrative analysis (schema work) again.

You will need a tape player to carry out your the narrative homework. If you have trouble arranging the privacy you may need, it may be helpful to use headphones. Try to find a comfortable place where you will not be disturbed.

During the narrative, try to relive the experience; smell, taste, and feel everything as if you are really there. Although this can be scary, in the back of your mind you will know that you are safe. Some people find it helpful to have a trusted family member or friend nearby in another room or available by phone the first time they do the narrative homework alone. If you feel you will not be able to follow through without support, you may make arrangements for someone to be present or easily available to you during the task.

Use the Trauma Narration Form to record your subjective units of distress (SUDs) immediately before and after the narrative. Also note the highest SUDs level you reached during the narrative. Next, jot down on the Interpersonal Schemas Worksheet II, the interpersonal schemas that you associate with this story. If possible, formulate an alternative schema that is more representative of the beliefs you wish to hold about yourself and your relationship with others in the present. If you cannot do this on your own, this work will be completed with your therapist in your next session.

CHAPTER 20

∿

SESSION 10

Narrative of First Memory

And suddenly it had come to her . . . that the voice she was hearing
was her own, for the first time in her life.
—ANNA QUINDLEN (1992, p. 393)

OVERVIEW

In Session 10, the client will complete her first trauma narrative. The therapist will help
put the client at ease by reviewing the rationale for NST, identifying the client's available
coping skills, and reminding the client of the therapist's presence as a support. The client
will first practice with a neutral memory, in order to become familiar with the structure
and pacing of the narration. The same structure and process are then implemented with a
selected abuse memory. The main goal of the session is for the client to experience mastery over the memory, so it is important for the client and therapist to titrate the intensity
of the client's emotions carefully during this process, according to the client's strengths.

When the narrative ends, client and therapist will conduct grounding exercises if
needed. The client will then identify feelings that emerged from the telling, including
what parts of the story elicited these feelings and how intense they were. Therapist and client will then listen to the tape together. This gives the client some familiarity with the task
before she listens to the tape at home. It also helps the therapist monitor and explore the
client's reaction to her own story. We have found that clients experience a range of reactions, many of which appear unavailable when they are engaged in the actual narration.
These often include sympathy for themselves and curiosity—as if they are experiencing
themselves as interesting people, with histories and stories to tell. Box 20.1 outlines the
theme and curriculum for Session 10 of treatment.

BOX 20.1
Goals and Curriculum for Session 10: Narrative of First Memory

THEME

The client's recollection of the trauma is only memory, and as such it cannot hurt the client. When the client is able to revisit the memory in a detailed and emotionally alive way, there is an opportunity to help her experience mastery over the traumatic memory. When the client listens to the tape, she often becomes aware of feelings that were not available in the telling of the story. These include sympathy for what she has been through, and curiosity about herself as a person with a story to tell.

PLANNING AND PREPARATION

Prepare two completed versions of the memory hierarchy, one for the client and one for therapist use. Bring tape recorder and blank tapes. Bring a copy of the Assessment of Postexposure Emotional State form (Handout 20.2), and several copies of the Interpersonal Schemas Worksheet II (Handout 15.1) and the SUDs during Trauma Narration handout (Handout 20.1).

AGENDA

- Begin with emotional check-in and review of between-session exercises.
- Review rationale for narrative work.
- Practice narrative of a neutral memory.
- Conduct first narrative of a trauma memory.
- Ground client to the present.
- Listen to the first taped narrative together.
- Explore beliefs about self and/or others in narrative.
- Assign between-session work:
    - Listen to tape daily; monitor distress with SUDs using Trauma Narration Form (Handout 20.1).
    - Initiate at least one interpersonal situation and practice alternative schema, using Interpersonal Schemas Worksheet II (Handout 15.1) to record; include emotion regulation skills as relevant to situation.
    - Practice focused breathing twice a day.

SESSION HANDOUTS

Several copies of Handout 20.1. SUDs during Trauma Narration
Additional copies of Handout 15.1. Interpersonal Schemas Worksheet II

REVIEW RATIONALE FOR NARRATIVE WORK

Before beginning the first narrative, the therapist should review in whatever detail is appropriate to the particular client the rationale for NST and the nature of the analysis that will follow. Also, the therapist should take the time to talk with the client about how she feels about starting NST. The client can be reminded that she has many more resources now than she did as a child, and that these resources will be available to her to conduct this task. She will revisit the past with the strengths and resources of the present. She will view the experiences of her childhood from the critical and more informed perspective of an adult. The therapist can say something like this:

> "When you experienced the abuse, you were just a child, alone, with limited coping skills, and the experience was overwhelming. Our goal is to create a different experience for you. You will not be alone this time; I will be with you every step of the way. Part of the rationale for the first phase of the treatment was to prepare you for trauma-focused work. As an adult, having gone through this treatment, you have skills and resources you didn't have as a child. You have the resources to confront these memories. Does this make sense to you?"

PRACTICE WITH A NEUTRAL MEMORY

In prolonged exposure (Foa & Rothbaum, 1998), prior to beginning work with traumatic memories, clients first practice with a narrative of a neutral memory. This practice is extremely useful in allowing the client to learn the process and structure of NST before having to confront intense emotions. The therapist can explain to the client:

> "Before focusing on your abuse memories, let's practice with a memory from your childhood that is not related to your abuse. Some people choose a memory of a birthday party, or vacation or friend they liked to play with, or their childhood room. Can you think of a memory like that? [The therapist should help the client choose a memory if she has difficulty. This memory should be neutral to positive in valence.] OK, so we will focus on this memory in the same way we will later with an abuse memory. Sit back in your chair in a comfortable position. Close your eyes, or let them rest on an object or location that is comfortable and where you will not get distracted. Tell about a particular incident in your life. The story should have a beginning, a middle, and an end. You should describe it in the first person, as if you are there right now—for example, 'When I wake up, I am happy because I remember it is Saturday, which means no school today.'"

As the client talks through the memory, the therapist probes her for details about what she sees, hears, smells, and touches. The therapist also asks her what she is feeling and what sensations she experiences in her body. If she forgets to stay in the first person, she should be reminded to do so. When the client has finished, the therapist can provide support and continued direction:

> "That was very good. That is exactly what we are going to do again, but this time you will narrate an abuse memory. We are going to start a memory that you think you can manage, but the most distressing one you can manage."

CONDUCT FIRST NARRATIVE OF A TRAUMA MEMORY

Selecting a Memory

The memory selected should be the one that elicits the most distress the client feels she can handle. This will ensure that processing for fear reduction is relevant, but that the client will succeed in experiencing distress reduction in the session. Our experience has been that when a client succeeds in managing a high-distress memory, those associated with less distress become very easy to narrate, and in fact may become uninteresting and irrelevant to the client in her recovery work.

If the client has more than one distressing memory of equal weight, she should pick the one that has the most relevance to problems she is dealing with in her day-to-day life. This also serves the purpose of enlivening the postnarrative schema analysis with particular value. Therapist and client should work together in the selection of the memory.

The client should be allowed to go through the memory once with no interruptions. The second time the client begins the memory, the therapist should reinforce his or her instructions as necessary. For example, the therapist may need to remind the client to stay in the first person if she has forgotten, to speak more slowly, or to provide more details. The clinician's goal is to help the client make the memory as real as possible, so questions should facilitate this process. How this works best depends on the client. For some clients, asking them to provide more detail about sensations (sights, smells) enables them to get deeper into the memory. If the therapist believes that the client is avoiding reexperiencing the feelings associated with the memory, she should be asked how she is feeling. Some general guidelines for the therapist during the session include the following:

1. *Active listening.* Since some clients will have their eyes closed or focused away from you, show that you are listening with vocalizations such as "Uh-huh," "Yes," or "I see."

2. *Be supportive.* If the client demonstrates strong emotions during narrative work, reinforce this by being empathic: "I know this is difficult. It takes courage to do this. I am listening. You are doing well."

3. *Clarification.* If the client moves out of the first person ("I"), rushes through the memory, or doesn't seem to be allowing herself to relive the experience, clarify the procedure before she begins the memory the next time.

4. *Details.* Help the client emotionally engage in the memory by asking her questions about details of her experience, particularly details about sensations (e.g., touch, smell).

5. *Encouragement.* Praise the client for her courage in confronting her abuse memories: "You can be proud of yourself. You have done something very difficult."

6. *Focus.* If the client becomes distracted (e.g., by noise outside the office), gently remind her about where she was in the memory: "You were falling asleep and you just said your stepfather came into the bedroom." Or sometimes the client will break out of the memory and ask a question. If she does, tell her you will make a note of it and answer it later. For now, ask her to return to the memory.

The therapist can begin the process by saying:

"Now we are going to focus on your abuse memory, just like we did a few minutes ago with the memory of your [the therapist describes the neutral memory]. Sit back in the chair, and close your eyes or focus on an image from the memory. We are going to travel back in time to when this memory occurred. Make the memory as real as possible. Talk slowly, in the first person, using 'I,' as if the events were happening to you right now. Describe what you are experiencing, feeling, thinking, tasting, and touching. I may ask you questions along the way to help you make the memory more real. It is sometimes tempting to avoid the memory by speaking quickly and trying to get it over with. If I think you are doing this, I will help slow down. Remember, I will be here next to you every step of the way. To keep in touch with how you are doing, I will be asking for SUDs ratings every few minutes. I will say, 'Rating,' and then you are to give me your SUDs for how you are feeling in that moment on a scale from 0 to 100. Does this make sense? When you have finished the memory, I will ask you to start over again. We will cycle through the narrative two or three times. Ready?"

The therapist should record the rating on the Subjective Units of Distress (SUDs) during Trauma Narration form (Handout 20.1) as the client revisits the abuse memory. How often to ask for a SUDs rating will depend on the length of the trauma memory. Often, in the beginning, these memories are very short, so the therapist may ask only once or twice during the memory, every few minutes. After the memories become more elaborate, we usually ask for ratings every 5 minutes or if a client is appearing very distressed. The use of SUDs ratings is an excellent way for the client and therapist to stay in touch with the client's emotional movement through the narrative. These ratings become a rapid, rather telegraphic way for the client to communicate her in-the-moment emotions as she narrates the event.

As the client goes through her memory, the therapist should note parts that seem particularly distressing. These parts provide clues to the meaning of the memory for the client, and also to which parts of the memory the therapist might choose to focus on in later sessions. In addition to SUDs ratings, the therapist should also record any relevant observations in the "Comments" section on Handout 20.1—for example, any physical reactions, facial expressions, or voice changes noted during the narrative.

When the client has gone through the memory once, the therapist asks her to go back to the beginning and start again. For instance, the therapist can say this: "Very good. I know that was hard to do the first time. Now we are going to go through the memory again. This time I am going to ask you more questions, to try to make the memory more real to you."

Number of Repetitions and Duration of Narrative Retelling

The therapist should have the client go through the memory two or three times. This can take between 10 to 20 minutes, depending on the length of the narrative. It is recommended that the client spend at least 10 minutes engaged in repeated narrations of the memory (or, if the telling of the memory is relatively lengthy, at least one repetition). If the memory takes longer than 20 minutes to describe, client and therapist can work on breaking the memory down into shorter, more emotionally focused, and more manageable narratives.

In later sessions, the narrative may need to be completed only once. This can happen when the SUDs levels are relatively low, or the intensity of the event is no longer as strong as it was when it was first rated. The initial narrative work can diminish fear reactions to other memories in the hierarchy that have not been described when they are related in content or theme. Sometimes rapid fear reduction occurs when the client experiences a significant insight about what she has described. Insight often demolishes fear. The client is much more likely to be experiencing excitement, curiosity or satisfaction.

Ending the Retelling of the Narrative

If the client's distress or anxiety decreases within this session of narrative work, the therapist should ask her if she notices a difference (in terms of SUDs ratings) between how she is feeling at the end and how she felt at the beginning of the session:

> "When we started today, you rated your distress at a [SUDs]; by the end of the session, you were at a [SUDs]. This is what we talked about: Your distress decreases if you allow yourself to face the memory."

In the circumstance that the client's distress does not decrease, the therapist should remind her that this happens when someone is struggling with a particularly difficult memory and praise her for sticking with it:

> "I know this was very difficult today. You showed a lot of courage sticking with the memories, even though it was very difficult. We will be discussing the meaning of the memory, and in doing that, we can identify what makes it so hard. Before that, let's do some distress reduction exercises."

If the therapist and client are interested in obtaining a more detailed picture of the client's emotional reactions at this stage, the Assessment of Postexposure Emotional State in-session form (Handout 20.2) can be used. After briefly describing the 1–10 rating scale, the therapist can ask the client about the intensity of her feelings in each domain following the initial telling. This form creates a more specific preliminary profile of the client's emotional state, and can also be used by the therapist and client in later sessions to guide the narrative work.

GROUND THE CLIENT TO THE PRESENT

The first activities in the transition from narration to analysis are simply stating that the narrative work portion of the session is finished and asking how the client is feeling. These comments or similar sentences signal that the narrative work is over, and that the client is ready for review, discussion, and exploration of the narrative experience. The therapist ensures that the client is clearly in the present, is physically comfortable, and is engaged with the therapist. While many feelings and thoughts from the narrative work may be resonating in the client, the client should also be able to maintain a comfortable distance from the experience.

If the client feels somewhat disoriented, there are several techniques the therapist and client can use to ground the client in the present. These can include having the client do breathing exercises, look around the room, drink a hot or cold beverage, rub her hands together, or rub her face on her hands. The client and therapist will at this point have identified the activities the client prefers to use to increase her physical comfort and awareness of the immediate environment.

Sometimes the therapist's voice can be very soothing to the client and orient her to the present. In addition, the therapist can make several comments that reinforce a sense of safety and of being grounded in the present. The therapist can state that the client is in a safe environment, and that the events described belong to the past.

The therapist can also congratulate the client for completing the narrative. The shift from narration to analysis is a passage from immersion in the traumatic past to engagement in the present. And this in itself is a therapeutic experience. It is a demonstration to the client that she has the skills to shift from the past to the present, and that the feelings elicited during the narrative work can be diminished at will. The therapist should comment on this by specifically identifying the ways in which the client has been able to manage her feelings and use coping skills—not only during the narration, but also in coming to successful closure on the task.

LISTEN TO THE FIRST TAPED NARRATIVE TOGETHER

Next, the therapist and client will listen to the recording together. Again, it is important to reiterate the purpose of this activity. The therapist can say something like this:

> "At this point, I would like us to listen to the tape together. This is what I will be asking you to do on your own between sessions. Listening to yourself detailing an

abuse narrative for the first time can be daunting, so doing it in session will hopefully be helpful in decreasing this initial anxiety and will give us a chance to talk about what it felt like to hear yourself. Often clients have very different reactions to telling the narrative of their abuse and listening to themselves tell it on the tape."

EXPLORE BELIEFS ABOUT SELF AND/OR OTHERS IN NARRATIVE

After the client has identified and labeled the central feelings emerging from the narration, the client can explore what beliefs about herself and others are embedded in the narrative. The client can use the feelings she has identified as a springboard for this. At this point in treatment, the therapist and client are aware of the client's core interpersonal schemas, based on their work in the STAIR phase. However, new or more detailed and precise beliefs often emerge from organizing the trauma narrative or from articulating details to which the client has never given thought. The central goal of the analysis is to clarify and repeatedly reinforce the fact that certain beliefs the client holds about herself as a traumatized child are no longer applicable to herself as an adult. Alternative and more adaptive schemas, along with supporting evidence from current experience, are discussed.

Below is a case illustration of a narrative analysis that occurred after the first telling of the abuse history. We have found that our clients are often full of thoughts, feelings, and observations after the first narrative experience. Clients experience relief, sadness, amazement, and curiosity about what might come next. It is very valuable to take an informal approach to the schema analysis after the first telling and follow a client's lead about important observations. In the example below, the most important observation for Tina was the difference between her therapist's reaction and her mother's reaction. The therapist helped Tina to summarize her insights at the end of the session, using two copies of the Interpersonal Schemas Worksheet I (Handout 14.1; see Examples 20.1 and 20.2).

Interpersonal situation	Feelings/beliefs about self	Expectations about other	Resulting action
• What happened? • Who was involved?	• What did I feel/believe about myself?	• How did I expect the other person to act/respond to me?	• What did I do? • What was the result?
Told my mother about the abuse.	Afraid, confused, wanting comfort.	Frightened, uncomfortable, angry at me.	Decided never to tell anyone else and not to bring it up again.

EXAMPLE 20.1. Tina's filled-in Interpersonal Schemas Worksheet I for her relationship with her mother (when Tina, at age 8, told her about the abuse).

Interpersonal situation	Feelings/beliefs about self	Expectations about other	Resulting action
• What happened? • Who was involved? Telling my therapist about the abuse.	• What did I feel/believe about myself? She asked me to tell. But she will still think less of me. Can she take it?	• How did I expect the other person to act/ respond to me? Maybe she will accept what I have to say.	• What did I do? • What was the result? I told her. She seemed concerned for me, not frightened. <u>Not everyone is like my mother.</u>

EXAMPLE 20.2. Tina's filled-in Interpersonal Schemas Worksheet I
for her relationship with her therapist
(when Tina described the abuse in session, in the present).

CASE EXAMPLE:
TELLING ABOUT THE ABUSE, THEN AND NOW

In the initial phase of treatment, Tina's therapist focused on skills training, particularly on helping her develop ways to manage her anxiety and to be more direct in communicating her distress with others. When presented with the rationale and description of the narrative work, Tina reacted strongly: "I feel like what you are saying goes against all of my natural human instincts. It's like you're suggesting I jump off of a cliff or put my hand on a hot stove." In addition, Tina had never told anyone the whole story of her abuse. The first and only occasion on which she had disclosed what had happened had been to her mother when she was 8 years old. Tina described her mother's reaction as "frightening": The mother repeatedly asked her about details, and would then become "hysterical" and go back to her room. After a week, Tina "couldn't take it any more" and told her mother that she had made it up. She decided never to tell anybody about the abuse again. Tina's therapist spent time discussing her fear of telling about her abuse and reiterated the connection among her symptoms, her problems in relationships, and her trauma experiences. Although Tina was hesitant and frightened to begin narrative work, her distress over her worsening symptoms and their impact on her functioning gave her incentive.

At the beginning of Session 10, Tina continued to express anxiety and skepticism. Her therapist repeated the treatment rationale and reviewed the reasons Tina had given for wanting to be in the treatment. At the end of the first narration, Tina saw the experience in a different way and felt much more comfortable with beginning to tell about herself. She had experienced some sense of mastery in the process, even during this first time. She compared the process of revisiting her abuse memories to trying to hold onto a handful of sand: "If you hold it tightly, it slips out through your fingers, but if you keep your grip loose, you can actually keep it in your hand."

Tina and her therapist also discussed her strongly held belief that talking about the abuse was dangerous and would have disastrous consequences. Tina linked this belief to her experience with her mother, and expressed the feeling that as a child she had to choose between telling the truth and protecting her mother. Tina's therapist focused with her on the fact that she no longer had to make this painful choice. She could tell about the abuse and still expect that at least some people would still be there for her—in fact, would feel closer to her than before. Neither Tina nor her therapist had fallen apart in the disclosure of her abuse.

ASSIGN BETWEEN-SESSION EXERCISES

At the end of the session, the therapist will give the client the audiotape of the narrative portion of the session and request that she listen to it once a day. The client should also be told to record her SUDs ratings and any comments or observations on the SUDs during Trauma Narration worksheet (Handout 20.1) after each listening. As with previous between-session assignments, the therapist should spend some time predicting any potential obstacles to the clients' completing this between-session work and suggesting ways to make it feasible.

The client will need to have a tape player available, and she may or may not want to listen with headphones. The therapist and client should also discuss when it makes the most sense to listen to the tape, taking into consideration the client's schedule and possible times when she is free and can have some privacy. Another consideration is the surrounding environment during tape listening. A client should not listen to the tape along with other people. However, if she has identified safe and supportive people, she might enlist these individuals in certain ways (such as calling them before and after listening to the tape, to check in). She might also make a social plan for later if this would be helpful.

As always, it is up the client to decide how much she would like to share with others. For example, some clients feel comfortable sharing with significant others about the treatment process; others want to make contact with others without directly involving them in the process; and others prefer to keep the process a private experience. Whereas some clients prefer to listen to tapes when nobody else is around, others prefer to do it in a place where they feel less isolated (e.g., using headphones at a coffee shop, or doing it at home when others are present in another room). As long as distractions are minimized and the client can devote time to concentrating on the tape, the context is of relatively minor importance.

Subjective Units of Distress (SUDs) during Trauma Narration

Brief description of memory: _____

_____

_____

Date _____	Preexposure SUDs ____ Highest SUDs ____ Postexposure SUDs ____	Comments:
Date _____	Preexposure SUDs ____ Highest SUDs ____ Postexposure SUDs ____	Comments:
Date _____	Preexposure SUDs ____ Highest SUDs ____ Postexposure SUDs ____	Comments:
Date _____	Preexposure SUDs ____ Highest SUDs ____ Postexposure SUDs ____	Comments:
Date _____	Preexposure SUDs ____ Highest SUDs ____ Postexposure SUDs ____	Comments:
Date _____	Preexposure SUDs ____ Highest SUDs ____ Postexposure SUDs ____	Comments:
Date _____	Preexposure SUDs ____ Highest SUDs ____ Postexposure SUDs ____	Comments:
Date _____	Preexposure SUDs ____ Highest SUDs ____ Postexposure SUDs ____	Comments:

Assessment of Post-Narrative Emotional State

Date:

Exposure #:   Session #:

Rating scale

1	2	3	4	5	6	7	8	9	10
Not at all		Mild		Moderate			Severe		Extreme

Fear/anxiety

1	2	3	4	5	6	7	8	9	10

Numbness

1	2	3	4	5	6	7	8	9	10

Anger

1	2	3	4	5	6	7	8	9	10

Sadness

1	2	3	4	5	6	7	8	9	10

Shame

1	2	3	4	5	6	7	8	9	10

Guilt

1	2	3	4	5	6	7	8	9	10

Strongest feeling: _____

CHAPTER 21

≈

SESSIONS 11–15

Narratives of Fear

> The patient reproduces instead of remembering . . . . This condition is shifted bit by bit within . . . the treatment . . . [W]hile the patient lives it through as something real and actual, we have to accomplish the therapeutic task, which consist chiefly in translating it back again into terms of the past.
>
> —FREUD (1914/1963, p. 163)

OVERVIEW

The sessions following the first narrative (Sessions 11–15) maintain essentially the same structure as Session 10. This includes a review of the feelings elicited by the narrative, an identification of the schemas embedded in the story, a critical analysis comparing the schemas of the traumatic past with the client's current situation, and applications of new schemas to current life difficulties. These procedures will become routine, and the sessions will move fluidly from one activity to the next. Clients will progress from one memory to the next, repeating this cycle of activities.

Some clients will have difficulty making progress, however, because they tend to react to fear with avoidance or dissociative responses to fear-laden memories. This chapter describes strategies for managing such reactions, to be used as needed. This chapter also describes the benefit of close and sensitive attention to, and possible revision of, schemas. In narration, as the particulars of abuse histories are told, a better understanding of critical interpersonal experiences emerges and can lead to more precise, "emotionally real" versions of established schemas. The strategies for management of fear-laden reactions, sustained emotional involvement in the narration, and the evolution of schemas all share in common the recognition that these experiences belong to the past. Although memories have extraordinary power to influence current behavior, they nevertheless have, by definition, one weakness: They belong to the past. The client, in contrast, has one major strength, which is that she lives in the present.

The client's capacity to live in and feel the power of the present will provide an important resource in putting distance between herself and her memories, and developing a per-

BOX 21.1
Theme and Curriculum for Sessions 11–15: Narratives of Fear

THEME

Clients quickly learn the structure and process of NST. The sessions that follow involve conducting repeated narratives of the most distressing aspects of a particular abuse event, or moving to other events that would have been too distressing to begin the narrative work with. The resolution of fear reactions results in large part from the realization that the trauma belongs to the past, and as such cannot hurt the client. The client begins to experience control over her memories and is actively working to organize them. She is also beginning to assess their influence over her current attitudes and behaviors. Consequently, the narrative work is a form of self-reflection and the beginning of the development of a historical sense of self. The repeated narration of an organized past, and identification of its relationship to the present, establish and reinforce an experience of continuity in the self.

PLANNING AND PREPARATION

Bring memory hierarchy, tape recorder, and blank tape. Bring at least one copy of the Assessment of Postexposure Emotional State form (Handout 20.2), and several copies each of the SUDs during Trauma Narration handout (Handout 20.1) and the Interpersonal Schemas Worksheet II (Handout 15.1).

AGENDA

- Begin with emotional check-in and review of between-session work.
- Select a memory.
- Conduct narrative.
- Identify feelings elicited by narrative.
- Work with avoidance behaviors.
- Manage dissociative reactions: Help clients face the worst fears.
- Use additional grounding techniques to orient client to present.
- Revisit and revise schemas (e.g., "I am my perpetrator").
- Conduct role plays.
- Apply relevant schemas to current life difficulties.
- Assign between-session work:
  - Listen to tape daily; monitor distress with SUDs during Trauma Narration form (Handout 20.1).
  - Initiate at least one interpersonal situation and practice alternative schema, using Interpersonal Schemas Worksheet II (Handout 15.1) to record; include emotion regulation skills as relevant to situation.
  - Practice focused breathing twice a day.

SESSION HANDOUTS

Additional copies of Handout 20.1. SUDs during Trauma Narration
Additional copies of Handout 15.1. Interpersonal Schemas Worksheet II

spective on the limited influence these events need to have. Accordingly, a basic principle of the work is to maintain the client's engagement in and appreciation for the present. The therapist and client can work together to maximize the resource of the here and now. This can be done through words, through sensory exercises, and through repeatedly contrasting the past with present living conditions and opportunities. Negative beliefs about self and others belonging to the traumatic past can be countered with alternative schemas and experientially based demonstrations that disconfirm these beliefs and support new formulations about the self. As this effort proceeds, the client will begin developing a sense of a historical self—a self with a past that is distinct from the present. Box 21.1 outlines the theme and curriculum for working with narratives of fear in Sessions 11–14 of treatment.

BEGIN WITH EMOTIONAL CHECK-IN AND REVIEW OF BETWEEN-SESSION WORK

During Sessions 11–15, the therapist begins each session by checking in with the client about her reaction to listening to the tape. This will help identify the next step in the narrative work. Often a client will identify parts of the narrative that were particularly difficult for her. A brief discussion will determine whether the memory should be further explored. The therapist can review the pattern of SUDs ratings with the client and determine whether they should go on to a new memory, repeat the memory, or focus on a particular aspect of the memory. Before this is decided, the therapist should elicit from the client any insights she might have had as a result of listening to the tape—about her feelings, views of herself, or schemas she has identified. This will also help inform the therapist whether the client feels "done" with the memory.

SELECT A MEMORY

The decision to move on to a new memory is determined by the amount of fear the client still experiences when revisiting the memory, as well as her satisfaction with her understanding of it. The therapist and client can review the SUDs ratings the client reported on each day she listened to the tape. Ratings of 30 or below indicate low fear responses, suggesting that the therapist and client can select a new memory. If there are particular areas of difficulties, indicated by the client's report and high SUDs ratings only for a section of the narrative, the next narrative can be a repetition and analysis of this "high-distress" section.

The selection procedure is the same for each new memory: The client and therapist select the memory that has the highest SUDs rating the client believes she can manage. The choice is also influenced by the relevance of particular memories in the client's day-to-day life. A memory with an initially low rating may become relevant to the further elaboration of a theme in a memory, or may become more significant due to life circumstances. For example, if a client identifies a theme of chronic fear of suffocation from narratives of adolescent sexual abuse memories, she may eventually recognize the same theme in a less intense memory of an early childhood molestation. Alternatively, a memory of physical abuse by the client's mother may be reactivated upon a visit from or some news about the mother. The memory thus becomes more salient to the client and should be addressed. SUDs ratings for this memory can be revised accordingly.

CONDUCT NARRATIVE

The procedures for conducting the narrative are identical to those described for the first narrative in Session 10 (see Chapter 20). This includes orienting the client to the task, recording the narrative on tape, following the client with SUDs ratings, occasionally inquiring about details, and determining the number of repetitions. When the client is done, the tape is shut off, and grounding exercises are conducted as needed. This is followed by postnarrative assessment of feelings in the narrative.

IDENTIFY FEELINGS ELICITED BY NARRATIVE

The therapist facilitates activities that label and contain the traumatic feelings and associated material. These include literally labeling the tape of the narrative with a title selected by the client. The title can provide clarity of feeling and some distance from the event via humor (albeit black humor)—for example, "Trapped in the Closet: Part III."

In addition, the therapist should inquire about the client's specific feeling states, such as fear/anxiety, numbness, anger, sadness, shame, and guilt. The Assessment of Postexposure Emotional State in-session worksheet (see Handout 20.2) can be used as a guide for this activity. After briefly reviewing the 1–10 rating scale, the therapist can inquire about the intensity of the client's feelings in each domain after the narrative work. As described in Chapter 20, this creates a specific profile of the client's feeling states and informs both client and therapist about the key feelings that have emerged as a result of this narrative work.

The therapist will be able to compare this profile to others that have been elicited from the same memory. It is likely that there will be reductions in the severity of feeling states of fear and anxiety in this first narrative. The therapist should identify these changes to the client as examples of the patient's growing mastery of the trauma memory. An essential part of narrative work includes explicit recognition of mastery over overwhelming reactions to the trauma memory. This highlights the client's progress in an essential aspect of trauma recovery.

WORK WITH AVOIDANCE BEHAVIORS

Avoidance behaviors are behaviors that distract the client from approaching a distressing aspect of the trauma. They are often evident in the client's speech or gestures. A client may hesitate before moving to the next word or sentence in her narrative, or may turn away or look down at certain segments of the narrative. Over time, the therapist will become familiar with these "clues." The therapist may initially simply observe these behaviors if the overall level of emotional engagement in the narrative is strong. However, if the client seems to have habituated to many fear-related elements of the story and seems to be going through the story in a rote fashion, the therapist can gently inquire at the moment he or she observes the behavior: "I noticed that you hesitated. Was there something you thought or felt?" This can be enough to orient the client to pursue a detail she would have otherwise discarded. The therapist can also prompt the client by asking her what particular feeling or image she is having, which can lead to better engagement in meaningful aspects of the trauma.

CASE EXAMPLE 1: IDENTIFYING A HIGH-DISTRESS MOMENT IN THE NARRATIVE

Avoidance behaviors can be "flags" for identifying aspects of a narrative that are particularly distressing and have not been addressed in sufficient detail or possibly at all. A therapist can facilitate identification of high-distress, high-conflict memories by becoming familiar with a client's particular patterns of avoidance and bringing them to the client's attention. Some of these patterns can be subtle.

This process is exemplified by a situation where a client, Jillian, was observed turning her body away when she described how her older brother slid into her bed before he raped her. Initially the therapist didn't comment, but this behavior continued in the repeated narrations. The therapist then called Jillian's attention to this behavior, and she was able to move further into the details of the story. It became clear that Jillian had been avoiding a key aspect of her trauma. Jillian described the moment when she turned around in her bed, looked into her brother's face, and saw "someone whom I did not know." This had been a very frightening moment. As she described it, her world completely crumbled. Her brother became a stranger to her. She felt she had "lost" her brother, who was the only member of the family still living in their abandoned household and on whom she depended in every way. She was able to describe this moment in detail in one of her final narrations of this event:

> "I am feeling mortified, dirty, scared, angry, revolted. My heart is absolutely pounding. Still, I am afraid of running away. I am paralyzed with fear. It is like moving through molasses. If I try to get up and leave, it will be acknowledging that this is really happening. And I can't do that. It will send me over the edge."

Jillian noted that from then on, she knew she was "pretty much alone in the world," although at the time she would not have identified the source of this belief as the assault by her brother. In reflecting on her experience at the time, she added an important postscript:

> "A few days later, I told him that I was moving out. At the time, I did not think it was because of what had happened. I was very shut down. If someone had told me it had happened, I would not have believed them, even though I knew it had."

Completing the narrative with access to a greater range of feelings led Jillian to recognize the devastating impact the assault had on her relationship with her brother, where she lived and why, and how she conducted herself in her adolescent years. This was difficult. But telling about this aspect of the trauma led to greater clarity about one of Jillian's principal schemas, which was "If you rely on someone, that person will just exploit and abandon you." This schema had previously been a free-floating belief that had been, to her, a self-evident truth about the world. Pinning the origins of this belief on this particular moment with her brother allowed her to consider limiting this belief to the context of the abuse. Once this schema was anchored in a particular episode in her life, she was able both to make sense of this belief and to consider that it might not be generally applicable to all relationships.

MANAGE DISSOCIATIVE REACTIONS: HELP CLIENTS FACE THE WORST FEARS

As the narrative work moves toward the client's more challenging memories, she will be facing her worst fears and worst experiences. Some clients respond to high stress material by dissociating. The information below will provide guidelines for managing, and ideally preventing, these kinds of reactions.

Dissociation and Trauma Narration

The best intervention for dissociation is prevention. A guiding principle of our narrative work is that the emotional intensity of the experience must be titrated so that the client always remains in the here and now and in control of the process, particularly in the modulation of her fear. The purpose of the narrative is for the client to confront the trauma and to experience mastery of the memory. A successful narrative exercise is an empirical demonstration of the client's mastery over her trauma and emotional experiences. A key aspect of the client's initial trauma (and indeed of the very definition of trauma) is loss of mastery and control. During the abuse, the client did not have the ability to control the event or its outcome. Narration of the traumatic memory is therapeutic because it demonstrates to the client that while she was helpless to stop the trauma as it happened, she can now regain control of the event via its influence on her memory and emotional reactivity. This success leads to remarkably rapid resolution of the symptoms of PTSD.

Dissociation, in contrast, indicates that the client has become overwhelmed by the traumatic material. This is countertherapeutic, as it reinforces the client's experience of herself as having little control over her memories—an experience similar to the loss of control during the trauma itself. Indeed, this type of experience can be retraumatizing or can become a new trauma in its own right. The battle between the client and her PTSD symptoms is the battle between the power of the memory and the power of the client to confront and manage the memory.

Strategies for Managing Dissociation

When working with a client who has a tendency to dissociate, the therapist should talk with the client about it, reassure her that he or she (the therapist) is aware of it, and identify specific strategies for dealing with it.

We have found it helpful if the therapist and client agree on a signal for indicating that the client is feeling vulnerable to dissociation. This can be as simple as having the client raise her hand. The client and therapist can use such a gesture as a signal to reduce the emotional intensity of the narrative or to back away from material.

In addition, clients may exhibit specific automatic behaviors indicating that they have reached their maximum coping capacity and may be at risk for breaking off emotional or cognitive engagement with the present. These include small gestures such as rubbing their fingers together, "pilling" the fabric of their clothing, rapid blinking, or other kinds of eye or hand movements.

Perhaps the most powerful intervention in reducing dissociative experiencing is to remind the client regularly that the traumatic event is in the past. This can be done in a straightforward statement at the end of the narrative, such as "All of this happened in the past." This reality will be elaborated in relation to the client's particular core fears, and reinforced through role play and experiential exercises outside of sessions.

USE ADDITIONAL GROUNDING TECHNIQUES TO ORIENT CLIENT TO PRESENT

Some childhood sexual and physical abuse survivors experience strong fears of physical injury or death, particularly if sustained and regular injury has been inflicted. More common are fears of the perpetrators' coming after them, intruding upon them, and violating their bodies. Perhaps most particular to abuse by caretakers and its chronic nature (often over years) are clients' fears that they will never "get away" from their perpetrators because the perpetrators "live inside" them. This is evidenced not only in nightmares and images, but in their own day-to-day emotional reactions and behaviors that remind them of their caretakers/perpetrators.

These fears are often effectively resolved through the repeated narration of the trauma and habituation to the fear associated with particular aspects of the traumas. After the narration, repeated reminders of differences between the conditions of a client's childhood and the present create a "life history" in which to contextualize the trauma as an event of the past. A client can be told, "You are no longer in your father's house. You have a home of your own," or "Your mother can't hurt you any more. She is old and feeble," or "Your grandfather can't get you any more. He is dead and buried."

Exercises in mastery that invite contrast to the traumatic memory can provide evidence supporting these statements. This may include visiting the old neighborhood or house that the client lived in during the abuse. Often the power of this environment is much diminished when actually viewed from the perspective of the adult survivor. Fears of being physically overwhelmed by the perpetrator can be addressed in a similar way, by looking at pictures of the abuser as that person is now or was in the past. The abuser's size and strength are usually much less impressive from the adult survivor's perspective. In addition, the client's own physical strength and adult size can be identified by the therapist. The client may also be encouraged to engage in activities that reinforce development and awareness of physical strength. This might include engagement in sports, exercises, or any activity that creates awareness of physical integrity and agency. Such an activity can be as simple as walking or stretching, or using focused breathing.

REVISIT AND REVISE SCHEMAS (E.G., "I AM MY PERPETRATOR")

Some schemas reflect patterns of behavior reminiscent of the perpetrator, or are patterned behaviors intended to create distance from memories of or identification with the perpetrator. A client often indicates that she feels there is no escape from the feared perpetrator even if the person is dead, because he or she "lives on inside" the client in the form of attitudes, emotional reactions, and behaviors identified with the perpetrator. The "internalization" of the perpetrator may be one of the distinguishing features of childhood abuse by a caretaker, as well as other types of interpersonal violence that occur for sustained periods of time under conditions of psychological vulnerability. This may result from the caretaker's long-term role in the client's life and the power of a caretaker to shape a child's attitudes, beliefs, and patterns of behavior. Clients often do not necessarily act or react to situations as their perpetrators did, but they live in chronic fear that they may.

Schemas identified during STAIR may be based solely on problematic behaviors and beliefs identified in day-to-day difficulties. Often very good progress can be made in the development of alternative schemas and their implementation in role plays and between-session exercises. However, sometimes alternative schemas and role plays do not elicit any significant change in a client's behaviors and are resisted by the client.

Under these circumstances, it is worthwhile to consider that the schema formulation is not quite accurate or conflicts with other fear-based schemas. Little progress may occur during this time, but it is worthwhile for the therapist to keep tracking the expression of behaviors claimed to be associated with this schema. Reformulation of the schema can occur during NST, where, in the context of narrative work, previously unidentified feelings and memories will inform the "grain of truth" that was in the first schema. The schema identified as embedded in the narrative may be a more accurate and precise formulation of the beliefs and feelings driving the client's problematic behaviors. A more substantial and relevant alternative schema can then be formulated, and shifts in behavior can be more easily accomplished. An example of this process is provided below.

CASE EXAMPLE 2: REFORMULATING SCHEMAS

Initial Schema Identification during STAIR

During the STAIR phase of treatment, Rose and her therapist had identified some maladaptive schemas that kept her from asking for things she wanted. The initial identified schema was "If I love you, then I put your needs first." The behaviors associated with this schema of putting others' needs before hers had created conflict in Rose's marital relationship. Her husband, a likeable and easygoing person, did not particularly share her beliefs. Thus he did not engage in giving things he needed to his wife; nor was he particularly observant of her efforts to "sacrifice her needs" as expressions of her love for him. Her husband's lack of response to her efforts made Rose angry and feel disregarded and uncared for.

This schema was critically examined, and an alternative was developed that explored an opposite principle: "If I love you, I share my feelings and needs with you." The therapist and client engaged in assertiveness role plays in which Rose asked her husband for things and sometimes simply told her husband she was going to do things in accord with her own wishes. Both in life and in role plays, the husband was agreeable to these changes and to the more equal sharing of responsibilities and resources. Still, these activities were only modestly successful and yielded little change in the relationship.

Schema Revision during NST

During NST, Rose described many different episodes of having been physically abused by her mother. The mother had in fact terrorized all of her children. Rose recalled her mother coming home in a drunken state in the middle of the night and rousing all of the children to look for her cigarettes or to clean out the bathroom. Rose also described some frightening scenes in her childhood home, which involved random demands by her mother that were enforced with physical violence. These demands included giving up food on their plates to their father. The narration of each of these stories was followed by an analysis of the schemas embedded in the narrative.

The schema that had first been articulated during STAIR was eventually, in the context of Rose's abuse history, developed and refined into a much more meaningful belief: "If I make demands, I am just like my cruel and crazy mother."

The therapist and client then discussed ways in which Rose was unlike her mother. Rose, having reached the age of 47 years, had never been physically abusive to her husband, nieces, and nephews. She was consistently kind and considerate of others. She was articulate and had a sense of humor, unlike her mother, who had been surly and had spoken rarely (and generally incoherently). Her mother had been an alcoholic; Rose was not. Her mother tended to like dark rooms, while Rose thrived in sunlight and open spaces. Distinguishing herself from her mother, and distinguishing appropriately assertive request behaviors from abusive demand behaviors, freed Rose to approach request behaviors in a more healthy and positive way.

CONDUCT ROLE PLAYS

During both the STAIR and NST phases of treatment, the therapist and client continue to engage in assertiveness role-play practice at the end of sessions. In Rose's case, one role play with particular relevance to the narrative described above concerned Rose's reported difficulty in distributing food on the table and uncertainty about how much to give herself compared to her husband. The client and therapist practiced scenarios (with appropriate language, tone of voice, and behavior) that allowed Rose to engage in a variety of exchanges with her husband. In one she gave all of the remaining food to her husband, and in another she shared the remaining food. Finally, in a third, Rose was to express her desire for the remaining items to her husband, make an explicit request to her agreeable husband ("I really would like those two baked potatoes"), and engage in the behavior of placing the food on her plate. The client was in fact unable to complete the third scenario in the initial tries. First she disavowed her desire ("You know what? I am really not that hungry. Why don't you have some more?"). In the second effort, when she began reaching for the platter, she asked her husband, "Do you want me to cook you up something else?" even when he stated he was already finished with his meal.

It was not until Rose and her therapist had elaborated the initial schema to include its relevance to her perceptions of her mother's behavior that she was able to participate in this role play effectively. The final alternative schemas generated from this effort were "I can ask for my needs to be met and still be a good person," and a more emphatic variation, "I must identify my needs to be a good person." In a complementary fashion, Rose's perceptions about her husband's view of her were also changing. Her earlier assumption that her husband would view her as selfish, mean, and abusive was altered to "He will still love me (may even respect me more) if I ask for what I want." (See Example 21.1.)

APPLY NEW SCHEMAS TO CURRENT LIFE DIFFICULTIES

Over time, Rose was able to view her some of her current beliefs as related to her childhood abuse experiences and consequently not particularly valuable or adaptive for living in the present. Through a review of some of her family history, and with the help of the therapist, it became apparent that her mother might have had a significant psychiatric illness; the mother had been hospitalized at least twice, according to the reports of her siblings. This information helped Rose create a way of understanding her mother's behavior and of seeing herself as quite different from her mother. The narrative work gave her a more organized, coherent, and understandable version of her childhood. It also helped her understand why she was "where she was at" in the present. Awareness of the particular ways that the past influenced her present—for example, her difficulty in expressing her needs—gave her the ability to critically analyze the necessity and value of this behavior. She also importantly recognized that she now had the skills and resources to change her current behavior and plan her future, guided by different expectations of herself and others.

Interpersonal situation	Feelings/beliefs about self	Expectations about other	Resulting action
• What happened? • Who was involved? There are only two potatoes left on the platter.	• What did I feel/ believe about myself? If I love you, I put your needs first If I make demands, I am just like my cruel and crazy mother.	• How did I expect the other person to act/ respond to me? If you do not attend to my needs, you are a selfish, mean, bad person.	• What did I do? • What was the result? Gave husband both potatoes.

Interpersonal goals	Alternative feelings about self	Alternative expectations	Alternative action
• What are my goals in this situation? Maintain loving relationship while asking for my needs to be met.	• What else could I feel/believe about myself? I can ask for my needs to be met and still be a good person. I am not my mother. I must identify my needs to be a good person.	• How else could I expect the other person to act/ respond to me? My husband is a grown man. He will tell me if he wants more to eat. He will still love me (may even respect me more) if I ask for what I want.	• What else could I do? Share the potatoes. Ask for potato and help myself.

EXAMPLE 21.1. Rose's filled-in Interpersonal Schemas Worksheet II for her relationship with her husband (specifically, the "potato incident" role play).

ASSIGN BETWEEN-SESSION WORK

In Rose's case, appropriate between-session work might include implementation of the new schema "I can ask for my needs to be met and still be a good person" with her husband in situations other than negotiating at the dinner table. The client, for example, had significant health problems that she had not even disclosed to her husband, let alone asked for his help in managing. The particular conversations and requests inviting him into her life would need to be titrated in a way that would not overwhelm him and disappoint her. Rose jotted down her successes on additional copies of the Interpersonal Schemas Worksheet II. She also continued to practice focused breathing, particularly to deal with her anxiety in confronting her health problems and making an appointment to see a doctor.

CHAPTER 22

~

SESSIONS 11–15
Narratives of Shame

If the client is ashamed of her past, she cannot create an integrated life history.
—JUDITH HERMAN (1992)

OVERVIEW

Shame is an inevitable and salient consequence of childhood sexual abuse, but it is rarely deeply explored in therapy. As one survivor wryly observed, "We have shame about feeling shamed." Clients often feel profound shame about their victimization because they think that they deserved or provoked it in some way. The ensuing feelings of shame often serve as self-confirmation of their own wrongdoing, creating a vicious cycle. The present chapter provides information to share with the client about how shame influences the survivor and reasons for telling about shameful experiences. It also includes suggestions about the therapist's reactions to disclosure of shaming events, the importance of the therapist's positive regard for the client, and guidelines for sensitively conducting narrative retelling and schema analyses with shame themes (see Box 22.1).

GUIDELINES FOR THERAPISTS' RESPONSE
TO DISCLOSURE OF SHAMING EVENTS

The aspects of the trauma about which the client is most ashamed tend to emerge only in the later part of the therapy, during NST, and even then, in the later part of the narrative work. Disclosure of shaming experiences creates a variety of risks and so a client may delay or avoid doing this. A client may fear that disclosing an experience in which she was diminished will lead the listener to view her in a diminished way. She may

286

BOX 22.1
Theme and Curriculum for Sessions 11–15: Narratives of Shame

THEME

Often the most difficult aspects of a story involve themes of shame. Effective work with shame involves several activities, the most important of which is repairing the client's diminished sense of worth. Ways in which this can be accomplished are the critical analysis of the sources for her sense of shame, building alternative schemas involving her competence and value, and developing opportunities for building competence and for having positive experiences with others who value the client. The therapist also accomplishes this through direct expressions of positive regard for the client.

PLANNING AND PREPARATION

Bring memory hierarchy, tape recorder, and blank tape. Bring at least one copy of the Assessment of Postexposure Emotional State Form (Handout 20.2), and several copies each of the SUDs during Trauma Narration form (Handout 20.1) and the Interpersonal Schema Worksheet II (Handout 15.1).

AGENDA

- Begin with emotional check-in and review of between-session exercises.
- Identify and explore reasons for telling about shameful events.
- Elicit and explore shame narratives.
- Identify alternative schemas and resources to support them.
- Conduct role play.
- Provide client with support: Express positive regard.
- Assign between-session exercise.
  - Listen to tape daily; monitor distress with SUDs during Trauma Narration form (Handout 20.1).
  - Initiate at least one interpersonal situation and practice alternative, schema, using Interpersonal Schemas Worksheet II (Handout 15.1) to record; include emotion regulation skills as relevant to situation.
  - Practice focused breathing once a day.

SESSION HANDOUTS

Additional copies of Handout 20.1. SUDs during Trauma Narration
Additional copies of Handout 15.1. Interpersonal Schemas Worksheet II

worry that the listener will be disgusted and repelled by the event, and so will be disgusted and repelled by her. She may worry that she will be stigmatized not only for the event, but also for not having stopped the event, not having had the capacity to do so, or for having maintained, provoked, or encouraged the abuse in some way. A client's disclosure of these events risks the revision of the therapist's view of her as "less than" she was before: of less value, interest, importance to the therapist. The client may assume that the human connection, so difficult to forge in the first place, will be broken and that she will be worse off than before.

A supportive, compassionate, and practical response to the client's shaming experience is integral to helping the client resolve negative attitudes about herself. In the experience of shame, a person fears the negative opinion and evaluation of another. The client expects that disclosing events in which she was demeaned will make the therapist think less of her. The repeated responses by a therapist of continued support and positive regard will help disconfirm this expectation, facilitating the client's capacity to think in other ways about her experiences and herself. This attitude will be reinforced as the therapist proposes alternative schemas that help the client identify her value, and as the therapist helps her identify opportunities for building competence and having positive experiences with others who value her.

LISTEN FOR AND ELICIT CLIENT'S REACTIONS TO NARRATIVES WITH SHAME THEMES

Any type of victimization leads to feelings of shame, because such events are often interpreted as signs of weakness, defeat, worthlessness, or inferiority (see Chapter 7). Childhood sexual abuse carries with it an added burden to the victim, because of the social stigma associated with sexual violation. The therapist can identify shame themes when stories involve the client's description of herself as feeling "small," "humiliated," "weak," "inferior," "worthless," "less than human," or "nonexistent." After a narrative, a client may judge herself in the story as a pathetic or despicable person.

IDENTIFY AND EXPLORE REASONS FOR TELLING ABOUT SHAMEFUL EVENTS

Though the client has already learned by this point in the treatment that avoiding emotions only makes them stronger and feel more out of control, she will often resist exploring feelings of shame. In fact, however, a powerful antidote to feelings of shame can be the satisfactory disclosure of these painful experiences.

There are several benefits in telling of shameful experiences, and the therapist should articulate them clearly to the client. The therapist should also be aware that his or her own reactions and comments will be relevant to the client's ability to benefit from this process. The therapist can note any of the benefits below that apply to a particular client.

Benefits of Telling

Reducing Feelings of Alienation

Shame burdens a person with a feeling of being different from others. The client may believe that "if you knew I was abused in this particular way, you would not connect with me." Telling about the abuse, and receiving a response of understanding and recognition, can dissipate the feeling of having an "outsider status." The client's belief that the experiences she has undergone are "beyond the range of normal" can be revised when the therapist conveys that what happened was terrible, but that she is not alone in her experience. Even when the particulars of the experience are felt to be unique, the client can know that her feelings are experienced and understood by many.

Reducing Strength of Bond to Perpetrator

The client's abuse has been one of the defining experiences of her life. Often, because of the secrecy in which sexual (and sometimes physical) abuse takes place, the reality of the abuse is shared only with the abuser. To the extent that the client's self-definition is reflected this shared reality, the client remains psychologically bonded to the perpetrator for a feeling of authenticity. The survivor may feel that the only person who knows everything or perhaps the worst about her, is the perpetrator, and thus that the perpetrator is the only person who knows the "real me." By telling about the abuse, the client is able to dissolve that link and become independent of the abuser for her sense of authentic personal history. The client becomes free to be herself in full, and authentically herself with others.

Enhancing Client's Compassion for Herself

A survivor's shame often arises from belief that the abuse or her inability to escape from it indicates that she was inherently weak, deserving of the abuse, or inviting of it. These beliefs are often the result of the client's childhood view of herself "frozen in time" and that she is responsible for the things that happen around her. Reevaluation of this conclusion, perhaps prompted by observation of children in day-to-day life, can lead the client to understand the essential vulnerability of children. In addition, listening to the tapes of her trauma can provide the client with sufficient distance from her own experience to give her sympathy for what she has lived through. Listening to the tape can also provide a different perspective about the locus of responsibilities and shame. The narrative is a story of what happened to the client, and it includes not only herself but the perpetrator. Shifting focus or widening the perspective of the story can help the client understand the active role of the perpetrator, the perpetrator's own motivations, and the powerful forces that the client was up against.

Allowing the Client to Appreciate and Know Herself Better

The experience of self-compassion is particularly beneficial if the client is able to appreciate her capacity to have survived as she did in very difficult circumstances. A more positive, more open, and less defensive attitude about herself will allow the survivor to understand her own motivations and vulnerabilities with greater clarity (e.g., schemas based in efforts to avoid shame, or in her perceptions of shaming behaviors). It will provide insight about the meaning of her feelings, actions, and reactions, and help the client map out strategies for effective change.

Improving Interpersonal Relationships

A survivor's negative and critical view of herself also affects her evaluation of others. The survivor who internalizes the view that vulnerability is weakness and weakness is bad not only views herself negatively, but often judges others in the same fashion. These attitudes diminish her opportunities for positive social experiences and the development of sustained interpersonal relationships. The growth of self-compassion allows the client to live much more easily with herself, and perhaps even to feel some pride and enthusiasm. This more positive and more generous process of self-evaluation may lead to more generous appraisal of others. Positive changes in self-regard go hand in hand with positive changes in regard for others. The client thus benefits in her relationships with others, as well as in relationship to herself.

Allowing Client to Experience Agency and Facilitate Growth

Narration is an action, and as such can be an effective antidote to shame. Shame, which often arises from a sense of being ineffectual, is countered by the experience of agency in the creation of the story. A common, immediate, and understandable reaction to shame is silence. But in silence, many aspects of a person's experience and identity are left misunderstood or are not understood at all. The client's personal history is reduced to a schematic and incomplete version of what she has experienced. In contrast, disclosure of the abuse story can liberate the client from the burden of secrecy that often paralyzes the capacity for self-expression and growth. If the client can tell about the abuse, even the shameful parts, she can tell about anything. The client's feelings and imagination are liberated and can be harnessed as resources for understanding her needs and for planning her present and future.

ELICIT AND EXPLORE SHAME NARRATIVES

In the way that narratives of fear must be titrated so that the client experiences mastery over fear rather than a reinstatement of it, so too narratives of shame should be titrated so that the client experiences dignity rather than humiliation in the telling.

Attention to feelings of shame can derive from the client's description of these feelings during the narrative or the postnarrative review (see Chapter 20). The therapist can suggest further exploration of events related to these feelings or support the client's interest in doing so.

In shame-based narrative work, the greater part of the effort, time, and energy is spent on the analysis of the narrative after it has been completed and an appraisal of its meaning. Repeated telling of the story is useful to elicit details of the experience that produced the critical moments of shame. However, the transformation of shame lies in an exploration of the client's understanding of what happened and why, and a purposeful designation of its value to the client now. A client's shame may arise from having engaged in reprehensible acts during the course of the abuse (such as active participation in one's own abuse or the abuse of others). The therapeutic task is to help the client realistically evaluate the context in which these events occurred, which often involve rather dire circumstances and limited choices. Shame also arises from the perceived lack of action or inability to act in ways that would have averted or ended the abuse. Here, too, the therapeutic goal is to help the client make a realistic and compassionate evaluation of his or her circumstances.

The transformation of shame requires continual reference to the essential worth of individuals as they confront the ways in which they have been humiliated and diminished. This cannot be done in a naive or simplistic way that directs the clients to attend to their "positive qualities." Rather, this process involves recognition of the psychological harm and accumulated losses that are a result of the abuse, and an attendant and emerging sense of compassion for the person in the narrative and for the person who tells the story. In this way, the client can more readily explore the past in a respectful way and simultaneously work toward seeing value in him- or herself now.

Perhaps the strongest feelings of shame emanate from circumstances in which a client reports that she obtained physical pleasure from sexual abuse, or actively participated in the abuse by initiating abuse events or engaging in the established sexual activities that constituted the abuse scenario.

When a client repeats that she felt compelled to submit to either sexual or physical abuse, the client's feelings of self-blame are often fairly easy for the therapist to counter. A child is outmaneuvered emotionally, cognitively, and physically by an abuser. However, in situations where the client reports initiating or clearly provoking events, the therapist may have more difficulty in articulating this reality. From our perspective, however, the child's active engagement in abuse scenarios typically represents the extreme end of the abuser's domination over the child's life and the child's effort to exert a sense of personal control—and, in some cases, to secure her own survival when other avenues are closed off. The following case provides an example of such a situation and describes the successful interventions made by her therapist.

CASE EXAMPLE 1:
CLIENT AS ACTIVELY ENGAGED IN HER OWN ABUSE

Shanique had completed three tellings of physical and sexual abuse committed by her older brother when she was between the ages of 4 and 8. She believed that before she was born, her brother had been physically and sexually abused by her father. Her father took off shortly after she was born, and all she knew of him was that he had spent a lot of time in jail for drug-related offenses. She now began telling of another period of abuse in her early teen years. At this time, her brother was in his mid-20s.

"When I was about 9, my brother enlisted in the armed forces. So the sexual abuse by my brother ended for a while. But things were still pretty bad for me at home. My mother was having long periods of depression where she stayed in bed for days, just staring at the ceiling. I'd have to take care of myself—borrow money from one of my aunts, and do the food shopping, cleaning, and cooking. When she was up and about, she just went out for days at a time, looking for drugs.

"About the time I was 12, my brother came back. The armed forces hadn't done much for his temper or attitude. He was just a lot bigger now. My mother did not seem to notice one way or the other that he was back. I was terrified. I thought I had escaped from his torture, but no. I thought about how he had sodomized and beat me until I was a bloody mess. I knew there was no one I could go to. Then (*Shanique started crying*)—I feel terrible to tell about this—I just gave up fighting him. It's worse. I started getting involved with him, anticipating his moods. He'd get this glassy-eyed look, and I knew it was time for me to give him a blow job. Sometimes I'd even bring it on more, doing the things he liked or telling him how I liked it.

"It makes me sick. It makes me hate myself. After about 5 months of this, I realized he was settling into the house for good. Seeing how things were going, I convinced my best girlfriend to let me move in with her family. When I turned 18, I joined the armed forces. I got out of there ASAP. I still hate myself, though. What I did was sick, and it makes me sick to my stomach to think about."

Admission of her active involvement in her own abuse was a shameful component of Shanique's story, and it took several narratives before this aspect of the experience emerged. The therapist knew Shanique fairly well at this point and was able to articulate several reasons for this behavior. She presented them to the Shanique, with compassion for her situation and support for how well she had done under those circumstances.

When her brother returned from his military service, Shanique had been thrown back into a situation she thought she had escaped. At that point, she literally feared for her life and knew, without a doubt, that she could not count on anyone (including her mother) to help her survive her brother's presence. After a few years of relative peace and independence, and just as she was entering her early teens, she was desperate for a sense of control over her body and her environment. Her active efforts in prompting and participating in the abuse was a way to experience control over being abused, so that she did not feel so dominated and terrified. It was a "counterphobic" response similar to the one many individuals engage in when confronted with a fear (such as heights or flying). Shanique hated being at the mercy of her fear and her brother. Her behavior gave her a sense of mastery. Unfortunately, in "matching" her brother, she also became, like him, a perpetrator of abuse—of her own abuse. This left her with feelings of self-loathing and an inescapable core belief in herself as evil and bad.

By emphasizing the purpose of Shanique's behavior, the therapist was able to provide a way for Shanique to be more sympathetic to herself. Shanique was not being masochistic; she was engaged in reaching a goal that most people wish for and attain relatively easily—self-control and mastery of her body. Shanique had few if any other options to reach this goal. The alternative for her risked complete physical dominance and subjugation.

In addition, Shanique's past experience with her brother had informed her that he was capable of severe violence. Now he was bigger and angrier. Shanique believed, probably accurately, that he could kill her. She protected herself by anticipating his needs, essentially acting like an external mood modulator. If he was not angry, he was less likely to hurt her. She took the situation into her own hands as best she could. Taking care of his needs kept her alive.

The therapist acknowledged the horrors that Shanique had gone through. She noted especially that Shanique had been a survivor in the most basic meaning of the word: She had probably saved her own life. Shanique had also effectively used the resources she had at hand. As soon as she was able, she found other accommodations for herself with a friend's family, again showing her resilience in this situation. In reviewing her story with the therapist, Shanique understood that she had done the best she could, which was very good. She had held on to her life, to emerge at another time and place where things were very different. She now had the gift of life and a choice about how to live her life in freedom and with future opportunity.

IDENTIFY ALTERNATIVE SCHEMAS AND PERSONAL RESOURCES TO SUPPORT THEM AND PRACTICE IN ROLE PLAY

To be successful, the development of alternatives to shame-driven schemas (and their role plays) requires the regular identification, development, and support of psychological, practical, and emotional resources that reinforce the client's sense of value. Active efforts to demonstrate the client's value and current competencies include explicit identification of latent positive characteristics in the client and the enhancement of these characteristics in the STAIR activities. The testing and application of this schema may utilize—and may in fact require—circumstances in which the client has confidence in an identified ability and the opportunity to share this skill with interested others. Role plays help the clients practice presenting themselves in ways previously unimagined.

PUTTING IT ALL TOGETHER: NARRATIVE ANALYSIS, ALTERATIVE SCHEMAS, RESOURCE IDENTIFICATION, AND ROLE PLAY

Clients who have experienced abuse can have long-held negative beliefs about themselves and deeply entrenched maladaptive behavioral patterns. Change is difficult and can be frightening. While there is a desire for new and better ways of living, there is also resistance to leaving behind the comfort of the familiar. This work can be very challenging for both the client and the therapist. Below we present a client whose life has been a series of victimizations. Her deep shame has been defensively organized into a paradoxical stance: She is good at being a victim. While this stance is a dysfunctional adaptation to her trauma history, it has given her a measure of pride and self-respect. Below we describe each intervention of the treatment toward the goal of reevaluating her history, resolving some of the shame she feelings about herself, reorganizing her view of herself and others, and exploring new behaviors and attitudes.

Case Example 2: Finding Power in Being a Victim

Ahmet had experienced childhood physical and verbal abuse by her mother, sexual abuse by a male relative, and a rape by a stranger who subjected her to extreme humiliation and denigration. After the rape, Ahmet had become more and more disparaging of herself, and highly functionally impaired because of her feelings of helplessness and shame. She desperately wanted to think well of herself, but she simply could not imagine behaviors and way of relating that did not include victimization. She believed that she was "fated" for a life of trauma. In fact, over the course of the treatment, it became clear that she viewed herself as having one source of strength from which she derived great pride, and that was her ability to withstand the abuse of others. Ahmet concluded: "My only strength is in understanding and accepting people whose inner turmoil leads them to be abusive." In her self-appraisal, wrought of desperation, she reversed the typical beliefs about consequences of chronic abuse to buoy herself up psychologically. In submission, she had found her strength.

One goal of the treatment was to provide Ahmet with alternative ways of experiencing herself as worthwhile and strong. This was a challenge, because her shame and self-blame beliefs served multiple functions: They provided a source of personal identity and stability in an otherwise chaotic life, a sense of control and mastery over herself and others, and a sense of meaning and purposefulness in life.

Ahmet believed that she was essentially a bad person, and that this was why she had experienced trauma throughout her life. She believed that something about her attracted violence, and that she was entirely responsible for the traumas and problems she had experienced. Several steps were taken to explore the source, viability, and adaptive nature of these beliefs. These steps included (1) listening to the tapes of her narratives, from the perspective of an adult listening to the story of a child and revising views of herself as "bad"; (2) engaging in critical analysis of schemas by evaluating the sources of blame for the traumatic events; and (3) proposing alternative interpersonal schemas and behaviors that would support connection to others and the development of healthy, nonabusive relationships. These activities helped motivate Ahmet to "give up" her identity as a victim by (4) building a base of experiences that support and gave life to the alternative schemas through role play and real-life practice, and (5) identifying personal and social resources consistent with effective use of new schemas.

Narrative Analysis: Beliefs about "Self as Bad"

Ahmet's view of her abuse was that she must have deserved it (i.e., been a bad child), or that she was bad because she had "let the abuse happen" to her. Sometimes these beliefs were toxically combined: In considering the possibility that she had not been deserving of abuse (i.e., not a bad child), then she became bad for letting it happen.

After the childhood abuse narratives were completed, the therapist explored the reasons for these beliefs. Ahmet's belief that she was a bad child derived from being told she was bad by her mother and other family members. This label organized her experience; it created consistency between what was happening to her (how she was treated) and who she was. Ahmet's belief that she was bad for letting herself be sexually abused as a child was maintained because of the distorted, unrealistic expectations she currently held concerning her own autonomy and mastery in her youth.

The therapist and client reviewed the logic of these beliefs from the perspective of an adult rather than a child. Ahmet's belief that she was bad because she had "let the abuse happen" was revised by moving out of the childhood perception that she was in control of the events of her early life to the adult understanding that children have relatively underdeveloped resources in cognitive and emotional domains to control events; rather, they depend on adults who are charged with the responsibility to care for and protect them. Of greatest impact, however, was engaging in the assignment to watch neighborhood children approximately the same age as she was (between 5 and 8 years) when she was abused. Watching them play and interact with adults provided very concrete and realistic information about the significant levels of dependency and trust children exhibited toward adults.

Ahmet's belief that she deserved the abuse because she was a "bad person" was challenged in a straightforward way by asking her to assess the quality and soundness of her mother's judgment. (She had described her mother in ways suggesting that the mother's functioning was globally impaired.) The therapist and Ahmet also searched for alternative sources of information: What bad things had she done lately? Had she ever done anything good? Positive responses in this area provided a small but accumulating foundation of "evidence" for the creation of positive self-regard, which was reinforced by the therapist.

Identifying Alternative Schemas

By the time Ahmet entered treatment, she was tired of the burden of shame, but could not extend her repertoire of behaviors beyond those defined in a victim role. This resulted in a desperate assertion that victim behaviors were reasons to be proud. Her core schema for relating to others was this: "If I am strong during someone's abusive rages, he will love and appreciate me."

More problematic was Ahmet's firm belief that she could not create relationships based in schemas other than variants of the victim–abuser dyad. She was convinced that "If I try to be with others who don't abuse me, they don't want me or don't accept me," "If I express feelings, then I will be punished," or "If I ask for my needs to be met, I will be abandoned." Stripped down to caricature, the schemas often expressed the relationship between self and other in all-or-nothing terms, particularly in regard to themes of power and control: the self as a victim (powerless and with no control), and the other as a perpetrator (with unmitigated power and control).

The therapist and client developed alternative schemas to directly combat those expressed above. These included, for example, "If I express feelings, people will find me interesting to talk to," or "If I express my needs, I will be recognized and given what I need."

Identifying Resources

Ahmet was well able to identify and monitor the mood of a potentially threatening person. This was an activity she had practiced extensively in childhood, in order to manage and subdue her mother's irritability and reduce the risk of a beating. This interpersonal sensitivity was identified as a skill ready for "translation" to current circumstances. Her ability to detect the pleasure or displeasure of others was keen. The reorganization of this skill required disconnecting her monitoring skills from the automatic behavior of acquiescence to the source of threat. The client and therapist were able to identify a few alternative uses for this "sensing device." When she felt a threat, she would ask herself, "Is this the kind of person I want to spend time with?" and use it as an opportunity to disengage from the situation or perhaps from the relationship.

Ahmet was also very intelligent and knowledgeable about the arts. This knowledge was viewed as a personal resource for her and was applied to building her self-esteem. The therapist reinforced this effort by expressing appreciation of her knowledge and describing it as a positive attribute. Her arts knowledge was also viewed as a resource for establishing new social relationships. It allowed Ahmet to consider building friendships based on mutual interests that gave both people pleasure and satisfaction. Looking at her love of art as a resource for living was a very new experience for Ahmet, who had previously dismissed it as irrelevant to her trauma problems. Lastly and fortunately, Ahmet was able to reconnect with professional friends she had dropped during her "helpless/hopeless" period. She tested schemas such as "If I express my feelings, people will be interested." She began understanding that friendships could be resources for coping with life difficulties and for experiencing life's pleasures.

Conducting a Role Play

An opportunity for Ahmet to test the alternative schemas emerged in a situation with her best friend. Ahmet really did not want to go to a party given by this friend, because he had been bullying her. She had no idea what to do. She brought the problem in to her session (see Example 22.1). When the therapist proposed that she call him to decline the invitation, her first reaction was "I am being selfish. Although he is a bully, he really needs me to go." The client and therapist developed new ways of thinking about the problem ("It's okay to say no to a friend sometimes"), and an alternative schema for understanding the potential contingencies of this relationship. ("If he cares about me, he will understand," and

Interpersonal situation	Feelings/beliefs about self	Expectations about other	Resulting action
• What happened? • Who was involved? I wanted to call a friend and decline an invitation to a party.	• What did I feel/believe about myself? I am bad. I am being selfish. Although he is a bully, he really needs me to go.	• How did I expect the other person to act/respond to me? Angry, rejecting.	• What did I do? • What was the result? Thought about what else I could do. Figured there might be an alternative, even though I could not think of it.

Interpersonal goals	Alternative feelings about self	Alternative expectations	Alternative action
• What are my goals in this situation? To stay home that night <u>and</u> to keep my friendship.	• What else could I feel/believe about myself? It's okay to say no to a friend sometimes. If he cares about me, he will understand. When I can convey my wishes to stay it's a way of being connected with him.	• How else could I expect the other person to act/respond to me? Disappointed but understanding.	• What else could I do? What I did: Called and said I did not want to go. Suggested we make plans to do something else. He agreed.

EXAMPLE 22.1. Ahmet's filled-in Interpersonal Schemas Worksheet II for her relationship with her friend (specifically, her wish not to attend his party).

"When I convey my wishes to stay, it is a way of being connected to him"). Ahmet and the therapist then conducted a role play for the client to find effective and comfortable words and emotional tone.

First, Ahmet role-played herself, and the therapist role-played the bullying friend. The client's initial role play immediately placed her in a position where she was overly apologetic. The therapist then reversed this role play, taking the role of Ahmet and explaining to the friend in a sensitive but unapologetic manner that she would not be able to attend the party but would want to meet with the friend at another time. Ahmet oriented herself to this language and tone, and practiced in an effective way. The role play was also useful because it facilitated identification and processing of conflicting beliefs about herself that might have emerged during the phone call itself ("I am being selfish" vs. "Friends recognize each others' needs").

PROVIDE CLIENT WITH SUPPORT: EXPRESS POSITIVE REGARD

The therapist's capacity to convey his or her continued perception of the client's positive value can counter incipient feelings of shame provoked by struggles in meeting the challenges in the treatment work. This includes difficulties completing the narratives, assimilating new schemas and practicing self-enhancing exercises. Make observations about what the client has felt, said, or done that supports the positive valuation of the client. It is reinforced by working steadfastly with the client on the tasks of the therapy with hope and vigor.

A therapist's positive regard for a client is generally viewed as a "nonspecific" positive aspect of the therapy. Some of our own research, however, suggests that the therapist's positive regard for the client does not exist in a vacuum but is part of a collaborative working relationship, which is expressed through active engagement in competency-enhancing activities (Cloitre et al., 2004). The experience of someone (in this case, a therapist) expending effort on her behalf and showing interest in her problems may contribute to persuading a client of her value.

CHALLENGE: WHEN CLIENTS DON'T TELL

Clients in short-term treatment may not have the opportunity, readiness, or inclination to reveal humiliating details of what has occurred. There is a risk that if clients withhold something important about themselves, they will discount the therapist's good opinion of them and the value of the work they have completed. A client may think, "If the therapist really knew who I was, he would not think well of me," or "If the therapist knew what happened then, she would realize I am permanently 'damaged goods.'" This outcome may be avoided by saying something to clients that acknowledges and "normalizes" the possibility that they may not be able to disclose particularly painful or humiliating aspects of their trauma:

> "I understand that there may be some things that are very difficult for you to say, and that you may in fact not be able to tell about them right now. Many people have this experience. This will not in any way reduce the value of your efforts here or the progress you have made. You can identify important trauma schemas without necessarily stating or even knowing all of the reasons you hold these beliefs. Similarly, the new schemas you have developed are valuable and consistent with who you are now and are becoming. You have gone through terrible things. You deserve to live a good life now, and as best you are able."

SUMMARY

The therapist's behavior plays a particularly important role in the client's recovery from shame. As described in some detail in the case of Ahmet, the therapist actively works with the client in implementing the interventions of the treatment to identify and revise shame-based schemas and behaviors. In addition, the therapist's *attitude* of compassion about what has been shaming for the client is itself a therapeutic intervention. It contradicts the expectation that when the client discloses events of gross humiliation, the therapist will be appalled, think less of her, or create distance or a break in the relationship. Shameful events engender a fear of rejection and, in the big picture, fear of permanent dislocation outside the mainstream of ordinary life. The positive interaction between the therapist and client upon disclosure of humiliating stories models for the client the possibility of acceptance by another. When the therapist describes the client's circumstances with respect and compassion, the client understands her own experience in a new way, through the therapist's eyes. The client's experience of shame is transformed into one of respect for herself.

CHAPTER 23

~

SESSIONS 11–15
Narratives of Loss

Grieving for . . . lost opportunities, for lost childhood, for lost innocence, for losses of
long ago and far away is quite difficult. . . . for traumatic losses that do not involve
immediate death, grieving is often an uncharted and socially unsupported wilderness.
—SANDRA L. BLOOM AND MICHAEL REICHERT (1998, p. 193)

OVERVIEW

The experience of loss is, like that of shame, rarely addressed in traditional trauma treatments. In part, this is because feelings of loss often emerge relatively late in the working
through of childhood abuse trauma. In order to truly understand and mourn losses suffered in the context of childhood trauma, one must first feel deserving of the care, protection, and resources that were not available. The belief among some clients that the abuse
was deserved or is in some way "normative" interferes with the development of self-
compassion and a healthy sense of entitlement, both of which are relevant to the grieving
process.

In addition, the grief for "what never was and never can be" is often very acute and
can amplify other negative trauma-related feelings, such as shame. Typically, survivors
have warded off feelings of sadness about their abuse histories through avoidance and
numbing, or through focusing solely on their anger. As one client put it, "If I let myself
really feel how sad my life has been, I would never stop crying. I would turn to mush, and
you would have to peel me off the floor."

However, until a client can conceptualize what her childhood might or should have
been, and can allow for sorrow associated with this recognition, it is likely that she will
remain stuck in her past. In contrast, helping the client to tolerate and process feelings of
sadness and grief associated with childhood abuse and its costs can, over time, serve to further decrease symptoms of numbing and avoidance. It can also increase the possibility of

BOX 23.1
Theme and Curriculum for Sessions 11–15: Narratives of Loss

THEME

Themes of loss tend to emerge during narrative work. This emergence provides a valuable opportunity to help the client initiate the grief process. Successful engagement in this effort can result in decreased avoidance and numbing symptoms, increased self-compassion, and increased intimacy and openness in relationships. The therapist listens for ways sadness and loss are expressed in narratives (e.g., loss of protective parent figure, loss of childhood, loss of time) and describes potential long-term benefits of tolerating and processing painful trauma-related loss experiences. The therapist provides support and containment while encouraging the client to elaborate on feelings and to mourn losses. The therapist also helps the client to identify the impact of loss experiences on current relationships through interpersonal schemas, and to generate and practice alternative schemas that will increase positive connections with others in the present.

PLANNING AND PREPARATION

Bring memory hierarchy, tape recorder, and blank tape. Bring at least one copy of the Assessment of Postexposure Emotional State form (Handout 20.2), and several copies each of the SUDs during Trauma Narration form (Handout 20.1) and the Interpersonal Schemas Worksheet II (Handout 15.1).

AGENDA

- Begin with emotional check-in and review of between-session work.
- Listen for and elicit client's reactions to taped narratives with loss themes.
- Identify and explore reasons for grieving.
- Conduct narrative.
- Identify and revise loss-related schemas from narrative.
- Identify ways of living in the present with a history of loss.
- Provide client with support: Share the burden of mourning.
- Conduct role plays.
- Assign between-session work:
  - Listen to tape daily; monitor stress with SUDs during Trauma Narration form (Handout 20.1).
  - Initiate at least one interpersonal situation and practice alternative schema, using Interpersonal Schemas Worksheet II (Handout 15.1) to record; include emotion regulation skills as relevant to situation.
  - Practice focused breathing (or other relevant coping skills) twice a day.

SESSION HANDOUTS

Additional copies of Handout 20.1. SUDs during Trauma Narration
Additional copies of Handout 15.1. Interpersonal Schemas Worksheet II

developing a more positive and meaningful personal identity and better connections with others. Box 23.1 outlines the theme and curriculum for working with narratives of loss in Sessions 11–15 of treatment.

LISTEN FOR AND ELICIT CLIENT'S REACTIONS TO NARRATIVES WITH GRIEF THEMES

The therapist needs to listen for how themes and layers of loss (e.g., loss of protective parental figure, loss of childhood, loss of time, etc.) are expressed in narratives, and observe these with the client. The therapist should elicit the client's own observations of these themes as she listens to tapes of narratives both in and outside of sessions. Often clients have been too busy recruiting their emotional and cognitive resources to manage fear reactions, which typically carry with them a sense of urgency and crisis, and have not attended to their experiences of loss.

As they often are with feelings of fear, clients may be somewhat avoidant of or reluctant to deal with feelings of sadness. If themes of loss are present in a narrative, the therapist may broach the theme by making comments such as "It sounds like such a sad and terrible thing to have happened." Sometimes a client's feelings of anger indicate an awareness or belief that the trauma has "cheated" her of what she should have had. If so, the therapist should ask the client to articulate what specifically makes her angry about what has happened.

Sometimes clients say they feel angry or sad when they think or tell about their abuse, but cannot specify what makes them feel that way. One exercise that can be helpful in this regard is to ask such a client between sessions to observe a child who is the same age she was when abused. The client should watch how "normal," nonabusive caretakers interact with the child, and then ask herself, "What does that child have or do that I did not?" This exercise often evokes powerful loss-related feelings.

IDENTIFY AND EXPLORE REASONS FOR GRIEVING

Why Grieve?

Though the client has already learned by this point in the treatment that avoiding emotions only makes the emotions feel stronger and more out of control, many questions and anxieties are still often raised: "Why do I have to feel sad about it?", "How is that going to help me?", "What good is feeling sorry for myself?" The therapist must acknowledge the pain and distress involved in this process, empathize with the client's fears about delving into feelings of sadness, and understand her skepticism about how this will be helpful. In response to the implicit or explicit question "Why should I grieve?", the therapist should be able to articulate clearly to the client potential important long-term benefits of doing this work, described below.

Benefits of Grieving

Liberating Emotional and Physical Energies

Giving voice to feelings of underlying sadness and grief can provide tremendous relief and decrease the level of mental energy the client has been consistently expending to avoid feelings and reminders of the past. This makes more energy available for the client to develop her life in the present. Since it is not possible to numb negative feelings selectively, allowing sadness to come to the surface also increases the possibility of experiencing more positive emotions, such as happiness. In this way, the grief process ultimately facilitates the availability of a fuller spectrum of feelings, where previously there was access to only a constricted range.

Disrupting Links between Loss/Grief and PTSD Symptoms

As appropriate, the therapist should help the client recognize ways that unprocessed loss feelings may be keeping her stuck and perpetuating PTSD symptoms. When difficult feelings from the past are expressed in the present, their power to disrupt the future may be decreased.

Cultivating Self-Compassion

Often even if a survivor is no longer in an abusive relationship, she is still perpetuating these experiences through self-blame, intolerance of her emotions, and invalidation of her life experiences. One of the main goals of grieving is to gain more compassion toward oneself and to cultivate respect for what one has endured.

Increasing Capacity for Meaningful Interpersonal Relationships

As self-compassion develops, a client also has the possibility of forming more meaningful interpersonal connections. Being dismissive of one's own emotional experiences can make it difficult to be understanding and remain open to those of others. Being locked in a self-protective mode breeds isolation and alienation. In contrast, being more empathic toward the self often translates into being more empathic toward others. The increase in openness and authenticity that often accompanies the grief process is likely to elicit more responsiveness and engagement on the part of others.

Finding Value in the Present

Developing a deeper understanding of what has been missing can allow a client to put more value on the things she does have in the present and could have in the future. The distress associated with loss can provide a powerful impetus for making life changes, so that at least some of what has been lost can be balanced by what can be had in the present.

The alternative—avoidance of grief—keeps the client emotionally paralyzed and prevents growth.

CONDUCT NARRATIVE

Although a client may accept the value of grieving and be aware of her sadness, she still may be very unclear about what exactly she has lost and feels sad about. By revisiting her childhood traumas, the client can experience greater clarity about what makes her sad. Telling about the losses will help clarify events that were significant to the client and the impact that these experiences have had on both her beliefs about herself and her current behaviors. Procedures for conducting loss narratives are the same as those described in Chapter 20.

Narratives of loss, like all trauma narratives, also provide the client with the opportunity to have someone be witness to the loss and share in remembrance of the child who once was before the trauma, or who never was and could have been. This may lead to ways of creating some aspects of the imagined but lost self or identified experiential losses through planned activities in the present.

IDENTIFY AND REVISE
LOSS-RELATED INTERPERSONAL SCHEMAS

Grieving for the losses engendered by childhood abuse requires that they first be recognized. This recognition is often hampered by a client's critical and self-blaming attributions about her history. The therapist can make efforts to promote respect and understanding of the experiences the client has endured. Often listening to tapes provides useful distance, which can be effective in helping the client develop self-compassion (e.g., "I felt sorry for that little girl"). If the client is still having difficulty accessing feelings of sadness, sharing the impact that hearing the narrative has had on the therapist can be an effective catalyst (e.g., "When I was listening, I was aware of how desperate and abandoned that little girl sounded, and it made me feel very sad that nobody was taking care of her").

In this context, the client will be able to identify interpersonal schemas that reflect themes of loss and that perpetuate painful feelings of loss, grief and disappointment in the present relationships. The therapist should help the client understand how her feelings of loss typically get reactivated and reenacted, and identify current relationships in which this is most likely to happen.

The development of alternative interpersonal schemas will emphasize changes that decrease the sense of loss and increase social connection. This may include the client's either extricating herself from or making changes in particular relationships that tend to trigger loss feelings. Covert modeling and role playing can be used in sessions to experiment with different ways of interacting, so as to identify how the client could increase feelings of connection and decrease feelings of detachment in interpersonal interactions. A description of this process is provided in the case example below.

IDENTIFY WAYS OF LIVING IN THE PRESENT WITH A HISTORY OF LOSS

Coming to terms with abuse-related losses can be more tolerable if clients can gain a sense that some good can come in the present from having had to endure such painful experiences in the past. Clients may benefit from considering how their loss experiences give them a unique ability to value and appreciate certain things others may waste or take for granted. Clients can also gain from realizing what they have lost by identifying areas in their lives where they want to make changes. For example, clients who feel they have lost time because of the abuse can work on turning that around by better valuing and making use of the time they still do have.

PROVIDE SUPPORT: SHARE THE BURDEN OF PAIN

The therapist needs to offer a consistent source of containment, support, and empathy while the client elaborates on loss experiences and begins mourning. This involves reminding the client that she does not have to bear her pain alone, and identifying ways she can keep this in mind between sessions (e.g., letting other trusted people in her life know what is going on; reading something written in the clinician's handwriting; or keeping a symbolic token from the clinician with her, such as a paperweight or stone). This also involves reminding the client of coping strategies she has learned earlier in the treatment (e.g., distress tolerance) to deal with intense feelings that may arise.

CONDUCT ROLE PLAYS

Role plays associated with grief usually reflect fears of intimacy and of abandonment. Role plays about building relationships are successful when a client is guided by strategies that allow her to go slowly and in an informed way ("Who is this person?", "What do I do?") in seeking out the companionship and friendship of others. The case example provided below illustrates this.

CASE EXAMPLE: LOSS THEMES, LOSS-RELATED SCHEMAS, AND ROLE PLAY

The case of Andrea, a 35-year-old single woman with a history of sexual abuse and long-standing PTSD symptoms, serves to illustrate some common ways loss themes emerge in narratives and can be worked with in the treatment.

Andrea's mother was a single parent who worked long hours to support the family. Andrea's uncle lived nearby and often helped out by doing repairs around the house and caring for the kids. When she was 10, her uncle began molesting her. After the first few times, Andrea told her mother that she no longer wanted to be left alone with him.

Andrea's mother found her change in attitude toward her uncle surprising, but did not make much of it and also felt that there was no alternative to relying on the uncle for help. Over the next few months, her uncle began forcing himself on her more frequently, and Andrea realized that she would have to explain what was going on if there was to be any change: "I didn't want to tell her about the things he was doing to me, because I knew she would be upset, but I wanted it to stop." According to Andrea, her mother initially dismissed it by saying, "Your uncle loves you and would never hurt you or me." Andrea persisted and got more specific about the abuse. In shock and disbelief, her mother asked Andrea for more details and began shaking upon hearing them. Andrea remembers her mother desperately grabbing her and sobbing as she said things like "How could he do this to me?" and "How could I not have known?"

Andrea felt incredibly guilty and frightened by her mother's reaction. In order to stop her own mounting anxiety and dread, she told her mother that she had made it all up. Andrea's mother accepted this explanation, asked no further questions, and never brought it up again. Andrea's uncle continued to spend time around the house and continued to molest her until she was 16, at which time he moved to another state. Andrea did not try to tell her mother or anyone else about the abuse again, figuring it would be in everyone's best interest if she pretended it never happened.

Identifying and Working with Loss Themes

Loss of Parental Protector

Andrea remembered idealizing her uncle prior to the abuse and viewing him as a surrogate father—someone she loved and could turn to if she needed help. The way she managed her feelings of bewilderment and anger at this betrayal by someone she had been raised to believe loved her and had her best interests at heart was to "turn off" all thoughts and feelings about it. The unprocessed anger and grief that emerged during the narrative process, though at times overwhelming, did not surprise Andrea: "I always knew it was there, but was afraid to face it." With the support of her therapist, and equipped with improved emotion regulation skills, Andrea was able to verbalize and move through some of these feelings. Over time, they lost some of their power over her.

What caught Andrea off guard were her intense and complicated feelings toward her mother, which also emerged through the narratives. Prior to this phase of the treatment, Andrea had remained protective of her mother, feeling that she had done her best with limited resources. Andrea said she had forgiven her mother for "not knowing" that abuse was going on, and felt that it was in large part her own fault for making the decision to take back her original report of the molestation.

During Andrea's telling of the abuse during NST, the deep loss she felt with regard to her mother became apparent to both the therapist and herself. It was Andrea's sense that after she disclosed the abuse, there was a change in her relationship with her mother. For example, she felt that her mother spent less time alone with her and avoided asking her what was going on when Andrea seemed upset. Andrea became very panicky as feelings about being abandoned by her mother came to the forefront in the treatment. The therapist worked with Andrea to integrate and accept her previously unexpressed feelings of anger and grief about her mother's absence and her failure to protect Andrea, allowing them to coexist with knowledge that her mother was fragile and depressed. It was important for Andrea to realize the extent of her losses: She had in effect been abandoned by not one but by both of her central caregivers. This knowledge and understanding allowed her to feel more tolerant of her continued difficulties in putting her childhood abuse behind her.

Loss of Childhood

In one of her narratives, Andrea vividly recalled being able to hear kids from the neighborhood laughing and playing outside while her uncle was having sex with her. This memory tapped into the reservoir of grief she felt about not being able to have a "normal," carefree childhood. Because she had been victimized and forced into having sex prematurely by a trusted adult, she was not afforded the period of dormant sexuality and innocence most children have during their early preadolescent years. Andrea went on to share how knowing more than she should about sex made her feel very different and isolated from other kids her age, which was another source of great sadness to her: "While other kids were playing tag with friends, I was inside having sex." Andrea described her transformation from a happy and trusting little girl to a scared, shy, and strange one. Prior to the narrative analysis, this dramatic shift in her demeanor had been incomprehensible and had been viewed by Andrea as further evidence of her "defectiveness." Being able to link these changes to her trauma experiences provided her with a way to challenge her belief that she had been at fault for taking back her original story. Instead, Andrea was able to see how she did in fact continue to try to communicate to others that something was very wrong. This understanding of events and their sequence also provided Andrea with a sense of order and meaning about what had previously felt confusing and mysterious to her.

Loss of Time

Symptoms of avoidance, as well as high levels of social discomfort, mistrust, and disappointment in others, continued to affect Andrea in numerous ways in adulthood. Though she was likeable and often sought out, Andrea had very few close relationships. The friends she did have, she kept at arm's length; she rarely socialized and did not invite anyone over to her house. She had been intimately involved with one man when she was in her mid-20s, but according to Andrea, this relationship was a constant source of pain. She described a cycle in which he often made plans and promises that he did not keep, which left Andrea feeling "needy" and "deserted." Andrea had trouble understanding why, instead of ending the relationship, she continued to hold out hope for so long that she would get what she wanted from him. After he eventually ended the relationship, Andrea made the decision that she would not give another person the power to hurt her so deeply.

Andrea's job progression also seemed to have been hurt by her difficulties in cultivating relationships. Andrea described that whenever people at her office got more personal, she wanted no part of it and often opted out of work-related gatherings. Feedback reports from her manager described her as having lack of enthusiasm and difficulty working collaboratively on a team.

Through narrative analysis, Andrea's growing awareness of the connection between her abuse experiences and current interpersonal difficulties compounded her anger and grief. She wondered how she would ever be able to make up for the time and life experiences she had lost. She also felt depressed that her early abuse experiences continued to have such an impact on her life. Andrea's therapist worked with her on accepting that what had been lost could not be reclaimed, but also on identifying ways these losses could be used to make meaningful changes in the present. Though it was quite distressing for Andrea to face just how much her trauma experiences were continuing to "rob" her in the present, this awareness ultimately provided tremendous motivation for her to finally make some important life changes, including taking more risks in relationships.

Andrea also began to recognize that though her trauma-related losses would always be there, they could become more manageable and ebb and flow at different times, rather than remain at such an intense and disorganizing level. Also critical was her belief in her therapist's rationale that grief related to the past would lessen as she became more engaged in the present.

Identifying and Revising Loss-Related Schemas

Accessing the extent of her loss and grief feelings in NST provided Andrea with more clarity about the emotional context in which her models of relationships were developed. Based on her experiences, Andrea learned to expect that people she trusted would use or abandon her, and that expressing her needs ultimately would lead to loss of relationships. In order to cope with these contingencies, Andrea learned to be extremely guarded and to maintain a façade of independence and self-sufficiency. Though this strategy had once served an adaptive function, it was no longer useful, as evidenced by her ongoing PTSD symptoms, depression, and isolation.

Andrea's clinician worked with her to identify the benefits and costs of this method of self-protection that had become so ingrained. Through continued use of Interpersonal Schemas Worksheets I and II, she could observe concretely how at present these schemas, rather than sparing her emotional pain, actually perpetuated her feelings of disappointment and abandonment and confirmed her belief that others could never fill the void created by earlier losses. Though she did not give others much opportunity and sent strong signals for others to keep their distance, she still often felt abandoned by others and believed that they should figure out what she was really needing or wanting.

Adopting and Practicing New Schemas through Role Play

An opportunity soon became available for Andrea to experiment with an alternative way of interacting. One consequence of Andrea's taking more social risks was that she began getting more invitations. When a long-time acquaintance, Ben, asked her out on a date, Andrea was taken off guard. She told him she would get back to him, but then avoided contacting him and stopped going to places they both frequented. She reported feeling guilty and "like a coward."

Using the Interpersonal Schemas Worksheet II (see Example 23.1), Andrea and her therapist were able to break down and examine her beliefs and expectations of the situation that drove her avoidance behavior. Andrea said that she was interested in Ben but felt she could not afford to risk being hurt: "He thinks he wants to get to know me better, but what if he does and then decides he doesn't like me?" In addition to prematurely preparing for a negative outcome, Andrea also assumed that if things did not work out, she would be unable to handle it. Andrea's automatic beliefs about Ben were that he probably did not know many other single women and was primarily interested in using her for sex: "Once he gets what he wants, he will be out of there."

When asked about her interpersonal goals, Andrea identified her desire to break her cycle of avoidance and stop basing her behavior on fear of negative expectations from the past. Andrea agreed that if nothing else, the situation with Ben could be a good practice opportunity. When asked about her alternative beliefs, she said she could believe it possible to take the risk to go out on a date and potentially get to know someone. She could also try to trust that if it did not work out, she would be able to cope. Andrea and her therapist discussed how this potential "loss" would be different from past losses, given that she was now an adult with coping skills who did not need to rely on others to take care of her. In terms of Ben's intentions, Andrea felt she could believe that he was not out to use her, but that maybe he was actually interested in getting to know her. Andrea and her clinician did some role playing of a scenario in which Andrea called Ben and expressed an interest in a date, as well as an apology for not getting back to him sooner. Also, the therapist and Andrea agreed that it would be important for her to determine the parameters that were comfortable for her, and to take it slowly by keeping the date brief and casual.

This example shows the importance of encouraging the client toward new behaviors in seemingly safe situations, while keeping in mind that other people's responses are not in her control. In this case, Andrea's alternative belief that she could handle it even if things did not work out kept the emphasis on her own role in the interaction. Luckily, Andrea's willingness to take this work outside of the session resulted in her getting positive feedback from Ben. Thus as Andrea was in the process of mourning past losses, she was also simultaneously building more opportunity for intimacy in the present. These therapeutic activities reinforced each other and provided needed momentum to push her work in treatment forward.

ASSIGN BETWEEN-SESSION EXERCISES

The client should listen to the tape of the latest narrative daily during the week and identify interpersonal schemas of loss she finds in the narrative. The therapist and client should have already identified some of these schemas and role-played some alternative formulations of the schemas. Now the client and therapist should determine a "real-life" circumstance in which to practice an alternative schema. Practice of emotion regulation skills should continue.

Interpersonal situation	Feelings/beliefs about self	Expectations about other	Resulting action
• What happened? • Who was involved?	• What did I feel/believe about myself?	• How did I expect the other person to act/respond to me?	• What did I do? • What was the result?
I was asked out on a date by Ben, someone I am very interested in.	I am really scared. I want to say no. I couldn't take it if I connected with him and then he just took off. If I depend on him, he will just take off. Maybe we can have sex just for fun, and I will leave him cold before anything else happens.	He is probably really immature and will vanish the first instant I need him. He probably just wants sex and doesn't know many single women. If we have sex, he will have gotten what he wanted and will then disappear.	Avoided giving him an answer, stopped going to places he might be. Felt like a coward.

Interpersonal goals	Alternative feelings/ beliefs about self	Alternative expectations about others	Alternative action
• What are my goals in this situation?	• What else could I feel/believe about myself?	• How else could I expect the other person to act/respond to me?	• What else could I do?
To take more social risks. To make an active decision rather than just avoid. Not to base decision on fear or negative expectations.	I am capable of taking the risk to get to know someone. If it does not work out, I will be able to handle it. I am a different person than I was in the past and now have coping skills and resources.	He is interested in actually getting to know me. He is not out to use me. Not everyone abandons people when they get scared.	Agree to go on date, but keep it casual and brief.

EXAMPLE 23.1. Andrea's filled-in Interpersonal Schemas Worksheet II for her potential relationship with Ben.

CHAPTER 24

~

SESSION 16

The Last Session

Freedom is what you do with what's been done to you.
—JEAN-PAUL SARTRE,
quoted by GLORIA STEINEM (1992, p. 63)

OVERVIEW

The goals of the last session are to summarize the client's progress, to plan the next steps, and to identify risks for relapse and associated recovery strategies. Above all, the therapist should give recognition to the survivor for her specific accomplishments in the treatment, and should convey a sincere appreciation for the courage and strength that this work has involved. Box 24.1 outlines the theme and curriculum for Session 16 of treatment.

ELICIT FROM CLIENT
HER EXPERIENCE OF CHANGE AND PROGRESS

The most important task of the last session is to identify and give positive recognition of the progress the client has made. The client will have her own ideas about which aspects of the work she is most proud of and most satisfied with, and the therapist should elicit these assessments. The therapist can prompt the client to consider changes in PTSD symptoms, emotion regulation skills, interpersonal functioning, general life functioning, and experience of self since the beginning of treatment, and to compare her overall past and present status.

BOX 24.1
Theme and Curriculum for Session 16: The Last Session

THEME

The goals of the last session are to summarize the client's progress, plan next steps, identify risk for relapse and associated recovery strategies. Most importantly, the therapist should give recognition to the survivor of specific accomplishments that have been achieved and a sincere appreciation of the courage and strength that this work has involved.

PLANNING AND PREPARATION

Create summary of client's progress. Create list of resources for next steps and relapse recovery. Bring final session handouts.

AGENDA

- Begin with emotional check-in and review of between-session work.
- Elicit from client her experience of change and progress.
- Elaborate on or add to identified progress.
- Identify plans for next steps.
- Review risks for relapse and associated recovery strategies.
- Indicate respect for pace of change process.
- Provide resources for transition and future needs.
- Say good-bye.

SESSION HANDOUTS

Handout 24.1. Posttreatment Goals and Strategies Sheet
Handout 24.2. Affirmation for Living
Resource list (to be compiled by therapist)

ELABORATE ON OR ADD TO IDENTIFIED PROGRESS

Typically, the client has done more work and has changed more than she is able to see and experience. The therapist, as an outside observer, has had the benefit of a different vantage point and thus may be able to identify further accomplishments, or to elaborate on and give depth to the changes the client has identified.

Severity of PTSD Symptoms

Pronounced changes are likely to have occurred in the frequency and severity of PTSD symptoms. In the week preceding the final session, it is useful to have the client fill out a PTSD symptom questionnaire identical to the one completed during the assessment. The client may have forgotten the significant distress she was experiencing when she entered treatment; if so, she is likely to discount the amount of symptom reduction there has been. A comparison of the total PTSD scores before and after treatment is an effective way to summarize and demonstrate this change.

Emotion Management Skills

The therapist should elicit, and participate with the client in, an enumeration of the improvements in emotion regulation and emotional experiences. Changes in emotional experiencing to inquire after include the following:

- Ability to face fear and anxiety
- Ability to manage angry feelings with specific strategies
- Ability to tolerate depression and reduce the amount of time spent in a depressed state
- Reduction in dissociative experiencing (less spacing out, derealization, and depersonalization)

Interpersonal Skills

Changes in interpersonal functioning are often best reviewed by reference to "experiential exercises" that were successfully completed. It is unrealistic to believe that interpersonal functioning can be entirely transformed within 4 months. Such behaviors are strongly ingrained habits. However, the therapy has provided three important interventions that will help the client maintain and continue the change process. These are the "triple A's" of awareness, alternatives, and action.

1. *Awareness* of interpersonal patterns is the first step in changing behavior. Interpersonal patterns of behavior have been clearly identified. They are no longer automatic behaviors, out of the client's awareness. The client has learned that with awareness comes the opportunity to intervene and choose alternative ways of thinking and alternative behaviors.

2. *Alternatives* to interpersonal patterns from the past have been formulated. An alternative template for ways of thinking about relationships has been developed in the form of interpersonal schemas ("If . . . then . . . " and "When . . . then . . . "). This template can be used to guide the client in analyzing difficult situations, identifying interpersonal goals, and organizing alternative behaviors to reach these goals.

3. *Action* has demonstrated capacity for change. The client has developed and practiced alternative behaviors with success. These new behaviors provide building blocks for new situations as they emerge. They have also demonstrated the client's capacity for successful change. Knowledge of this capacity should give the client confidence in experimenting with new behaviors and seeking out new people.

A New Experience of Self

The therapist should elicit from and explore with the client her subjective experiences with each component of the treatment: How did she feel about herself during each phase of treatment? Were there times when she felt the treatment was just right for her, resonated with her goals? Were there times when she disliked the treatment? Felt alienated from the tasks, methods, or goals? How did she experience each of the components as a change or growth experience? Below are some characterizations of the treatment that may help guide this discussion.

The STAIR interventions have provided the client with tools for behaving, thinking, and feeling in more positive and competent ways. As such, this phase of treatment lays the groundwork for the possibility of continued positive change. In contrast, the narrative work has required going back to the past and telling about distant events with emotional depth and intensity. The process has returned the client to a traumatic early life history and led to the recognition of the far-reaching influence these formative experiences have had on the trajectory of her life. Together, the two phases of treatment have helped the client integrate the past with the present and with a sense of the future, giving the client a sense of a coherent self that was not possible before.

Honest grappling with the pain, shame, and loss generated from these experiences deepens a person's inner emotional life. Recognizing and experiencing a gamut of feelings, and surviving them, lead to renewed emotional strength. Increased capacity for openness in emotional experiencing also provides the opportunity for authentic connection with others. These connections are supported by the very necessary skills of self-management and social competence that have been in practice during the STAIR treatment. In this way, the STAIR and the NST components of treatment are necessary partners in the recovery process. The client has completed both parts of treatment. The client can continue to use these skills to express who she is and who she hopes to become.

IDENTIFY PLANS FOR NEXT STEPS

There will inevitably be many tasks remaining for the survivor as she moves out of this treatment. The client and therapist should identify the client's goals during this transition and for the near future. This can include emotional and interpersonal goals such as "being kinder to myself when I make mistakes" or "being more assertive with friends about what I like to do with them." For each of these goals, it is useful to clarify which skills or resources the client has that will allow to her to reach and maintain these goals. Therapist and client can take some time to jot down these goals and potential strategies for reaching these goals (see Handout 24.1). During periods of depression or demoralization, the client may forget the goals she has set for herself, and may not recall that she does have the basic capacity and the knowledge to tackle new challenges. Handout 24.1 can serve as a reminder and morale booster during such periods.

In addition, the client may have concerns about dealing with the exacerbation and management of symptoms—particularly PTSD symptoms, feelings of anger and depression, and dissociation. Here again, the therapist and client should review which strategies they have learned work best to negotiate these difficulties.

REVIEW RISKS FOR RELAPSE AND ASSOCIATED RECOVERY STRATEGIES

It is likely that the client has ongoing life stressors, and it is inevitable that the client will experience additional stressful life events in the future. It is therefore useful to identify any such events that seem likely, particularly those the client is fearful of managing. These may include confronting the abuser, disclosing abuse to friends or family members, becoming a parent, or making a relationship commitment. Again, written guidelines for effective management of these stressors are useful to create now, so that they will be available when the client needs them but may be less able to formulate them effectively.

Other practical preparations for management of setbacks should be made ahead of time. These may include keeping medication prescriptions up to date or checking regularly with a physician, and identifying which friends are best at helping with which type of crisis and reaching out for help accordingly.

General principles for coping with setbacks should be articulated. First, the client should accept and remember that relapses to old behaviors and symptom exacerbations are inevitable. A second general guideline is for the client to avoid putting energy into self-criticism or languishing in humiliation. The client needs to be encouraged that a healthy response to relapse is to begin (or prepare to begin) the process of recovery. The client can be reminded of her accomplishments in the therapy, and can be told that these successes demonstrate her capacity to manage difficult and emotionally demanding situations.

INDICATE RESPECT FOR PACE OF CHANGE

Some clients may feel unsure of their readiness to continue their recovery without the therapy. The therapist should convey that this is a natural and understandable anxiety. Often a client's anxiety about making the transition out of therapy is effectively responded to by repeating the many successes that the client has achieved. In addition, the therapist should provide a summary of the results of follow-up research interviews with clients who have participated in STAIR/NST. These indicate that after treatment ends, clients continue to improve even further—generalizing the gains they have made, as they encounter new opportunities to put their skills and mastery into practice.

For other clients, especially those with multiple traumas, the work accomplished during the therapy may seem like a "drop in the bucket." Such a client and her therapist should concretely evaluate outstanding problem areas. If there is opportunity in the clinical setting to extend treatment and the client is willing to do so, this option may be considered. Alternatively, the therapist may be able to make recommendations for continuing treatment in a program or modality that best suits the client at this point in her recovery.

PROVIDE RESOURCES FOR TRANSITION AND FUTURE NEEDS

The therapist should provide a "resource list" of local services or programs that the client may find useful in the transition or in the near future. This can include information about programs related to the client's identified goals or continued recovery needs, such as Twelve-Step groups, legal services, employment skills training programs, or other community services. It can also include basic resources, such as telephone numbers for the client's local emergency room, domestic violence bureau, or crisis hotline. In addition, the therapist can provide the client with an affirmation of life goals as a reminder (see Handout 24.2).

SAY GOOD-BYE

At some point in this session (perhaps toward the end), the therapist should summarize his or her appreciation of the client's hard work, and extend a message of hope and good wishes for the client's next steps.

The issue of future contact with the therapist is likely to be brought forward by the client. If it is not, the therapist should address this issue, as the client is likely to be thinking (if not talking) about it. There is no "right" decision in this situation. It depends on many factors, including the nature of the treatment setting, the client's needs and preferences, and the therapist's own guidelines in work. The discussion should be guided, however, by the therapist's awareness that the client has shared some of the most intimate details of her life. The therapist has given witness to this history and is also now a guardian of it. Therefore, whatever the particulars of the ensuing discussion, it is important for the therapist to express respect for the client's history, appreciation for having learned about her life, and gratitude for having had the opportunity to learn from her.

Posttreatment Goals and Strategies Sheet

GOALS	STRATEGIES

Affirmation for Living

With all your heart
say out loud,

I want to live a happy life. Listen to what you just said, take notice of things, surround yourself with people you love, listen to the wind, imagine, let everything change all the time, let go of the why, welcome miracles, thank God constantly, breathe, tell the truth about how you feel, make choices, want what you want, let animals reach you, have children teach you, take good care of your body, love passionately, share your dreams, spread your gifts, check it out, forgive the past, dive in, eat it up, take chances, be real.

APPENDIX A

~

Resources

EMOTION REGULATION STRATEGIES

Benson, H., with Klipper, M. Z. (2000). *The relaxation response.* New York: HarperColllins.

Bernstein, D. A., Borkovec, T. D., & Hazlett-Stevens, H. (2000). *New directions in progressive relaxation training: A guidebook for helping professionals.* Westport, CT: Praeger.

Harvey, J. (1998). *Total relaxation: Healing practices for body, mind and spirit.* New York: Kodansha America.

Kabat-Zinn, J. (1994). *Wherever you go, there you are: Mindfulness meditation in everyday life.* New York: Hyperion Books.

Kabat-Zinn, J. (1995). *Mindfulness meditation: Cultivating the wisdom of your body and mind* [Audiotape]. New York: Simon & Schuster Audio/Nightingale.

Lazarus, J. (2000). *Stress relief and relaxation techniques.* Lincolnwood, IL: Keats.

Sapolsky, R. (2004). *Why zebras don't get ulcers* (3rd ed.). New York: Owl Books.

Wilson, P. (1995). *Instant calm: Over 100 easy-to-use techniques for relaxing mind and body.* New York: Penguin Books.

THERAPIST SELF-CARE

Books and Articles

Baker, E. K. (2003). *Caring for ourselves: A therapist's guide to personal and professional well-being.* Washington, DC: American Psychological Association.

Courtois, C. A. (1993). Vicarious traumatization of the therapist. *NC-PTSD Clinical Newsletter, 3*(2), 8–9.

Kottler, J. A. (1998). *The therapist's workbook: Self-assessment, self-care, and self-improvement exercises for mental health professionals.* San Francisco: Jossey-Bass.

McCann, L., & Pearlman, L. A. (1990). Vicarious traumatization: A framework for understanding the psychological effects of working with victims. *Journal of Traumatic Stress, 3,* 131–149.

Pearlman, L. A., & Saakvitne, K. W. (1995). *Trauma and the therapist.* New York: Norton.

Pope, K. S., & Vasquez, M. J. T. (2005). *How to survive and thrive as a therapist: Information, ideas, and resources for psychologists in practice.* Washington, DC: American Psychological Association.

Ruzek, J. I. (1993). Professionals coping with vicarious trauma. *NC-PTSD Clinical Newsletter, 3*(2), 12–13, 17.

Websites

www.ncptsd.va.gov./publications/cq/v8/n1/V8N1.pdf
kspope.com/therapistas/index.php

~

Examples of Assessment Measures by Domain

TRAUMA HISTORY

Interviews

Child Interpersonal Violence Inventory (CIVI; Briere, 1992; Briere & Runtz, 1990).—The CIVI is used to assess a wide range of childhood experiences, including physical, sexual, and emotional abuse and neglect.

Sexual Assault and Additional Interpersonal Violence Schedule (Foa, Rothbaum, Riggs, & Murdock, 1991; Resick & Schnicke, 1992).—This instrument is used to assess exposure to rape and other forms of interpersonal violence in adolescence and adulthood.

Self-Report

Life Stressor Checklist—Revised (LSC-R; Wolfe & Kimerling, 1997).—The LSC-R is used to assess a wide range of traumatic experiences, including exposure to natural disaster and sudden unexpected death of a close friend or relative. The LSC-R is available at no cost from the National Center for PTSD (see the website URL given below).

POSTTRAUMATIC STRESS DISORDER

Interview

Clinician-Administered PTSD Scale (CAPS; Blake et al., 1995).—The CAPS is the "gold-standard" structured clinical interview for PTSD diagnosis. It is available at no cost from the National Center for PTSD.

Self-Report Scales

PTSD Checklist—Civilian Version (PCL-C; Blanchard, Jones-Alexander, Buckley, & Forneris, 1996). The PCL-C is a widely used self-report measure of PTSD symptoms. It too is available at no cost from the National Center for PTSD.

Posttraumatic Diagnostic Scale (PDS; Foa, 1995; Foa, Cashman, Jaycox, & Perry, 1997). The PDS is a self-report scale for PTSD symptoms that corresponds to DSM-IV diagnostic criteria.

For information on other trauma exposure and PTSD assessment measures, go to the "Assessment Instruments" section of the National Center for PTSD website (www.ncptsd.va.gov/publications/assessment).

Therapists may also find a book edited by Antony, Orsillo, and Roemer (2001) very helpful. This book discusses 24 measures for PTSD and acute stress disorder in detail (with original citations, descriptions, administration and scoring information, and psychometric properties) and 18 briefly. Source and contact information are given for all instruments. The book also includes the content of 11 instruments.

EMOTION REGULATION

Difficulties in Emotion Regulation Scale (DERS; Gratz & Roemer, 2004).—The DERS assesses modulation of emotional arousal, awareness, understanding, and acceptance of emotions, and the ability to act in desired ways regardless of emotional state.

Generalized Expectancy for Negative Mood Regulation (NMR) Scale (Catanzaro & Mearns, 1990, 1999).—The NMR Scale (see Appendix A) is a 30-item Likert scale measuring generalized expectancy that some overt behavior or cognition will alleviate a negative state or induce a positive one. Expectations concerning negative feelings include the ability to change a negative state (" I can usually find a way to cheer myself up") as well as to tolerate a negative state ("It won't be long before I can calm myself down").

State–Trait Anger Expression Inventory (STAXI; Spielberger, 1988).—The STAXI consists of 44 items that are administered in three parts and distributed across the five main scales—State Anger, Trait Anger, and Anger Expression—broken down into three constructs—In, Out, and Control.

State–Trait Anxiety Inventory (STAI; Spielberger, 1983).—The STAXI consists of 40 items distributed across the two main scales that differentiate between trait and state anxiety.

Beck Depression Inventory–2nd Edition Revised (BDI-II, Beck, Ward, Mendelsohn, Mock & Erbaugh, 1961; Beck & Steer, 1984; Beck, Rial, & Rickets, 1974).—The BDI-II is a 21-item self-report measure of cognitive and vegetative symptoms that is widely used to assess depression.

INTERPERSONAL AND ROLE FUNCTIONING

Inventory of Interpersonal Problems (IIP; Horowitz, Rosenberg, Baer, Ureno, & Villasenor, 1988).—The IIP is a 127-item self-report measure that examines difficulties in six dimensions of interpersonal functioning: assertiveness, sociability, intimacy, submissiveness, responsibility, and control.

Social Adjustment Scale—Self Report (SAS-SR; Weissman & Bothell, 1976).—The SAS-SR is a 54-item questionnaire that assesses either instrumental or expressive role performance in six major areas: work, leisure, extended family, romantic relationships, parental, and family unit.

Interpersonal Support Evaluation List (ISEL; Cohen, Kamarack, & Mermelstein, 1983).—The ISEL consists of 40 statements concerning the perceived availability of social support in four domains: self-esteem, tangible support, appraisal support, and sense of belonging support.

RESILIENCE AND POSITIVE COPING

Coping Orientation to Problems Experienced (COPE; Scheier & Carver, 1985).—The COPE is a 60-item inventory that measures five problem-focused coping styles: active coping, planning, suppression of competing activities, restraint coping, and seeking instrumental social support.

The Posttraumatic Growth Inventory (PGI; Tedeschi & Calhoun, 1996).—The PGI was designed to assess positive outcomes of traumatic experiences. The 21-item scale includes factors of New Possibilities, Relating to Others, Personal Strength, Spiritual Change, and Appreciation of Life.

Multidimensional Trauma Recovery and Resiliency Scale (MTRRS; Harvey et al., 2003).—The MTRRS is a Likert-type scale used by therapists to assess client resilience across multiple domains of functioning.

References

Ackerman, P. T., Newton, J. E. O., McPherson, W. B., Jones, J. G., & Dykman, R. A. (1998). Prevalence of posttraumatic stress disorder and other psychiatric diagnoses in three groups of abused children (sexual, physical, and both). *Child Abuse and Neglect, 22*, 759–774.

Adam, B. S., Everett, B. L., & O'Neal, E. (1992). PTSD in physically and sexually abused psychiatrically hospitalized children. *Child Psychiatry and Human Development, 23*, 3–8.

Agosti, V., & Stewart, J. W. (1998). Social functioning and residual symptomatology among outpatients who responded to treatment and recovered from major depression. *Journal of Affective Disorders, 47*, 207–210.

Alaggia, R. (2002). Balancing acts: Reconceptualizing support in maternal response to intrafamilial child sexual abuse. *Clinical Social Work Journal, 30*(1), 41–56.

Allen, J. G. (1995). *Coping with trauma: A guide to self-understanding.* Washington, DC: American Psychiatric Press.

American Psychiatric Association. (1980). *Diagnostic and statistical manual of mental disorders* (3rd ed., text rev.). Washington, DC: Author.

Andrews, B. (1997). Bodily shame in relation to abuse in childhood and bulimia. *British Journal of Clinical Psychology, 36*, 41–50.

Andrews, B., Brewin, C. R., Rose, S., & Kirk, M. (2000). Predicting post-traumatic stress disorder symptoms in victims of violent crime: The role of shame, anger and childhood abuse. *Journal of Abnormal Psychology, 109*, 69–73.

Andrews, B., & Hunter, E. (1997). Shame, early abuse and course of depression in a clinical sample: A preliminary study. *Cognition and Emotion, 11*, 373–381.

Antony, M. M., Orsillo, S. M., & Roemer, L. (Eds.). (2001). *Practitioner's guide to empirically based measures of anxiety.* New York: Kluwer Academic/Plenum.

Baker, E. K. (2003). *Caring for ourselves: A therapist's guide to personal and professional well-being.* Washington, DC: American Psychological Association.

Beck, A. T., Rial, W. Y., & Rickets, K. (1974). Short form of depression inventory: crossvalidation. *Psychological Reports, 34*, 1184–1186.

Beck, A. T., & Steer, R. A. (1984). Internal consistencies of the original and revised Beck Depression Inventory. *Journal of Clinical Psychology, 40*, 1365–1367.

Beck, A. T., Ward, C. H., Mendelsohn, M., Mock, J., & Erbaugh, J. (1961). An inventory for measuring depression. *Archives of General Psychiatry, 4*, 561–571.

Beckham, J. C., Roodman, A. A., Barefoot, J. C., Haney, T. L., Helms, M. J., Fairbank, J. A., et al. (1996). Interpersonal and self-reported hostility among combat veterans with and without posttraumatic stress disorder. *Journal of Traumatic Stress, 9*, 335–342.

Benjamin, J. (1988). *The bonds of love: Psychoanalysis, feminism, and the problems of domination.* New York: Pantheon Books.

Benson, H., with Klipper, M. Z. (2000). *The relaxation response.* New York: HarperCollins.

Bernstein, D. A., Borkovec, T. D., & Hazlett-Stevens, H. (2000). *New directions in progressive relaxation training: A guidebook for helping professionals.* Westport, CT: Praeger.

Blake, D. D., Weathers, F. W., Nagy, L. M., Kaloupek, D.

G., Gusman, F. D., Charney, D. S., et al. (1995). The development of a Clinician-Administered Posttraumatic Stress Disorder Scale. *Journal of Traumatic Stress, 8,* 75–90.

Blanchard, E. B., Jones-Alexander, J., Buckley, T. C., & Forneris, C. A. (1996). Psychometric properties of the Posttraumatic Stress Disorder Checklist—Civilian Version (PCL). *Behaviour Research and Therapy, 34,* 669–673.

Blieberg, K. L. (2000). *The disclosure of childhood sexual abuse and post-traumatic stress disorder and related symptoms of cognitive and affective impairment.* New York: Adelphi University.

Bloom, S. L., & Reichert, M. (1998). *Bearing witness: Violence and collective responsibility.* Binghamton, NY: Haworth Press.

Boudewyns, P. A., & Hyer, L. A. (1990). Physiological response to combat veterans and preliminary treatment outcome in Vietnam veteran posttraumatic stress disorder patients treated with direct therapeutic exposure. *Behavior Therapy, 21,* 63–87.

Bourne, E. J. (1999). *The anxiety and phobia workbook.* Oakland, CA: New Harbinger.

Bouton, M. E., & Swartzentruber, D. (1991). Sources of relapse after extinction in Pavlovian and instrumental learning. *Clinical Psychology Review, 11,* 123–140.

Bowlby, J. (1969). *Attachment and loss: Vol. 1. Attachment.* New York: Basic Books.

Brewin, C. R. (2003). *Posttraumatic stress disorder: Malady or myth?* New Haven, CT: Yale University Press.

Brewin, C. R., Andrews, B., & Rose, S. (2000). Fear, helplessness, and horror in posttraumatic stress disorder. *Journal of Traumatic Stress, 13,* 499–509.

Brewin, C. R., Andrews, B., & Valentine, J. D. (2000). Meta-analysis of risk factors for posttraumatic stress disorder in trauma-exposed adults. *Journal of Consulting and Clinical Psychology, 68,* 748–766.

Brewin, C. R., Dalgleish, T., & Joseph, S. (1996). A dual representation theory of post-traumatic stress disorder. *Psychological Review, 103,* 670–686.

Briere, J. (1988). The long term clinical correlates of childhood sexual victimization. *Annals of the New York Academy of Sciences, 528,* 327–334.

Briere, J. (1992). *Child abuse trauma: Theory and treatment of the lasting effects.* Newbury Park, CA: Sage.

Briere, J., & Runtz, M. (1987). Post sexual abuse trauma: Data and implications for clinical practice. *Journal of Interpersonal Violence, 2,* 367–379.

Briere, J., & Runtz, M. (1990). Differential adult symptomology associated with three types of child abuse histories. *Child Abuse and Neglect, 14,* 357–364.

Brodsky, B., Cloitre, M., & Dulit, R. (1995). The relationship of dissociation to self-mutilation and childhood abuse in borderline personality disorder. *American Journal of Psychiatry, 12,* 1788–1792.

Brown, E. J., & Kolko, D. J. (1999). Child victims' attributions about being physically abused: An examination of factors associated with symptom severity. *Journal of Abnormal Child Psychology, 27,* 311–322.

Browne, A., & Finkelhor, D. (1986). Impact of child abuse: A review of the research. *Psychological Bulletin, 99,* 66–77.

Burnstein, A. (1986). Treatment noncompliance in patients with posttraumatic stress disorder. *Psychosomatics, 27,* 37–40.

Burroughs, A. R. (2003). *Dry: A memoir.* New York: St. Martin's Press.

Carlson, V., Cicchetti, D., Barnett, D., & Braunwald, K. (1989). Disorganized/disoriented attachment relationships in maltreated infants. *Developmental Psychology, 25,* 525–531.

Carson, R. C. (1969). *Interaction concepts of personality.* Chicago: Aldine.

Catanzaro, S. J., & Mearns, J. (1990). Measuring generalized expectancies of negative mood regulation: Initial scale development and implications. *Journal of Personality Assessment, 54,* 546–563.

Catanzaro, S. J., & Mearns, J. (1999). Mood-related expectancy, emotional experience, and coping behavior. In J. Kirsch (Ed.), *How expectancies shape experience* (pp. 67–91). Washington, DC: American Psychological Association.

Chaffin, M., Kelleher, K., & Hollenberg, J. (1996). Onset of physical abuse and neglect: Psychiatric, substance abuse, and social risk factors from prospective community date. *Child Abuse and Neglect, 20,* 191–203.

Chaplin, T. C., Rice, M. E., & Harris, G. T. (1995). Salient victim suffering and the sexual responses of child molesters. *Journal of Consulting and Clinical Psychology, 63*(2), 249–255.

Chemtob, C. M., Novaco, R. W., Hamada, R. N., & Gross, D. (1997a). Cognitive-behavioral treatment of severe anger in posttraumatic stress disorder. *Journal of Consulting and Clinical Psychology, 65,* 184–189.

Chemtob, C. M., Novaco, R. W., Hamada, R. S., Gross, D. M., & Smith, G. (1997b). Anger regulation deficits in combat-related posttraumatic stress disorder. *Journal of Traumatic Stress, 10,* 17–35.

Cicchetti, D., & White, J. (1990). Emotion and developmental psychopathology. In L. N. L. Stein & T. Trabasso (Eds.), *Psychological approaches to emotion* (pp. 359–382). Hillsdale, NJ: Erlbaum.

Cloitre, M. (1997). Comorbidity of DSM-IV disorders among women experiencing traumatic events. *NC-PTSD Clinical Quarterly, 7,* 52–53.

Cloitre, M. (1998). Sexual revictimization: Risk factors and prevention. In V. M. Follette, J. I. Ruzek, & F.

R. Abueg (Eds.), *Cognitive-behavioral therapies for trauma* (pp. 278–304). New York: Guilford Press.

Cloitre, M., Cohen, L. R., & Scarvalone, P. (2002a). Understanding revictimization among childhood sexual abuse survivors: An interpersonal schema approach. *Journal of Cognitive Psychotherapy: An International Quarterly, 16*, 91–111.

Cloitre, M., & Koenen, K. C. (2001). The impact of borderline personality disorder on process group outcome among women with posttraumatic stress disorder related to childhood abuse. *International Journal of Group Psychotherapy, 51*, 379–397.

Cloitre, M., Koenen, K. C., Cohen, L. R., & Han, H. (2002b). Skills training in affective and interpersonal regulation followed by exposure: A phase-based treatment for PTSD related to childhood abuse. *Journal of Consulting and Clinical Psychology, 70*, 1067–1074.

Cloitre, M., Levitt, J., Davis, L., & Miranda, R. (2003, November). Bringing a manualized treatment for PTSD to the community. In R. Bryant (Chair), *Improving treatment of posttraumatic stress disorder.* Symposium presented at the 19th annual meeting of the International Society for Traumatic Stress Studies, Chicago, IL.

Cloitre, M., Miranda, R., Stovall-McClough, C., & Han, H. (2005). Beyond PTSD: Emotion regulation and interpersonal problems as predictors of functional impairment in survivors of childhood abuse. *Behavior Therapy, 36*, 119–124.

Cloitre, M., Scarvalone, P., & Difede, J. A. (1997). Posttraumatic stress disorder, self and interpersonal dysfunction among sexually retraumatized women. *Journal of Traumatic Stress, 10*, 437–452.

Cloitre, M., Stovall-McClough, C., Miranda, R., & Chemtob, C. M. (2004). Therapeutic alliance, negative mood regulation, and treatment outcome in child abuse-related posttraumatic stress disorder. *Journal of Consulting and Clinical Psychology, 72*, 411–416.

Cloitre, M., Stovall-McClough, C., & Zorbas, P. (2005). *Childhood maltreatment, adult attachment status, and psychosocial adjustment.* Manuscript in preparation.

Cloitre, M., Tardiff, K., Marzuk, P. M., Leon, A. C., & Portera, L. (1996). Childhood abuse and subsequent sexual assault among female inpatients. *Journal of Traumatic Stress, 9*, 473–482.

Cohen, S., Kamarack, T., & Mermelstein, R. (1983). A global measure of perceived stress. *Journal of Health and Social Behavior, 24*, 385–398.

Conte, J., Wolfe, R. R., & Smith, T. (1989). What sexual offenders tell us about prevention strategies. *Child Abuse and Neglect, 13*, 293–301.

Conway, M. A., & Pleydell-Pearce, C. W. (2000). The construction of autobiographical memories in the self-memory system. *Psychological Review, 107*(2), 261–288.

Cooper, N., & Clum, G. (1989). Imaginal flooding as a supplementary treatment for PTSD in combat veterans: A controlled study. *Behavior Therapy, 10*, 381–391.

Coryell, W., Scheftner, W., Keller, M., Endicott, J., Maser, J., & Klerman, G. (1993). The enduring psychological consequences of mania and depression. *American Journal of Psychiatry, 150*, 720–726.

Courtois, C. A. (1993). Vicarious traumatization of the therapist. *NC-PTSD Clinical Newsletter, 3*(2), 8–9.

Courtois, C. A. (1996). *Healing the incest wound.* New York: Norton.

Courtois, C. A., & Watts, D. L. (1982). Counseling adult women who experienced incest in childhood or adolescence. *Personnel and Guidance Journal*, 275–279.

Cummings, E. M., Hennessy, K., Rabideau, G., & Cicchetti, D. (1994). Responses of physically abused boys to interadult anger involving their mothers. *Developmental Psychopathology, 6*, 31–41.

Davis, M., Eshelman, E. R., & McKay, M. (1995). *The relaxation and stress reduction workbook.* Oakland, CA: New Harbinger.

DeVries, A. P. J., Kassam-Adams, N., Cnaan, A., Sherman Slate, E., Gallagher, P., & Winston, F. K. (1999). Looking beyond the physical injury: Post-traumatic stress disorder in children and parents after pediatric traffic injury. *Pediatrics, 104*, 1293–1299.

Diaz, A., Simatov, E., & Rickert, V. I. (2000). The independent and combined effects of physical and sexual abuse on health: Results of a national survey. *Journal of Pediatric and Adolescent Gynecology, 13*, 89.

Dubner, A. E., & Motta, R. W. (1999). Sexually and physically abused foster care children and posttraumatic stress disorder. *Journal of Consulting and Clinical Psychology, 67*, 367–373.

Edwards, V. J., Holden, G. W., Felitti, V. J., & Anda, R. F. (2003). Relationship between multiple forms of childhood maltreatment and adult mental health in community respondents: Results from the adverse childhood experiences study. *American Journal of Psychiatry, 160*, 1453–1460.

Ehlers, A., Clark, D., Winton, E., Jaycox, L., Meadows, E., & Foa, E. B. (1998). Predicting response to exposure treatment in post-traumatic stress disorder: The role of mental defeat and alienation. *Journal of Traumatic Stress, 11*, 457–471.

Erickson, M. F., Egeland, B., & Pianta, R. (1989). The effects of maltreatment on the development of young children. In D. Cicchetti & V. Carlson (Eds.), *Child maltreatment: Theory and research on the causes and consequences of child abuse and neglect* (pp. 674–684). New York: Cambridge University Press.

Fanning, P., & O'Neill, J. T. (1996). *The addiction workbook.* Oakland, CA: New Harbinger.

Feiring, C., Taska, L., & Chen, K. (2002). Trying to understand why horrible things happen: Attribution, shame, and symptom development following sexual abuse. *Child Maltreatment, 7,* 25–39.

Feiring, C., Taska, L., & Lewis, M. (1998). The role of shame and attributional style in children's and adolescents' adaptation to sexual abuse. *Child Maltreatment, 3,* 129–142.

Finkelhor, D. (1980). Sex among siblings: A survey on prevalence, variety and effects. *Archives of Sexual Behavior, 9,* 171–194.

Finkelhor, D. (1994). Current information on the scope and nature of child sexual abuse. *The Future of Children, 4,* 31–53.

Fischer, A., Sananbenesi, R., Schrick, C., Spiess, J., & Radulovic, J. (2004). Distinct roles of hippocampal *de novo* protein synthesis and actin rearrangement in extinction of contextual fear. *Journal of Neuroscience, 24,* 1962–1966.

Foa, E. B. (1995). *The Posttraumatic Diagnostic Scale manual.* Minneapolis, MI: National Computer Systems.

Foa, E. B., Cashman, L., Jaycox, L., & Perry, K. J. (1997). The validation of a self-report measure of posttraumatic stress disorder: The Posttraumatic Diagnostic Scale. *Psychological Assessment, 9,* 445–451.

Foa, E. B., Dancu, C. V., Hembree, E. A., Jaycox, L. H., & Meadows, E. A. (1999). A comparison of exposure therapy, stress inoculation training, and their combination for reducing posttraumatic stress disorder in female assault victims. *Journal of Consulting and Clinical Psychology, 67,* 194–200.

Foa, E. B., Keane, T. M., & Friedman, M. J. E. (Eds.). (2000). *Effective treatments for PTSD: Practice guidelines from the International Society for Traumatic Stress Studies.* New York: Guilford Press.

Foa, E. B., & Meadows, E. A. (1997). Psychological treatments for posttraumatic stress disorder: A critical review. *Annual Review of Psychology, 48,* 449–480.

Foa, E. B., Molnar, C., & Cashman, L. (1995). Change in rape narratives during exposure therapy for posttraumatic stress disorder. *Journal of Traumatic Stress, 8,* 675–690.

Foa, E. B., Riggs, D. S., Massie, E. D., & Yarczower, M. (1995). The impact of fear activation and anger on the efficacy of exposure treatment for posttraumatic stress disorder. *Behavior Therapy, 26,* 487–499.

Foa, E. B., & Rothbaum, B. O. (1998). *Treating the trauma of rape: Cognitive-behavioral therapy for PTSD.* New York: Guilford Press.

Foa, E. B., Rothbaum, B. O., Riggs, D. S., & Murdock, T. B. (1991). Treatment of posttraumatic stress disorder in rape victims: A comparison between cognitive-behavioral procedures and counseling. *Journal of Consulting and Clinical Psychology, 59,* 715–723.

Ford, J. D., Fisher, P., & Larson, L. (1997). Object relations as a predictor of treatment outcome with chronic posttraumatic stress disorder. *Journal of Consulting and Clinical Psychology, 65,* 547–559.

Ford, J. D., & Kidd, P. (1998). Early childhood trauma and disorders of extreme stress as predictors of treatment outcome with chronic posttraumatic stress disorder. *Journal of Traumatic Stress, 11,* 743–761.

Fosha, D. (2000). *The transforming power of affect: A model for accelerated change.* New York: Basic Books.

Freud, S. (1955). Beyond the pleasure principle. In J. Strachey (Ed. & Trans.), The standard edition of the complete psychological works of Sigmund Freud (Vol. 18, pp. 3–64). London: Hogarth Press. (Original work published 1920)

Freud, S. (1963). Further recommendations in the technique of psychoanalysis: Recollection, repetition and working through. In P. Reiff (Ed.), *Therapy and technique.* New York: Macmillan. (Original work published 1914)

Freyd, J. J. (1996). *Betrayal trauma: The logic of forgetting childhood abuse.* Cambridge, MA: Harvard University Press.

Funari, D., Piekarski, A., & Sherwood, R. (1991). Treatment outcomes of Vietnam veterans with posttraumatic stress disorder. *Psychological Reports, 68,* 571–578.

Garnefski, N., & Diekstra, R. F. (1997). Child sexual abuse and emotional and behavioral problems in adolescence: Gender differences. *Journal of the American Academy of Child and Adolescent Psychiatry, 36,* 323–329.

Gergely, G. (2004). The role of contingency detection in early affect-regulative interactions and in the development of different types of infant attachment. *Social Development, 13*(3), 468–478.

Gergely, G., & Watson, J. (1996). The social biofeedback theory of parental affect-mirroring: The development of emotional self-awareness and self-control in infancy. *International Journal of Psycho-Analysis, 77,* 1181–1212.

Giaconia, R. M., Reinherz, H. Z., Silverman, A. B., Pakiz, B., Frost, A. K., & Cohen, E. (1995). Traumas and posttraumatic stress disorder in a community population of older adolescents. *Journal of the American Academy of Child and Adolescent Psychiatry, 34,* 1369–1380.

Gidycz, C. A., Hanson, K., & Layman, M. J. (1995). A prospective analysis of the relationships among sexual assault experiences. *Psychology of Women Quarterly, 19,* 5–29.

Gilmore, M. (1994). *Shot in the heart.* New York: Doubleday.

Gold, S. N. (2000). *Not trauma alone: Therapy for child abuse survivors in family and social context.* Philadelphia: Brunner/Routledge.

Golden, O. (2000). The federal response to child abuse and neglect. *American Journal of Psychiatry, 55,* 1050–1053.

Goleman, D. (1995). *Emotional intelligence.* New York: Bantam Books.

Gratz, K. L., & Roemer, L. (2004). Multidimensional assessment of emotion regulation and dysregulation: Development, factor structure, and initial validation of the difficulties in emotion regulation scales. *Journal of Psychopathology and Behavioral Assessment, 26,* 41–54.

Greenberg, J. R., & Mitchell, S. A. (1983). *Object relations in psychoanalytic theory.* Cambridge, MA: Harvard University Press.

Grossman, F. K., Cook, A., Kepkep, S., & Koenen, K. C. (1999). *With the phoenix rising: Ten resilient survivors of child abuse.* San Francisco: Jossey-Bass.

Gurewitsch, B. (Ed.). (1998). *Mothers, sisters, resisters: Oral histories of women who survived the Holocaust.* Tuscaloosa: University of Alabama Press.

Harvey, J. (1998). *Total relaxation: Healing practices for body, mind and spirit.* New York: Kodansha America.

Harvey, M. R. (1996). An ecological view of psychological trauma and trauma recovery. *Journal of Trauma and Stress, 9,* 3–23.

Harvey, M. R., Liang, B., Harney, P., & Koenen, K. C. (2003). A multidimensional approach to the measurement of trauma recovery and resiliency. *Journal of Aggression, Maltreatment and Trauma, 6,* 87–109.

Heffernan, K., & Cloitre, M. (2000). A comparison of PTD with and without borderline personality disorder among women with childhood sexual abuse: Etiological and clinical characteristics. *Journal of Nervous and Mental Disease, 188,* 589–595.

Heriot, J. (1996). Maternal protectiveness following the disclosure of intrafamilial child sexual abuse. *Journal of Interpersonal Violence, 11,* 181–194.

Herman, J. (1992). *Trauma and recovery.* New York: Basic Books.

Hien, D., & Honeyman, T. (2000). A closer look at the drug abuse—maternal aggression link. *Journal of Interpersonal Violence, 15*(5), 503–522.

Hill, C. R., & Safran, J. D. (1994). Assessing interpersonal schemas: Anticipated responses of significant others. *Journal of Social and Clinical Psychology, 13,* 366–379.

Hofer, M. A. (2003). The emerging neurobiology of attachment and separation: How parents shape their infant's brain and behavior. In S. W. Coates, J. L. Rosenthal, & D. S. Schechter (Eds.), *September 11: Trauma and human bonds* (pp. 191–209). Hillsdale, NJ: Analytic Press.

Holmes, J. (2001). *The search for the secure base: Attachment theory and psychotherapy.* Philadelphia: Brunner/Routledge.

Horowitz, K., Weine, S., & Jekel, J. (1995). Posttraumatic stress disorder symptoms in urban adolescent girls: Compounded community trauma. *Journal of the American Academy of Child and Adolescent Psychiatry, 34,* 1353–1361.

Horowitz, L. M., Rosenberg, S. E., Baer, B. A., Ureno, G., & Villasenor, V. S. (1988). Inventory of Interpersonal Problems: Psychometric properties and clinical applications. *Journal of Consulting and Clinical Psychology, 56,* 885–892.

Horowitz, M. J. (1976). *Stress response syndromes.* New Tork: Aronson.

Horvath, A. O., & Symonds, D. B. (1991). Relation between working alliance and outcome in psychotherapy: A meta-analysis. *Journal of Counseling Psychology, 36,* 223–233.

"How America Defines Child Abuse." National survey conducted by Penn, Schoen & Berland for Los Angeles-based Children's Institute International, http://www.childrensinstitute.org/publications.html. Results released June 3, 1999.

Jacobs, W. J., & Nadel, L. (1985). Stress induced recovery of fears and phobias. *Psychological Review, 92,* 512–531.

Janoff-Bulman, R. (1992). *Shattered assumptions: Towards a new psychology of trauma.* New York: Free Press.

Kabat-Zinn, J. (1994). *Wherever you go, there you are: Mindfulness meditation in everyday life.* New York: Hyperion Books.

Kabat-Zinn, J. (1995). *Mindfulness meditation: Cultivating the wisdom of your body and mind* [Audiotape]. New York: Simon & Schuster Audio/Nightingale.

Kagan, J. (1980). In O. G. Brin, Jr., & J. Kagan (Eds.), *Constancy and change in human development: Perspectives on continuity* (pp. xx–xx). Cambridge, MA: Harvard University Press.

Karen, R. (1998). *Becoming attached: First relationships and how they shape our capacity to love.* New York: Oxford University Press.

Keane, T. M., Fairbank, J., Caddell, J., & Zimmering, R. (1989). Implosive (flooding) therapy reduces symptoms of PTSD in Vietnam combat veterans. *Behavior Therapy, 20,* 246–260.

Keenan, K. (2000). Emotion dysregulation as a risk factor for child psychopathology. *Clinical Psychology: Science and Practice, 7,* 418–434.

Keppel-Benson, J. M., Ollendick, T. H., & Benson, M. J. (2002). Post-traumatic stress in children following motor vehicle accidents. *Journal of Child Psychology and Psychiatry, 43,* 203–212.

Kessler, R. C. (2000). Posttraumatic stress disorder: The burden to the individual and to society. *Journal of Clinical Psychiatry, 61*(Suppl. 5), 4–14.

Kiesler, D. J. (1983). The 1982 interpersonal circle: A taxonomy for complementarity in human transactions. *Psychological Review, 90,* 185–214.

Kilpatrick, D. G., Edmunds, C., & Seymour, A. (1992). *Rape in America: A report to the nation.* Arlington, VA: National Center for Victims of Crime; Charleston, SC: Medical University of South

Carolina, Crime Victims Research and Treatment Center.

Kilpatrick, D. G., Ruggiero, K. J., Acierno, R., Saunders, B. E., Resnick, H. S., & Best, C. L. (2003). Violence and risk of PTSD, major depression, substance abuse/dependence, and comorbidity: Results from the National Survey of Adolescents. *Journal of Consulting and Clinical Psychology, 71*(4), 692–700.

Klein, M. (1937). Love, guilt and reparation. In *Love, hate and reparation* (with J. Riviere). London: Hogarth.

Koenen, K. C. (1998). The impact of trauma training for graduate students. *NC-PTSD Clinical Quarterly, 8,* 12–13.

Kolko, D. J., Brown, E. J., & Berliner, L. (2002). Children's perceptions of their abusive experience: Measurement and preliminary findings. *Child Maltreatment, 7,* 41–53.

Kottler, J. A. (1998). *The therapist's workbook: Self-assessment, self-care, and self-improvement exercises for mental health professionals.* San Francisco: Jossey-Bass.

Krahe, B., Sheinberger-Olwig, R., Waizenhofer, E., & Koplin, S. (1999). Childhood sexual abuse revictimization in adolescence. *Child Abuse and Neglect, 4,* 383–394.

Kubany, E. S., Ownes, J. A., McCaig, M. A., Hill, E. E., Iannce-Spencer, C., & Tremayne, K. J. (2004). Cognitive trauma therapy for battered women with PTSD (CTT BW). *Journal of Consulting and Clinical Psychology, 72,* 3–18.

Lam, J. N., & Grossman, F. K. (1997). Resiliency and adult adaptation in women with and without self-reported histories of childhood sexual abuse. *Journal of Traumatic Stress, 10,* 175–196.

Lattal, K. M., & Abel, T. (2004). Behavioral impairments caused by injections of the protein synthesis inhibitor anisomycin after contextual retrieval reverse with time. *Proceedings of the National Academy of Sciences USA, 101,* 4667–4672.

Lazarus, J. (2000). *Stress relief and relaxation techniques.* Lincolnwood, IL: Keats.

Laor, N., Wolmer, L., Mayes, L. C., Gershon, A., Weizman, R., & Cohen, D. J. (1997). Israeli preschool children under Scuds: A 30–month follow-up. *Journal of American Academy of Child and Adolescent Psychiatry, 36,* 349–356.

Leary, T. (1957). *Interpersonal diagnosis of personality.* New York: Ronald Press.

LeDoux, J. E. (1998). *The emotional brain.* London: Weidenfeld & Nicolson.

Levitt, J., & Cloitre, M. (2005). A clinician's guide to STAIR/MPE: Treatment for posttraumatic stress disorder related to childhood abuse. *Cognitive and Behavioral Practice, 12,* 40–52.

Levitt, J., Malta, L., Martin, A., Davis, L., & Cloitre, M.

(in press). The flexible application of a manualized treatment for PTSD in survivors of the 9/11 World Trade Center attack. *Behavior Research and Therapy.*

Lieberman, A. F., & Amaya-Jackson, L. (2005). Reciprocal influences of attachment and trauma: Using a dual lens in the assessment and treatment of infants, toddlers, and preschoolers. In L. Berlin, Y. Ziv, L. Amaya-Jackson, & M. T. Greenberg (Eds.), *Enhancing early attachments: Theory, research, intervention, and policy.* New York: Guilford Press.

Lieberman, D. J. (2000). *Get anyone to do anything and never feel powerless again: Psychological secrets to predict, control, and influence every situation.* New York: St. Martin's Press.

Lifton, R. J. (1993). *The protean self: Human resilience in an age of fragmentation.* New York: Basic Books.

Lindy, J. (1996). Psychoanalytic psychotherapy of posttraumatic stress disorder: The nature of the therapeutic relationship. In B. van der Kolk, A. C. McFarlane, & I. Weisaeth (Eds.), *Traumatic stress: The effects of overwhelming experience on mind, body, and society* (pp. 525–536). New York: Guilford Press.

Linehan, M. M. (1993a). *Cognitive-behavioral treatment of borderline personality disorder.* New York: Guilford Press.

Linehan, M. M. (1993b). *Skills training manual for treating borderline personality disorder.* New York: Guilford Press.

Lipschitz, D. S., Rasmusson, A. M., Anyan, W., Comwell, P., & Southwick, S. M. (2000). Clinical and functional correlates of posttraumatic stress disorder in urban adolescent girls at a primary care clinic. *Journal of the American Academy of Child and Adolescent Psychiatry, 39,* 1104–1111.

Lipschitz, D. S., Winegar, R. K., Hartnick, E., Foote, B., & Southwick, S. M. (1999a). Posttraumatic stress disorder in hospitalized adolescents: Psychiatric comorbidity and clinical correlates. *Journal of the American Academy of Child and Adolescent Psychiatry, 38,* 385–392.

Lipschitz, D. S., Winegar, R. K., Nicolaou, A. L., Hartnick, E., Wolfson, M., & Southwick, S. M. (1999b). Perceived abuse and neglect as risk factors for suicidal behavior in adolescent inpatients. *Journal of Nervous and Mental Disease, 187,* 32–29.

Litz, B. T., & Gray, M. J. (2002). Emotional numbing of posttraumatic stress disorder: Current and future research directions. *Australian and New Zealand Journal of Psychiatry, 36,* 198–204.

Litz, B. T., Schlenger, W. E., Weathers, F. W., Fairbank, J. A., & LaVange, L. M. (1997). Predictors of emotional numbing in posttraumatic stress disorder. *Journal of Traumatic Stress, 10,* 607–618.

Lorde, A. (1984). *Sister outsider: Essays and speeches.* Trumansburg, NY: Crossing Press.

Lyons-Ruth, K., Alpern, L., & Repacholi, B. (1993). Disorganized infant attachment classification and maternal psychosocial problems as predictors of hostile–aggressive behavior in the preschool classroom. *Child Development, 63*, 572–585.

MacKinnon, C. A. (2005, April 16). Who was afraid of Andrea Dworkin? *The New York Times*, p. 13.

Main, M., Kaplan, N., & Cassidy, J. (1985). Security in infancy, childhood, and adulthood: A move to the level of representation. In I. Bretherton & E. Waters (Eds.), Growing points of attachment theory and research. *Monographs of the Society for Research in Child Development, 50*(1–2, Serial No. 209), 66–104.

Malatesta, C. Z., & Haviland, J. M. (1982). Learning display rules: The socialization of emotion expression in infancy. *Child Development, 53*, 991–1003.

Malmquist, C. P. (1986). Children who witness parental murder: Posttraumatic aspects. *Journal of the American Academy of Child and Adolescent Psychiatry, 25*, 320–325.

Mandoki, C. A., & Burkhart, B. D. (1989). Sexual victimization: Is there a vicious cycle? *Violence and Victims, 4*, 179–190.

March, J. (1999). Assessment of pediatric posttraumatic stress disorder. In P. A. Saigh & J. D. Bremner (Eds.), *Posttraumatic stress disorder: A comprehensive text*. Boston: Allyn & Bacon.

Markowitsch, H. J. (1995). Which brain regions are critically involved on the retrieval of old episodic memory? *Brain Research Reviews, 21*, 117–127.

Martin, D. J., Garske, J. P., & Davis, M. K. (2000). Relation of the therapeutic alliance with outcome and other variables: A meta-analytic review. *Journal of Consulting and Clinical Psychology, 58*, 438–450.

Matsakis, A. (1998). *Trust after trauma: A guide to relationships for survivors and those who love them*. Oakland, CA: New Harbinger.

McCann, L., & Pearlman, L. A. (1990b). Vicarious traumatization: A framework for understanding the psychological effects of working with victims. *Journal of Traumatic Stress, 3*, 131–149.

McDonagh, A., Friedman, M., McHugo, G., Ford, J., Sengupta, A., Mueser, K., et al. (2005). Randomized trial of cognitive behavioral therapy for chronic posttraumatic stress disorder in adult female survivors of childhood sexual abuse. *Journal of Consulting and Clinical Psychology, 73*(3), 515–524.

McEwen, B. S. (1992). Re-examination of the glucocorticoid hypothesis of stress and aging. *Progress in Brain Research, 93*, 365–378.

McFall, M. E., Marburg, M. M., Ko, G. N., & Veith, R., C. (1990). Autonomic responses to stress in Vietnam combat veterans with PTSD. *Biological Psychiatry, 27*, 1165–1175.

McGloin, J. M., & Widom, C. S. (2001). Resilience among abused and neglected children grown up. *Developmental Psychopathology, 12*, 1021–1038.

McLeer, S. V., Callaghan, M., Henry, D., & Wallen, J. (1994). Psychiatric disorders in sexually abused children. *Journal of the American Academy of Child and Adolescent Psychiatry, 33*, 313–319.

McLeer, S. V., Deblinger, E., Henry, D., & Orvaschel, H. (1992). Sexually abused children at high risk for PTSD. *Journal of the American Academy of Child and Adolescent Psychiatry, 31*, 875–879.

McLeer, S. V., Dixon, J. F., Henry, D., Ruggiero, K., Escovitz, K., Neidda, T., et al. (1998). Psychopathology in non-clinically referred sexually abused children. *Journal of the American Academy of Child and Adolescent Psychiatry, 37*, 1326–1333.

McNally, R. J. (2003). Progress and controversy in the study of posttraumatic stress disorder. *Annual Review of Psychology, 54*, 229–252.

Messman, T. L., & Long, P. J. (1996). Child sexual abuse and its relationship to revictimization in adult women: A review. *Clinical Psychology Review, 5*, 397–420.

Miller, D. (1994). *Women who hurt themselves: A book of hope and understanding*. New York: Basic Books.

Mongrain, M. (1998). Parental representations and support-seeking behaviors related to dependency and self-criticism. *Journal of Personality, 66*, 151–173.

Monnier, J., & Hobfoll, S. E. (2000). Conservation of resources in individual and community reaction to traumatic stress. In A. Y. Shalev, R. Yehuda, & A. C. McFarlane (Eds.), *International handbook of human response to trauma* (pp. 325–336). New York: Kluwer Academic/Plenum.

Monson, C. M., Schnurr, P. P., Stevens, S. P., & Guthrie, K. A. (2004). Cognitive-behavioral couples treatment for posttraumatic stress disorder: Initial findings. *Journal of Traumatic Stress, 17*, 341–344.

Muran, J. C., Segal, Z. V., Samstag, L. W., & Crawford, C. E. (1994). Patient pretreatment interpersonal problems in therapeutic alliance in short-term cognitive therapy. *Journal of Consulting and Clinical Psychology, 62*, 185–190.

Nader, K. (2003). Memory traces unbound. *Trends in Neurosciences, 26*, 65–72.

Najavits, L. M., Weiss, R. D., & Shaw, S. R. (1997). The link between substance abuse and posttraumatic stress disorder in women. *American Journal of Addictions, 6*, 273–283.

Nash, M. R., Hulsey, T. L., Sexton, M. C., Harralason, T. L., & Lambert, W. (1993). Perceived family environment, psychopathology, and dissociation. *Journal of Consulting and Clinical Psychology, 61*, 276–283.

Nichols, K., Gergely, G., & Fonagy, P. (2001). Experimental protocols for investigating relationships among mother–infant interaction, affect regulation, physiological markers of stress responsiveness, and attachment. *Bulletin of the Menninger Clinic, 65*(3), 371–379.

Norris, F. H., Perilla, J. L., & Murphy, A. D. (2001). Postdisaster stress in the United States and Mexico: A cross-cultural test of the multicriterion conceptual model of posttraumatic stress disorder. *Journal of Abnormal Psychology, 110,* 553–563.

O'Neill, K., & Gupta, K. (1991). Post-traumatic stress disorder in women who were victims of childhood sexual abuse. *Irish Journal of Psychological Medicine, 8,* 1224–1227.

Pearlman, L. A., & Saakvitne, K. W. (1995). *Trauma and the therapist.* New York: Norton.

Pitman, R. K., Altman, B., Greenwald, E., Longpre, R. E., & Macklin, M. L. (1991). Psychiatric complications during flooding therapy for posttraumatic stress disorder. *Journal of Consulting and Clinical Psychology, 52,* 17–20.

Pitman, R. K., Orr, S. P., Forgue, D. F., de Jong, J. B., & Claiborn, J. M. (1987). Psychophysiologic assessment of post-traumatic stress disorder imagery in Vietnam combat veterans. *Archives of General Psychiatry, 44,* 970–975.

Polusny, M., & Follette, V. (1995). Long-term correlates of child sexual abuse: Theory and review of the empirical literature. *Applied and Preventive Psychology: Current Scientific Perspectives, 4,* 143–166.

Pope, K. S., & Vasquez, M. J. T. (1998). *Ethics in psychotherapy and counseling: A practical guide* (2nd ed.). San Francisco: Jossey-Bass.

Pope, K. S., & Vasquez, M. J. T. (2005). *How to survive and thrive as a therapist: Information, ideas, and resources for psychologists in practice.* Washington, DC: American Psychological Association.

Putnam, F. W. (2004). *The costs and consequences of child abuse.* Paper presented at the annual meeting of the American Association for the Advancement of Science, Seattle, WA.

Pynoos, B., Frederick, C. J., Nader, K., Arroyo, W., Steinberg, A., Nunez, F., et al. (1987). Life threat and posttraumatic stress in school age children. *Archives of General Psychiatry, 44,* 1057–1063.

Quindlen, A. (1992). *Object lessons.* Branson, MO: Ivy Books.

Quirk, G. J., Repa, J. C., & LeDoux, J. E. (1995). Fear conditioning enhances auditory short-latency responses of single unites in the lateral nucleus of the amygdala: simultaneous mutlichannel recordings in freely behaving rates. *Neuron, 15,* 1029–1039.

Rapaport, M. H., Endicott, J., & Clary, C. M. (2002). Post-traumatic stress disorder and quality of life: Results across 64 weeks of sertraline treatment. *Journal of Clinical Psychiatry, 63,* 59–65.

Ray, K. C., Jackson, J. L., & Townsley, R. M. (1991). Family environments of victims of intrafamilial and extrafamilial child sexual abuse. *Journal of Family Violence, 6,* 365–374.

Resick, P. A., Jordan, C. G., Girelli, S. A., Hutter, C. H., & Marhoefer-Dvorak, S. (1988). A comparative outcome study of behavioral group therapy for sexual assault victims. *Behavior Therapy, 19,* 385–401.

Resick, P. A., Nisith, P., & Griffin, M. G. (2003). How well does cognitive-behavioral therapy treat symptoms of complex PTSD? An examination of child sexual abuse survivors within a clinical trial. *CNS Spectrums, 8,* 340–355.

Resick, P. A., Nisith, P., Weaver, T. L., Astin, M. C., & Feuer, C. A. (2002). A comparison of cognitive-processing therapy with prolonged exposure and a waiting condition for the treatment of chronic posttraumatic stress disorder in female rape victims. *Journal of Consulting and Clinical Psychology, 70,* 867–879.

Resick, P. A., & Schnicke, M. K. (1992). Cognitive processing therapy for sexual assault victims. *Journal of Consulting and Clinical Psychology, 60,* 748–756.

Resick, P. A., & Schnicke, M. K. (1996). *Cognitive processing therapy for rape victims: A treatment manual.* Newbury Park, CA: Sage.

Rodriguez, N., Ryan, S. W., Rowan, A. B., & Foy, D. W. (1996). Posttraumatic stress disorder in a clinical sample of adult survivors of childhood sexual abuse. *Child Abuse and Neglect, 20,* 943–952.

Rogers, C. R. (1951). *Client-centered therapy.* Boston: Houghton Mifflin.

Roth, S., Newman, E., Pelcovitz, D., van der Kolk, B., & Mandel, F. S. (1997). Complex PTSD in victims exposed to sexual and physical abuse: Results from the DSM-IV field trial for posttraumatic stress disorder. *Journal of Traumatic Stress, 10,* 539–555.

Rothbaum, B. O., & Foa, E. B. (1999). *Reclaiming your life after rape: Cognitive behavioral therapy for posttraumatic stress disorder.* New York: Oxford University Press.

Rowan, A. B., & Foy, D. W. (1993). Posttraumatic stress disorder in child sexual abuse survivors: A literature review. *Journal of Traumatic Stress, 6,* 3–20.

Russell, D. (1983). The incidence and prevalence of intrafamilial and extrafamilial sexual abuse of female children. *Child Abuse and Neglect, 7,* 133–146.

Ruzek, J. I. (1993). Professionals coping with vicarious trauma. *NC-PTSD Clinical Newsletter, 3,* 12–17.

Safran, J. D. (1990a). Towards a refinement of cognitive therapy in light of interpersonal theory: 1. Theory. *Clinical Psychology Review, 10,* 87–105.

Safran, J. D. (1990b). Towards a refinement of cognitive therapy in light of interpersonal theory: II. Practice. *Clinical Psychology Review, 10,* 107–121.

Safran, J. D., & Segal, Z. V. (1990). *Interpersonal process in cognitive therapy.* New York: Basic Books.

Saigh, P. A., & Bremner, J. (1999). The history of posttraumatic stress disorder. In P. A. Saigh & J. Bremner (Eds.), *Posttraumatic stress disorder: A comprehensive text* (pp. 18–43). Needham Heights, MA: Allyn & Bacon.

Sapolsky, R. (2004). *Why zebras don't get ulcers* (3rd ed.). New York: Owl Books.

Scheeringa, M. S., & Zeanah, C. H. (2001). A relational

perspective on PTSD in early childhood. *Journal of Trauma and Stress, 1,* 799–815.

Scheier, M. F., & Carver, C. S. (1985). Optimism, coping and health: Assessment and implications of generalized outcome expectancies. *Health Psychology, 4,* 219–247.

Schoen, C., Davis, K., & Collins, S. (1997). The Commonwealth Fund Survey of the Health of Adolescent Girls. Available online at www.cmwf.org/publications/pulbications_show.htm?doc_id=221230

Schwartz, D., & Proctor, L. J. (2000). Community violence exposure and children's social adjustment in the school peer groups: The mediating roles of emotion regulation and social cognition. *Journal of Consulting and Clinical Psychology, 68,* 670–683.

Scott, M. J., & Stradling, S. G. (1997). Client compliance with exposure treatments for posttraumatic stress disorder. *Journal of Traumatic Stress, 10,* 523–526.

Serretti, A., Cavallino, M. C., Macciardi, F., Namia, C., Franchni, L., Souery, D., et al. (1999). Social adjustment and self-esteem in remitted patients with mood disorders. *European Psychiatry, 14,* 137–142.

Shalev, A. Y. (1997). Treatment of prolonged post traumatic stress disorder learning from experience. *Journal of Traumatic Stress, 10,* 415–423.

Shalev, A. Y. (2002). Acute stress reactions in adults. *Biological Psychiatry, 51,* 532–543.

Shalev, A. Y., Tuval-Mashiach, R., & Hadar, H. (2004). Posttraumatic stress disorder as a result of mass trauma. *Journal of Clinical Psychiatry, 65,* 4–10.

Shear, K., Frank, E., Houck, P., & Reynolds, C. F. (2005). Treatment of complicated grief: A randomized controlled trial. *Journal of the American Medical Association, 293*(21), 2601–2608.

Shearer, S. L., Peters, C. P., Quaytman, M. S., & Ogden, R. L. (1990). Frequency and correlates of childhood sexual and physical abuse histories in adult female borderline inpatients. *American Journal of Psychiatry, 147,* 214–216.

Sheridan, M. J. (1999). A proposed intergenerational model of substance abuse, family functioning, and abuse/neglect. *Child Abuse and Neglect, 19,* 519–530.

Shields, A. M., & Cicchetti, D. (1998). Reactive aggression among maltreated children: The contributions of attention and emotion dysregulation. *Journal of Clinical Child Psychology, 27,* 381–395.

Shields, A. M., Ryan, R. M., & Cicchetti, D. (1994). The development of emotional and behavioral self-regulation and social competence among maltreatment school age children. *Developmental Psychopathology, 6,* 57–75.

Shipman, K. L., & Zeman, J. (2001). Socialization of children's emotion regulation in mother–child dyads: A developmental psychopathology perspective. *Developmental Psychopathology, 13,* 317–336.

Shipman, K. L., Zeman, J., Penza, S., & Champion, K.

(2000). Emotion management skills in sexually maltreated and nonmaltreated girls: A developmental psychopathology perspective. *Developmental Psychopathology, 12,* 47–62.

Singer, M. (2005, February 14–21). The misfit. *The New Yorker,* pp. 192–205.

Solomon, J., George, C., & DeJong, A. (1995). Children classified as controlling at age six: Evidence of disorganized representational strategies and aggression at home and at school. *Developmental Psychopathology, 73,* 447–463.

Spaccarelli, S. (1994). Stress, appraisal, and coping in child sexual abuse: A theoretical and empirical review. *Psychological Bulletin, 116,* 340–362.

Spielberger, C. D. (1983). *Manual for the State–Trait Anxiety Inventory (STAI).* Palo Alto, CA: Consulting Psychologists Press.

Spielberger, C. D. (1988). *State–Trait Anger Expression Inventory (STAXI), Research Edition. Professional Manual.* Odessa, FL: Psychological Assessment Resources.

Spielberger, C. D., Jacobs, G., Russell, S., & Crane, R. (1983). Assessment of anger: The State–Trait Anger Scale. In J. D. Butcher & C. D. Spielberger (Eds.), *Advances in personality assessment* (Vol. 2, pp. 159–187). Hillsdale, NJ: Erlbaum.

Spinazzola, J., Blaustein, M., & van der Kolk, B. A. (2005). Posttraumatic stress disorder treatment outcome research: The study of unrepresentative samples? *Journal of Traumatic Stress, 18,* 425–436.

Stedman's medical dictionary (27th ed.). (2000). Philadelphia: Lippincott Williams & Wilkins.

Steinem, G. (1992). *Revolution from within: A book of self-esteem.* Boston: Little, Brown.

Stern, D. N. (1985). *The interpersonal world of the infant.* New York: Basic Books.

Stiles, W. B., Agnew-Davis, R., Hardy, G. E., Barkman, M., & Shapiro, D. A. (1998). Relations of the alliance with psychotherapy outcome: Findings in the second Sheffield psychotherapy project. *Journal of Consulting and Clinical Psychology, 67,* 13–18.

Stoddard, F. J., Norman, D. K., Murphy, J. M., & Beardslee, W. R. (1989). Psychiatric outcome of burned children. *Journal of the American Academy of Child and Adolescent Psychiatry, 28,* 589–595.

Stupp, H. H., & Binder, J. L. (1984). *Psychotherapy in a new key: A guide to time-limited dynamic psychotherapy.* New York: Basic Books.

Sullivan, H. S. (1970). *The psychiatric interview.* New York: Norton.

Tarrier, N., Pilgrim, H., Sommerfield, C., Faragher, B., Reynolds, M., Graham, E., et al. (1999). A randomized trial of cognitive therapy and imaginal exposure in the treatment of chronic posttraumatic stress disorder. *Journal of Consulting and Clinical Psychology, 67,* 13–18.

Tedeschi, R. G., & Calhoun, L. G. (1996). The Posttraumatic Growth Inventory: Measuring the positive legacy trauma. *Journal of Traumatic Stress, 9,* 455–471.

Turner, S. W., McFarlane, A., C., & van der Kolk, B. (1996). The therapeutic environment and new explorations in the treatment of posttraumatic stress disorder. In B. A. van der Kolk, A. C. McFarlane, & L. Weisaeth (Eds.), *Traumatic stress: The effects of overwhelming experience on mind, body, and society* (pp. 537–596). New York: Guilford Press.

van der Kolk, B. (1996). The complexity of adaptation to trauma: Self-regulation, stimulus discrimination, and characterological development. In B. A. van der Kolk, A. C. McFarlane, & I. Weisaeth (Eds.), *Traumatic stress: The effects of overwhelming experience on mind, body, and society* (pp. 182–213). New York: Guilford Press.

van der Kolk, B. (2003, April 3). *Resilience in the face of trauma: Adolescent mental health and youth development.* Presentation at the Mount Sinai Adolescent Health Center, Mount Sinai Medical Center.

van der Kolk, B., Roth, S., Pelcovitz, D., & Mandel, F. S. (1993). *Complex posttraumatic stress disorder: Results of the posttraumatic stress disorder field trials for DSM-IV.* Washington, DC: American Psychiatric Association.

Weissman, E., & Bothell, S. (1976). Assessment of patient social adjustment by patient self-report. *Archives of General Psychiatry, 33,* 1111–1115.

Widom, C. S. (1999). Posttraumatic stress disorder in abused and neglected children grown up. *American Journal of Psychiatry, 156,* 1223–1229.

Wilson, J. P., & Keane, T. M. (Eds.). (2004). *Assessing psychological trauma and PTSD* (2nd ed.). New York: Guilford Press.

Wilson, P. (1995). *Instant calm: Over 100 easy-to-use techniques for relaxing mind and body.* New York: Penguin Books.

Wolfe, D. A., Sas, L., & Wekerle, C. (1994). Factors associated with the development of posttraumatic stress disorder among child victims of sexual abuse. *Child Abuse and Neglect, 18,* 37–50.

Wolfe, J., & Kimerling, R. (1997). Gender issues in the assessment of posttraumatic stress disorder. In J. P. Wilson & T. M. Keane (Eds.), *Assessing psychological trauma and PTSD* (pp. 192–238). New York: Guilford Press.

Wyatt, G. E., Guthrie, D., & Notgrass, C. M. (1992). Differential effects of women's child sexual abuse and subsequent sexual revictimization. *Journal of Consulting and Clinical Psychology, 60,* 167–173.

Wyatt, G. E., Loeb, T. B., Solis, B., & Carmona, J. V. (1999). The prevalence and circumstances of child sexual abuse: Changes across a decade. *Child Abuse and Neglect, 23*(1), 45–60.

Yang, Q., Khoury, M. J., Rodriguez, C., Calle, E. E., Tathan, L. M., & Flanders, W. D. (1998). Family history score as a predictor of breast cancer mortality: Prospective data from the Cancer Prevention Study II, United States, 1982–1991. *American Journal of Epidemiology, 147,* 652–659.

Yeomans, F. E., Gutfreund, J., Selzer, M. A., Clarkin, J. F., Hull, S. W., & Smith, T. E. (1994). Factors related to drop-outs by borderline patients: Treatment contract and therapeutic alliance. *Journal of Psychotherapy Practice and Research, 3,* 16–24.

Zlotnick, C., Zakriski, A. L., Shea, T. M., Costello, E., Begin, A., Pearlstein, T., et al. (1996). The long-term sequelae of sexual abuse: Support for a complex posttraumatic stress disorder. *Journal of Traumatic Stress, 9,* 195–205.

Index